Handbook of Pediatric Epilepsy Case Studies, Second Edition

Research in the field of epilepsy will continue at a rapid pace, with the ultimate hope of curing many intractable epilepsy syndromes. Fully updated, this new edition is organized chronologically, from neonate through adolescence, and the handbook is the culmination of a group effort involving leading physicians and researchers whose contributions constitute a concise and practical reference for health professionals in training. Here the contributors review the recent flood of new information on the pathophysiology, genetics, and treatment of the various epilepsy syndromes, and the volume is distilled into an easy-to-use guide.

- Fully updated text reviewing the latest research on the pathophysiology, genetics, and treatment of the various epilepsy syndromes.
- Thorough descriptions of the different syndromes commonly encountered in clinical practice across the pediatric range.
- Extensive resource section provided.
- Contributors describe why they chose each particular case, what they learned, and how it changed their practice.
- The book includes the most recent classification and nomenclature published by the International League Against Epilepsy.

Handbook of Pediatric Epilepsy Case Studies, Second Edition

Edited by

Maria Augusta Montenegro
UC Sand Diego School of Medicine

Jong M. Rho
UC San Diego School of Medicine

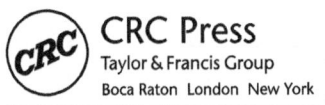

CRC Press
Taylor & Francis Group
Boca Raton London New York

CRC Press is an imprint of the
Taylor & Francis Group, an **informa** business

Second edition published 2023
by CRC Press
6000 Broken Sound Parkway NW, Suite 300, Boca Raton, FL 33487-2742

and by CRC Press
4 Park Square, Milton Park, Abingdon, Oxon, OX14 4RN

CRC Press is an imprint of Taylor & Francis Group, LLC

© 2023 selection and editorial matter, Maria Augusta Montenegro and Jong M. Rho; individual chapters, the contributors

First edition published by CRC Press | Taylor and Francis, LLC 2008

Library of Congress Cataloging-in-Publication Data
Names: Rho, Jong M., editor. | Montenegro, Maria Augusta, editor.
Title: Handbook of pediatric epilepsy case studies, second edition / edited by Jong M. Rho,
University of California, San Diego, Maria Augusta Montenegro,
Department of Neurology, University of Campinas/UNICAMP, Campinas, Brazil.
Other titles: Pediatric epilepsy case studies.
Description: Second edition. | Boca Raton, FL : CRC Press, 2023. | Revised
edition of: Pediatric epilepsy case studies / edited by Kevin Chapman,
Jong M. Rho. c2009. | Includes bibliographical references and index. |
Identifiers: LCCN 2022057002 | ISBN 9781032283548 (hbk) | ISBN
9781032283586 (pbk) | ISBN 9781003296478 (ebk)
Subjects: LCSH: Epilepsy in children—Case studies.
Classification: LCC RJ496.E6 P42 2023 | DDC 618.92/853—dc23/eng/20221214
LC record available at https://lccn.loc.gov/2022057002

ISBN: 9781032283548 (hbk)
ISBN: 9781032283586 (pbk)
ISBN: 9781003296478 (ebk)

DOI: 10.1201/9781003296478

Typeset in Times
by codeMantra

Contents

SECTION I   The Basics

SECTION II   The Neonate

SECTION III   The Infant

SECTION IV   The Child

SECTION V   *The Adolescent*

Preface

Epilepsy encompasses a wide variety of clinical syndromes characterized by heterogeneous etiologies, presentations, and prognoses. Accurate diagnosis is critically important for the proper care of patients with epilepsy, especially since some forms of epilepsy have a benign and self-limited course, while others are associated with progressive neurocognitive decline.

Advances in neuroimaging and genetics have improved our diagnostic abilities and our fundamental understanding of epilepsies. In addition, newer medications have offered patients better tolerability than traditional agents, but unfortunately, no significant improvements in overall seizure control have been afforded. Many epileptic conditions remain intractable to currently available medications. However, other nonpharmacological treatment options (such as the ketogenic diet and vagus nerve stimulator) have provided hope for improved seizure control in these patients with medically intractable epilepsy.

Since the publication of the first edition, there have been remarkable scientific and clinical advances in the field of pediatric epilepsy, the most notable of which has been our understanding of the genetic underpinnings of many disordered encountered in clinical practice. While we are still far from transforming the therapeutic landscape with precision therapies based on the unique neurobiology of an individual patient's epileptic condition, we have learned that the molecular mechanisms underlying seizure genesis (and indeed, epileptogenesis) are far more complex than previously realized. Nevertheless, with current efforts to explore and validate innovative gene therapies and a new generation of antiseizure medications with unique and somewhat unexpected mechanisms of action, the future remains promising.

For the physician or allied health professional in training, grasping the complexity and nuances associated with various epileptic syndromes can be daunting. The goal of this book remains the same – to help trainees at all levels and healthcare professionals understand the different epilepsies encountered in the clinical setting across the pediatric age range. The intent is to provide a readily digestible reference that introduces the novice to the remarkable and at times bewildering array of epilepsies in neonates, infants, children, and adolescents.

The initial section forms an introduction to the fundamentals of epilepsy, and subsequent sections include succinct case presentations and salient discussions of the more common epilepsy syndromes affecting each age group. There are other rarer forms of epilepsy that have not been included, such as seizures arising from certain metabolic-genetic and neurodegenerative conditions. Suggested references are also provided to guide the reader toward more detailed studies of a specific topic of interest.

This book is the culmination of a group effort involving many of the leading physicians and researchers in the field of pediatric epilepsy. We believe that their individual contributions together constitute a concise and practical reference for health professionals in training. Research in the field of epilepsy continues to grow at a rapid pace, with the ultimate hope of curing many patients with refractory epilepsy. We further hope that this book may spark the interest of residents, trainees, and other healthcare professionals in joining the international fight against epilepsy.

Maria Augusta Montenegro, MD, PhD
Rady Children's Hospital
University of California San Diego

Jong M. Rho, MD
Rady Children's Hospital
University of California San Diego

Authors

Maria Augusta Montenegro is a pediatric neurologist and epileptologist currently working at Rady Children's Hospital/University of California San Diego School of Medicine. Her clinical expertise is in pediatric epilepsy, with an emphasis on epileptic encephalopathy and EEG. She completed medical school, residency, and Ph.D. at the University of Campinas (Brazil) and a postdoctorate research fellowship at Columbia University (NY). Prior to her current position, she held an academic faculty appointment at the University of Campinas (Brazil) where she was the head of Pediatric Neurology.

Dr. Jong M. Rho is a Professor of Neurosciences, Pediatrics and Pharmacology at the University of California San Diego, and Division Chief of Pediatric Neurology at the Rady Children's Hospital San Diego. He received a bachelor's degree in molecular biophysics and biochemistry at Yale University, and an M.D. from the University of Cincinnati. He has held prior faculty appointments at the University of Washington (Seattle), the University of California at Irvine, the Barrow Neurological Institute (Phoenix), and most recently, the University of Calgary. His main research interests are the mechanisms underlying the antiseizure and neuroprotective effects of metabolism-based treatments such as the ketogenic diet. His research activities have been sponsored by research grants from the U.S. National Institutes of Health, Canadian Institutes of Health Research, and other public and private sector sources.

Abbreviations & Acronyms

AAN	American Academy of Neurology
ACMG	American College of Medical Genetics and Genomics
ACTH	adrenocorticotropic hormone
ADHD	attention deficit hyperactivity disorder
ADME	absorption, distribution, metabolism, and excretion
ADNFLE	autosomal dominant nocturnal frontal lobe epilepsy
ANT	anterior nucleus of the thalamus
ASM	antiseizure medication
BECTS	benign epilepsy with centrotemporal spikes
BIPDs	bilateral independent periodic discharges
BOLD	blood-oxygen-level-dependent
CAE	childhood absence epilepsy
CBT	cognitive-behavioral therapy
CBZ	carbamazepine
CEEG	continuous EEG monitoring
CI	confidence interval
CIV	continuous intravenous
CIVASM	continuous intravenous antiseizure medication
CMA	chromosomal microarray analysis
CNS	central nervous system
CNVs	copy number variants
COVE	childhood occipital visual epilepsy
CSE	convulsive *status epilepticus*
CSTB	cystatin B
CSWS	continuous spike-and-wave during sleep
CYP	cytochrome P450
DBS	deep brain stimulation
DEE	developmental and/or epileptic encephalopathy
DEE-SWAS	developmental epileptic encephalopathy with spike-and-wave activation in sleep
DEND	developmental delay, epilepsy, and neonatal diabetes
DNA	deoxyribonucleic acid
DNT	dysembryoplastic neuroepithelial tumor
EAF	epilepsy with auditory features
ECoG	electrocorticography
ED	emergency department
EEG	electroencephalogram
EIDEE	early infantile developmental and epileptic encephalopathy
EIMFS	epilepsy of infancy with migrating focal seizures
EMAS	epilepsy with myoclonic-atonic seizures
EME	early myoclonic epilepsy
ES	exome sequencing

ESES	electrical *status epilepticus* of sleep
ESET	*status epilepticus* treatment trial
ESI	electrical source imaging
ETC	Electron transport chain
ER	emergency room
FAME	familial adult myoclonic epilepsy
FCD	focal cortical dysplasia
FDA	food and drug administration
FDG-PET	2-Deoxy-2-[18F] fluoro-D-glucose positron emission tomography
FIRES	febrile infection-related epilepsy syndrome
FLAIR	fluid-attenuated inversion recovery
fMRI	functional magnetic resonance imaging
FSE	febrile *status epilepticus*
GABA	gamma-aminobutyric acid
GEFS+	genetic epilepsy with febrile seizures plus
GGE	genetic generalized epilepsies
GLUT1DS	glucose transporter 1 deficiency syndrome
GnRH	gonadotropin-releasing hormone
GS	genome sequencing
GTC	generalized tonic clonic
GTCA	epilepsy with generalized tonic-clonic seizures alone
HH	hypothalamic hamartoma
HIE	hypoxic-ischemic encephalopathy
HR	hazard ratio
HSE	herpes simplex encephalitis
HSV	herpes simplex virus
ICU	intensive care unit
IESS	infantile epileptic spasms syndrome
IGE	idiopathic generalized epilepsy
ILAE	International League Against Epilepsy
IVIG	intravenous immunoglobulin
JAE	juvenile absence epilepsy
JME	juvenile myoclonic epilepsy
JS	Jeavons syndrome
KD	ketogenic diet
LD	Lafora disease
LEAT	Low-grade developmental, epilepsy-associated brain tumor
LEV	levetiracetam
LGS	Lennox–Gastaut syndrome
LITT	laser interstitial thermal therapy
LKS	Landau–Kleffner syndrome
LPD	lateralized periodic discharges
MAD	modified Atkins diet
MAE	myoclonic astatic epilepsy
MAS	myoclonic-atonic seizures
MCD	malformation of cortical development

MEG	magnetoencephalography
MEI	myoclonic epilepsy of infancy
MELAS	mitochondrial encephalomyopathy, lactic acidosis, and stroke-like episodes
MERRF	myoclonus, epilepsy, with ragged red fibers
mFCD	minimal focal cortical dysplasia
MgFUS	MRI-guided focused ultrasound
MgLITT	MRI-guided laser interstitial thermal therapy
MGP	multigene panels
MHD	monohydroxy derivative
MOGHE	mild malformation of cortical development with oligodendroglial hyperplasia and epilepsy
MRI	magnetic resonance imaging
MRS	magnetic resonance spectroscopy
MS	myoclonic
MS-MLPA	methylation-sensitive multiplex ligation-dependent probe amplification
mtDNA	mitochondrial DNA
MTLE-HS	mesial temporal lobe epilepsy with hippocampal sclerosis
mTOR	mammalian target of rapamycin
MTS	mesial temporal sclerosis
nAChR	neuronal nicotinic acetylcholine receptor
NCS	nonconvulsive seizures
NCSE	nonconvulsive *status epilepticus*
NDDs	neurodevelopmental disorders
nDNA	nuclear DNA
NGS	next-generation sequencing
NICU	neonatal intensive care unit
NLSTEPSS	North London *Status Epilepticus* Surveillance Study
NMDA	N-methyl-D-aspartate
NMDAR	N-methyl-D-aspartate receptor
NORSE	new-onset refractory status epilepticus
NREM	nonrapid eye movement
OCP	oral contraceptives
OSA	obstructive sleep apnea
PCR	polymerase chain reaction
PDMS	patient data management system
PHACE	posterior fossa anomalies, hemangioma, arterial anomalies, cardiac anomalies, and eye anomalies
PICU	pediatric intensive care unit
PLEDs	periodic lateralizing epileptiform discharges
PME	progressive myoclonus epilepsy
PNES	psychogenic nonepileptic seizures
POLE	photosensitive occipital lobe epilepsy
POLG	polymerase gamma
ppm	parts per million

PPR	photoparoxysmal response
PWS	port-wine stain
REM	rapid eye movement
RFTC	radiofrequency thermocoagulation
RNS	responsive neurostimulation
RSE	refractory *status epilepticus*
SE	*status epilepticus*
sEEG	stereo-EEG
SeLEAS	self-limited epilepsy with autonomic seizures
SeLECTS	self-limited epilepsy with centrotemporal spikes
SeLIE	self-limited (familial) infantile epilepsy
SHE	sleep-related hypermotor epilepsy
SISCOM	subtraction ictal SPECT co-registered to MRI
SMAP	sulfamoyolacetylphenol
SMEI	severe myoclonic epilepsy of infancy
SPECT	single photon emission computed tomography
SRSE	super refractory *status epilepticus*
SSEPs	somatosensory evoked potentials
SUDEP	sudden unexpected death in epilepsy
SWI	spike–wave index
SWS	Sturge–Weber syndrome
TIRDA	temporal intermittent rhythmic delta
TLE	temporal lobe epilepsy
TMS	transcutaneous magnetic stimulation
TSC	tuberous sclerosis complex
UDP	uridine diphosphate
UGT	glucuronosyltransferase
ULD	Unverricht–Lundborg disease
VAP	valproic acid (VPA)
V_d	volume of distribution
VNS	vagus nerve stimulation
VZV	varicella zoster virus
WNV	west Nile virus

Contributors

Samiya Ahmad
Baylor College of Medicine
Houston, Texas

Danielle M. Andrade
University of Texas Southwestern
    Medical Center
Dallas, Texas

Juan Ignacio Appendino
Hospital Italiano de Buenos Aires
Buenos Aires, Argentina

Juan Pablo Appendino
University of Calgary
Calgary, Canada

Stéphane Auvin
Université Paris-Cité & Institut
    Universitaire de France (IUF)
Paris, France

Melissa Barker-Haliski
University of Washington
Seattle, Washington

Christie Becu
Barrow Neurological Institute at
    Phoenix Children's Hospital
Phoenix, Arizona

A. G. Christina Bergqvist
University of Pennsylvania
Philadelphia, Pennsylvania

Frank M. C. Besag
Neurodevelopmental Team
London, England

Michaela Castello
UC San Diego School of Medicine
San Diego, California

Kevin Chapman
University of Arizona College of
    Medicine
Phoenix, Arizona

Nitish Chourasia
The University of Tennessee Health
    Science Center
Memphis, Tennessee

Harry T. Chugani
NYU School of Medicine
New York, New York

Dave F. Clarke
The University of Texas at Austin
Austin, Texas

Danielle deCampo
Children's Hospital of Philadelphia
Philadelphia, Pennsylvania

Guillermo Delgado-García
University of Calgary
Calgary, Canada

Anita M. Devlin
Newcastle University
Newcastle upon Tyne, United Kingdom

Cornelia Drees
University of Colorado
Aurora, Colorado

Aliya Frederick
UC San Diego School of Medicine
San Diego, California

Daniel A. Freedman
The University of Texas at Austin
Austin, Texas

Andrew J. Gienapp
The University of Tennessee
Memphis, Tennessee

Jeffrey J. Gold
UC San Diego School of Medicine
San Diego, California

Jennifer Graves
Rady Children's Pediatric MS Center
San Diego, California

Marilisa M. Guerreiro
University of Campinas
Campinas, Brazil

Ajay Gupta
Neurological Institute Cleveland Clinic
Cleveland, Ohio

Shaun A. Hussain
UCLA Mattel Children's Hospital and
    David Geffen School of Medicine
Los Angeles, California

Ann Hyslop
Stanford University
Stanford, California

Kaitlin C. James
Monroe Carell Jr Children's Hospital at
    Vanderbilt
Nashville, Tennessee

Colin B. Josephson
University of Calgary
Calgary, Canada

Olivia Kim-McManus
UC San Diego School of Medicine
San Diego, California

Joerg Klepper
Children's Hospital Aschaffenburg
Aschaffenburg, Germany

Eric H. Kossoff
The Johns Hopkins Hospital
Baltimore, Maryland

Linda Laux
Northwestern University
Chicago, Illinois

Aimee F. Luat
Central Michigan University
Mount Pleasant, Michigan
and
Wayne State University
Detroit, Michigan

Eric Marsh
Children's Hospital of Philadelphia and
    University of Pennsylvania
Philadelphia, Pennsylvania

Sara Matricardi
Children's Hospital "G. Salesi"
Ancona, Italy

Berge A. Minassian
University of Texas Southwestern
    Medical Center
Dallas, Texas

Kenneth A. Myers
Montreal Children's Hospital - McGill
    University Health Centre
Montreal, Canada

Rima Nabbout
University of Paris cite
Paris, France

Yu-tze Ng
The Children's Hospital of San Antonio
    and Baylor College of Medicine
Houston, Texas

Douglas R. Nordli, Jr.
University of Chicago Medicine
Chicago, Illinois

Douglas R. Nordli, III
Mayo Clinic
Jacksonville, Florida

James W. Owens
University of Washington
Seattle, Washington

Heather Pekeles
McGill University Health
  Center
Montreal, Canada

Elia Pestana Knight
Cleveland Clinic
Cleveland, Ohio

Jesus Eric Pina-Garza
Centennial Children's Hospital
Nashville, Tennessee

Annapurna Poduri
Boston Children's Hospital
Boston, Massachusetts

Reega Purohit
Northwestern University Feinberg
  School of Medicine
Chicago, Illinois

James J. Riviello, Jr.
Baylor College of Medicine
Houston, Texas

Russell P. Saneto
University of Washington
Seattle, Washington

Harvey B. Sarnat
University of Calgary
Calgary, Canada

Shifteh S. Sattar
UC San Diego School of Medicine
San Diego, California

Morris H. Scantlebury
University of Calgary
Calgary, Canada

Sonali Sen
Baylor College of Medicine
Houston, Texas

Jerry Shih
UC San Diego School of Medicine
San Diego, California

Sabrina Tavella-Burka
Cleveland Clinic
Cleveland, Ohio

Mayank Verma
University of Texas Southwestern
  Medical Center
Dallas, Texas

James W. Wheless
The University of Tennessee
Memphis, Tennessee

Angus Wilfong
Barrow Neurological Institute at
  Phoenix Children's Hospital
Phoenix, Arizona

Korwyn Williams
Phoenix Children's Hospital
Phoenix, Arizona

Kimberly Wiltrout
Harvard Medical School
Boston, Massachusetts

Jennifer Yang
UC San Diego
San Diego, California

Steven Yang
UC San Diego School of Medicine
San Diego, California

June Yoshii-Contreras
UC San Diego School of Medicine
San Diego, California

Ifrah Zawar
UVA Health
Charlottesville, Virginia

Mary L. Zupanc
UC Irvine
Orange County, California

Section I

The Basics

1 A Pediatric Epilepsy Primer

James W. Owens
University of Washington

CONTENTS

Epilepsy is a common, and often misunderstood, chronic medical condition of childhood. As frequently encountered as childhood asthma, seizures (inclusive of febrile seizures) occur in up to 5% of all children in the United States and 1% of children are diagnosed with epilepsy. Appropriate diagnosis and management are crucial given the potential for life-long consequences to the developing brain.

Not all seizures need to be treated, as there are differences in the management of true epileptic conditions vs. reactive or isolated seizures. An example of the former would be recognizing the clinical phenotype of infantile spasms, a particularly devastating type of developmental brain disorder. An illustration of the latter would be refraining from the use of antiseizure medications (ASMs) for children with febrile seizures, even if recurrent. This common form of acute provoked seizure does not reflect an enduring epileptic condition, and, typically, daily preventative treatment is not warranted. Furthermore, there are many paroxysmal disorders affecting children, such as parasomnias and behavioral problems, which are frequently mistaken for epileptic phenomena.

The epilepsies of childhood differ significantly both from each other as well as from those encountered in adulthood; the pediatric brain is not just a smaller adult brain. The key, then, is to understand what epilepsy is and what it is not, and to appreciate the unique age-dependent – and syndrome-dependent – nature of epileptic conditions to guide proper diagnosis and management. In this introductory chapter, a few key points regarding pediatric epilepsy will be highlighted and expanded upon in the remainder of this book.

DOI: 10.1201/9781003296478-2

PEDIATRIC EPILEPSY IS COMMON

Within the first two decades of life, approximately 5% of children will have experienced some form of seizure. A significant majority of these seizures will be acutely provoked events, often in the context of a febrile illness, and not spontaneous recurrent seizures (SRSs) which are the hallmark of epilepsy. Among all children who have a single unprovoked seizure, only about 40% of them will ever have a second. This rate of recurrence varies greatly depending on such factors as what type of seizure occurred and whether there is other evidence of neurological dysfunction. For example, a patient who, at baseline, has an abnormal neurological examination, abnormal electroencephalogram (EEG), and abnormal brain MRI may have a risk of recurrence of approximately 90%. Of course, this does not indicate when a subsequent seizure might actually occur.

Approximately 20% of patients experiencing a seizure of some type will later develop epilepsy: by 20 years of age, approximately 1% of the population will have been diagnosed with this condition. Published studies of incidence vary greatly, which may be partly due to the inclusion of single unprovoked seizures as well as acute symptomatic seizures in some studies. With respect to age-specific incidence, it seems clear that the onset of epilepsy most frequently occurs at the two extremes of the lifespan. That is, several studies have shown that the incidence of epilepsy is high in the first year of life, lowest in middle age, and rises again in the elderly. In a population of patients aged 70 years or more, the incidence is as high as 3%. As one might imagine, the causes, types, and outcomes differ significantly between these two populations, although there is certainly some overlap.

PEDIATRIC EPILEPSY ENCOMPASSES A WIDE RANGE OF DISORDERS

Imagine sitting in the waiting room of a pediatric epilepsy clinic and observing the variety of patients awaiting their turn to be evaluated. A 6-year-old child, initially referred for "staring spells", is now here for a follow-up appointment with well-controlled childhood absence epilepsy. In a wheelchair, you see a 13-year-old child with spastic quadriparetic cerebral palsy and poorly controlled structural focal-onset epilepsy. She is here to have the settings on her vagus nerve stimulator (VNS) adjusted with the hope that her focal seizures, some of which spread to both hemispheres, might become less frequent. An 8-month-old infant has been worked into the schedule with continued clusters of infantile spasms despite completing a trial of adrenocorticotropic hormone (ACTH). A new patient is here for a second opinion about whether his brief stereotyped events of generalized shaking with partial loss of awareness are epileptic in nature. Finally, there is an 8-year-old for a 6-month postoperative follow-up visit after a focal neocortical resection to remove an area of cortical dysplasia and who happily remains seizure free. As different as these patients may be in age, clinical phenomenology, and response to therapy, they all have epilepsy. Clearly, this is a heterogeneous collection of distinct disorders, which may more appropriately be referred to as "epilepsies". To understand this clinical spectrum, one must be familiar both with what unifies these conditions as well as what makes each distinct.

The traditional definition of epilepsy is deceptively simple: having two or more unprovoked seizures separated by more than 24 hours. A couple of recent modifications have become increasingly accepted as meeting criteria for the diagnosis of epilepsy, specifically one unprovoked (or reflex) seizure and a probability of further seizures similar to the general recurrence risk (at least 60%) after two unprovoked seizures occurring over the next 10 years, or the diagnosis of an epilepsy syndrome. Each component of these definitions is important to bear in mind. Seizures are paroxysms of abnormally hyperexcitable and hypersynchronous cortical activity, which results in a change in sensation, motor function, behavior, or sensorium. If the seizure occurs immediately following a precipitating event, then it is referred to as an acutely provoked/reactive seizure or acute symptomatic seizure.

As mentioned above, a common example of such an event would be a febrile seizure: 2%–4% of all children between the ages of 6 months and 5 years' experience a generalized tonic–clonic seizure lasting less than 15 minutes in association with a fever not caused by a central nervous system (CNS) infection. In this case, the acute provoking event – the fever – is immediately followed by the seizure. Other examples of acute symptomatic seizures would include those which occur at the time of trauma, in the context of hyponatremia, or in association with a withdrawal syndrome (e.g., alcohol).

In contrast, with epilepsy, there is no immediate provoking event for the seizure. At times, the seizure may arise from an old injury such as from a prior stroke. Because the precipitating event precedes the seizure by weeks to years, such an event is considered unprovoked and is often referred to as a "remote symptomatic seizure", or structural/metabolic in origin. Finally, in order to meet the traditional definition of epilepsy, two or more unprovoked seizures must be separated by more than 24 hours. The reason for this is that rapidly recurrent seizures occurring close together carry the same epidemiological risk of eventual recurrence as a single seizure.

As stated above, another definition of epilepsy has been added: a single unprovoked seizure with a recurrence risk of at least 60%. The threshold of 60% reflects the risk of seizure recurrence after two unprovoked seizures. Findings on EEG, MRI, and neurological examination as well as other factors such as family history and the presence of a defined epilepsy syndrome determine the likelihood of recurrence. For example, if a patient has a single absence seizure, then one would not need to see a second in order to make the diagnosis of childhood absence epilepsy as this syndrome is known to be associated with frequent seizures.

If a patient has two or more unprovoked seizures (or a risk of recurrence of greater than 60%), then they may justifiably be labeled as having epilepsy. Given the broad nature of this definition, many different types of clinical phenotypes fall under the cover of this one large umbrella. It is a bit like stating that one lives in North America – helpful information but not very specific! Nowhere is this more evident than in pediatric epilepsies in which cause, clinical phenomenology, and outcome vary greatly.

Like the epilepsies which arise in adulthood, children may suffer from seizures as a consequence of trauma, CNS infections, strokes, and other brain insults. A particular example of this would be children who suffer injuries *in utero* or during the process of birth. Largely unique to childhood are seizures that arise from developmental brain malformations such as disorders of neuronal migration leading to focal cortical dysplasia. It is interesting to note, however, that although the abnormally formed cortex is present from birth, an epileptic disorder may not develop for many years. The reasons for this remain unclear.

To bring some semblance of order to this landscape, the epilepsies have historically been categorized or classified based on electroclinical features. Clinically, this is accomplished using a schema developed by the International League Against Epilepsy (ILAE), which utilizes etiology and seizure type. If the patient's epilepsy arises from an evident cause, such as a remote symptomatic seizure due to an old brain injury, then the epilepsy is referred to as *structural* (Figure 1.1). In general, the abnormal area of brain will be evident on MRI or other imaging modalities. Another example of a structural epilepsy would be one arising from a focal cortical dysplasia. However, some epilepsies are caused, not by a clear anatomic abnormality, but are instead inherited – either as a single mutation or, more commonly, as a collection of interacting mutations on different genes. Predictably, epileptologists refer to such epilepsies as *genetic*. Several common epilepsies of childhood, such as childhood absence epilepsy and self-limited epilepsy with centrotemporal spikes, are considered genetic.

Other etiological categories of epilepsy include infectious, metabolic, and immune mediated. Finally, some epilepsies occur in patients without an evident cause: the brain MRI is normal, there is no clear heritability, and no aspect of the workup reveals a potential etiology. These epilepsies were once labeled "*cryptogenic*" – literally meaning that the cause is hidden – but now are more straightforwardly referred to as "unknown" or "idiopathic" (equated with a likely genetic cause). One of the primary goals for the epilepsy research community is to abolish the need for this category by increasing our understanding of what causes epilepsy as well as expanding our repertoire of tools available for diagnosis.

In addition to etiology, the present classification scheme utilizes seizure type as a criterion. Seizures that arise from a particular region of the brain are labeled *focal* while seizures that involve both hemispheres from the onset are referred to as *generalized*. It should be noted that seizures may begin focally and then spread to involve the other hemisphere. Such a seizure is said to have evolved from focal to bilateral tonic–clonic expression (what were formerly called "*secondarily generalized seizures*"). Although not utilized in the classification scheme, focal seizures are further divided into those with loss of awareness and those without loss of awareness. They are also categorized as having motor onset (like clonic jerking on one side of the body) or nonmotor onset (like a visceral sensation or visual phenomenon). Putting the etiologic and phenomenological criteria together yields the appropriate classification. For example, epilepsies may be "structural focal" (a clear anatomic cause affecting just one part of the brain), "genetic generalized" (an inherited epilepsy producing seizures which affect both hemispheres at the outset-like childhood absence epilepsy), or any other combination of terms. As will become clear in the chapters to follow, utilizing this scheme is helpful in determining an appropriate evaluation and management strategy.

Another peculiarity of pediatric epilepsy is the concept of an epilepsy syndrome: a constellation of a particular type of seizure (or seizures), EEG features, and other

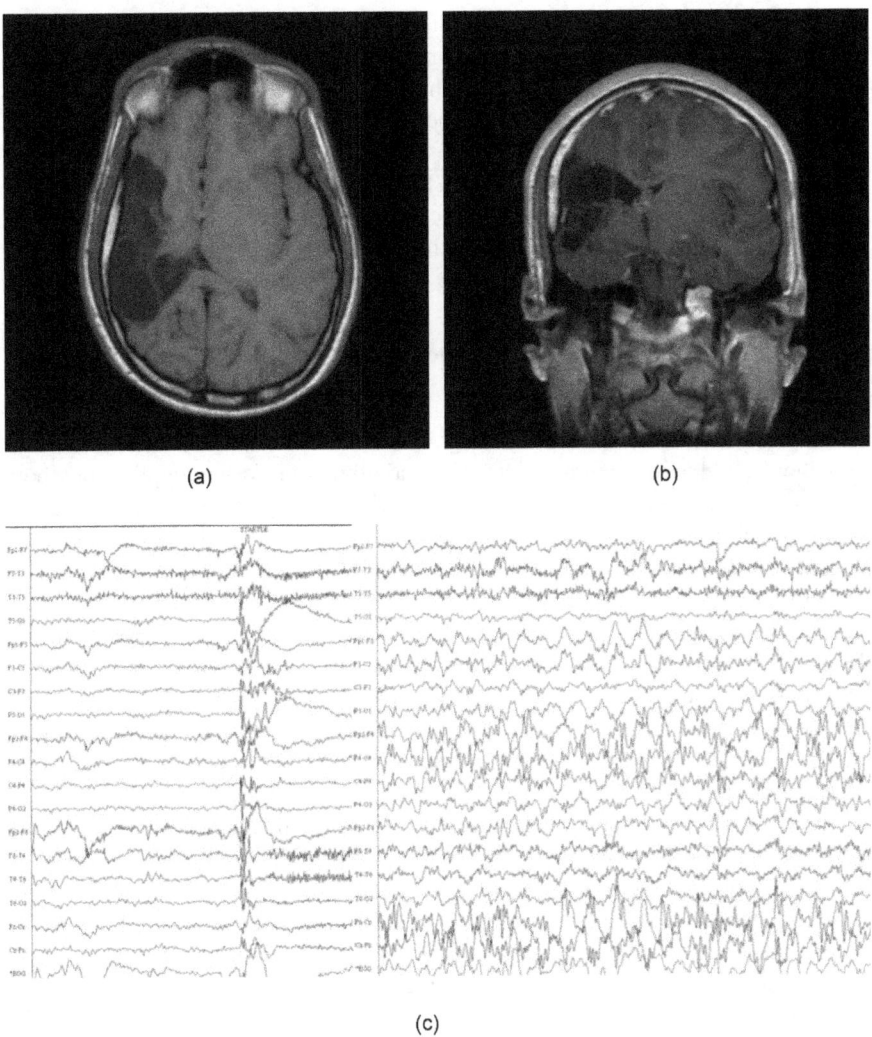

(a)   (b)

(c)

FIGURE 1.1 MRI images and EEG data from a teenager with structural focal epilepsy. This 15-year-old right-handed boy had left-sided hemiplegic cerebral palsy and startle-induced focal impaired awareness (previously referred to as complex partial) seizures. Panels A and B are representative T1-weighted postcontrast MRI images (axial and coronal planes, respectively) demonstrating the damage caused by an *in utero* right middle cerebral artery territory infarction (the left side of the image corresponds to the right side of the brain). Panel C shows the patient's EEG immediately prior to and following an auditory startle as well as several seconds into his typical electrographic ictal discharge. Note the high-amplitude slow activity with superimposed faster frequencies in the leads labeled Fp2–F4, F4–C4, and C4–P4 indicating that the seizure is arising from the right frontocentral region (by convention, EEG leads with even numbers are on the right and those with odd numbers are on the left; Fp, frontal polar; F, frontal; C, central; and P, parietal). The patient underwent definitive surgical resection and became seizure free.

clinical phenomena – often associated with a particular age of onset. For example, West syndrome represents the combination of epileptic spasms (a particular type of seizure), an interictal EEG pattern called hypsarrhythmia, and developmental arrest or regression with a peak age of onset between 3 and 7 months of age. Although still clinically diverse, epilepsy syndromes seem to represent a more homogeneous clinical population than is afforded by the ILAE classification scheme. For example, childhood absence and juvenile myoclonic epilepsy are both categorized as genetic generalized epilepsies, but they differ significantly in their age of onset, predominant seizure type, and rate of remission.

PEDIATRIC EPILEPSY VIEWED FROM A DEVELOPMENTAL CONTEXT

The CNS is unique in that its development extends from early embryonic life, throughout childhood, and even into early adulthood. This has implications both for the causes and the consequences of pediatric epilepsy as well as its treatment. An important determinant of the effects of a developmental insult is the ontogenetic stage at which it occurs. For example, failure of the anterior neuropore to close in the fourth embryonic week would cause anencephaly while an insult in the second trimester might cause a focal cortical dysplasia. For reasons that remain incompletely understood, the immature nervous system seems to be uniquely susceptible to developing seizures. Another way to state this is that the "seizure threshold" of the developing nervous system seems to be lower than that of the adult nervous system. At least part of this susceptibility may be secondary to the ongoing ontogenetic processes of the immature brain.

One possible contributor to the decreased seizure threshold of the immature nervous system is a physiologic imbalance of excitation and inhibition. In general, excitatory synaptic connections develop before inhibitory ones. Further, very early in development, it appears that inhibitory neurotransmission is actually depolarizing and therefore, possibly excitatory. This appears to be due to the developmental expression of a particular type of cation chloride cotransporter, which produces a more positive (depolarized) chloride reversal potential than what is found in the mature nervous system. This is a potentially clinically relevant physiological phenomenon since most first-line ASMs used to treat neonatal seizures – barbiturates and benzodiazepines – act by increasing inhibition. Maturation of the GABAergic system also involves expression of different receptor isoforms and unique modulatory neuropeptides (such as somatostatin). Overall, relatively late emergence of functional inhibition may increase the propensity of the CNS toward excessive excitation, which increases the likelihood of seizures.

The process of synaptogenesis involves abundant synapse formation followed by activity-dependent pruning of ineffective, aberrant, or unnecessary connections. Such developmental plasticity requires the developing nervous system to be uniquely responsive to environmental effects. Because of this, insults can have pervasive and persistent effects. Excessive activity during critical periods of development may strengthen neuronal pathways, which subsequently form a seizure focus or pathways of seizure propagation. Indeed, this may be one important component of the process of developmental epileptogenesis. Relative immaturity of cortical connections is also important for the clinical appearance of seizures. For example, neonates, who physiologically lack extensive well-formed intercortical and interhemispheric connectivity, do not exhibit generalized seizures.

Formation of the cerebral cortex is an intricate and remarkable process which begins with cells becoming neurons near the ventricles followed by migration of these new neurons to their appropriate location in the cortex. Interestingly, this process proceeds in an "inside-out" fashion – with the most recently generated neurons migrating through cells forming the more inner cortical layers. This choreographed relocation of cells involves glial cells, called radial glia, upon which the neurons migrate, as well as morphological cues to guide their entrance to and exit from this pathway. As might be expected, given the inherent complexity of this process, not all cells successfully reach their designated location.

Such "heterotopic" neurons are likely of little consequence if found in isolation as they are a common incidental finding in the brains of normal individuals without epilepsy. However, in some patients, a collection of neurons fails to completely migrate and may become a focal cortical dysplasia. The extent of dysplastic cortex can range from quite restricted to very extensive. For reasons that are incompletely understood, such foci of abnormally formed cortex are often highly epileptogenic and are commonly found in children with structural focal epilepsy.

In addition to the developmental causes of epilepsy, clinicians caring for children with epilepsy must always be mindful of the potential developmental consequences of our treatments. ASMs, in general, act by increasing inhibition or decreasing excitation; some have dual and opposing actions, such as felbamate. Such therapeutic manipulations interact with the ongoing process of synaptogenesis and may alter cognitive processes. This is one important reason to be judicious in the use of medical therapy since it can carry its own set of potential morbidities.

A WIDE RANGE OF TREATMENT OPTIONS ARE AVAILABLE

Once the diagnosis of epilepsy has been made, consideration turns to appropriate treatment. Some forms of childhood epilepsy may not require any intervention other than education and reassurance. For example, self-limited epilepsy with centrotemporal spikes is a common genetic focal epilepsy of childhood, which spontaneously resolves by the age of 16 years, and was previously referred to as Benign Rolandic Epilepsy and Benign Epilepsy with Centro-Temporal Spikes (BECTS). Approximately 60% of patients with this condition experience very few seizures. When seizures do occur under such circumstances, an abortive therapeutic option – such as a rectally administered form of diazepam – is often prescribed *in lieu* of daily medical therapy.

For those children with SRS, which are sufficiently frequent and/or severe to require intervention, there are many different medications from which to choose. Factors such as type of epilepsy, age of the patient, and comorbidities are important considerations in deciding which medication to use. Perhaps, the single most important factor in medication choice is the specific side-effect profile of the drug and its suitability for a particular patient.

Overall, approximately 60% of patients will become seizure free with one of the first two ASMs prescribed. Unfortunately, for those whose epilepsy does not respond, the chance of treatment success with subsequent medication trials becomes progressively less. For this reason, patients who do not respond to one of the first two or three medications are referred to as "pharmaco-resistant", "drug-resistant", "medically refractory", and "medically intractable". Fortunately, there is an ever-increasing range of options for patients with medically intractable epilepsy. One possibility is the use of the ketogenic diet: a high-fat and low-carbohydrate therapy which results in increased ketone body production by the liver and produces improved seizure control through as yet undefined mechanisms.

For certain carefully selected patients, the best option is epilepsy surgery: e.g., neurosurgical removal of the epileptogenic zone in the cortex. Examples of such procedures range from focal neocortical resection for patients with an area of cortical dysplasia, to removal of the anterior temporal lobe in patients with temporal lobe epilepsy, and to hemispherectomy in patients with hemimegaloencephaly. Epilepsy surgery candidates undergo an extensive presurgical evaluation that includes neuroimaging, EEG monitoring, and detailed neuropsychological studies, as well as other ancillary tests. Given the irreversible nature of surgical intervention, it is vital to determine whether potential functional deficits might result from the proposed resection. Still, for excellent candidates, the chance of becoming seizure-free following surgery is as high as 65%–70% depending principally on location of the focus and whether or not there exist clear imaging findings related to that focus. At times, surgical procedures are conducted with a goal of decreasing seizure frequency or for palliation. This may involve, for example, partial resection of a lesion, if the presence of eloquent cortex prevents complete removal, or corpus callosotomy to prevent generalization of seizure activity from one hemisphere to the other.

Another surgical option used to decrease seizure frequency is implantation of a VNS device. This device consists of a generator implanted subcutaneously over the pectoral muscle and is connected via leads wrapped around the left vagus nerve. The VNS has an adjustable stimulation cycle, which delivers pulses of defined intensity and duration to the vagus nerve. For unknown reasons, such stimulation significantly decreases seizure frequency in approximately 50% of patients.

Although unlikely to make a patient seizure free, the VNS may significantly improve seizure control. A unique responsive neurostimulator (RNS), which detects seizure activity and utilizes cortical stimulation to abort focal seizures, is now in routine use in adult epilepsy and is being used with greater frequency in children. Deep brain stimulation of targets in the thalamus is similarly being employed to treat severe pharmacoresistant epilepsy. As the range of therapeutic interventions for medically intractable epilepsy expands, it becomes ever more vital to refer such patients to a comprehensive epilepsy center where the possible use of such therapies can be considered.

PEDIATRIC EPILEPSY IS NOT JUST ABOUT SEIZURES

While seizures are surely the most dramatic aspect of epileptic disorders, they are far from the only clinical manifestation. Compared to children with other chronic medical conditions, patients with epilepsy have a lower rate of successful educational completion, employment, marriage, and other important quality-of-life measures. Rates of affective disorders and behavioral problems are also much higher than in the general population. Interestingly, this remains true even for patients with epilepsy that readily comes under medical control, as well as patients who undergo successful epilepsy surgery.

Certainly, many patients with epilepsy do extremely well, yet it remains troubling that there are those who do not. For some, frequent seizures can result in an encephalopathy that interferes with psychosocial function. Also, as ASMs generally work by increasing inhibition or decreasing excitation, cognitive dysfunction is not an infrequent side effect. Also, there are psychiatric problems such as depression and anxiety, and attentional deficits. Still, another aspect of this multifactorial phenomenon is the fact that epilepsy reflects, at some level, neuronal dysfunction. It is therefore perhaps not surprising that patients with epilepsy also may have difficulties with other cortically and subcortically mediated processes. This possibility is further suggested by the finding that neurobehavioral problems in children with epilepsy precede the diagnosis of epilepsy approximately 25% of the time. Regardless of the underlying pathophysiology, it is crucial that we consider such comorbidities in caring for our patients with epilepsy.

SUMMARY

Given the relatively high incidence of epilepsy, all physicians who work with children, regardless of specialty, will encounter patients afflicted with this heterogeneous disorder (more accurately termed, "epilepsies"). Appropriate care of these patients is crucial given the potential developmental consequences of both the underlying epileptogenic process, as well as those of the treatments we employ. The therapeutic armamentarium available to neurologists and epileptologists continues to expand as does our understanding of the basic neurobiology of these conditions. Yet, as we work with our patients to make them seizure free, we must also be continually cognizant of the wide-ranging effects of the epilepsies and avoid focusing solely on the seizures themselves.

SUGGESTED REFERENCES

Austin J., Harezlak J., Dunn D., Huster G., Rose D., Ambrosius W. Behavior problems in children before first recognized seizures. *Pediatrics* 2001; 107:115–22.

Baker G. Depression and suicide in adolescents with epilepsy. *Neurology* 2006; 66 (Suppl 3):S5–S12.

Bender R., Baram T. Epileptogenesis in the developing brain: What can we learn from animal models? *Epilepsia* 2007; 48(Suppl 5):2–6.

Devinsky O., Vezzani A., O'Brien T.J., Jette N., Scheffer I.E., de Curtis M., Perucca P. Epilepsy. *Nat Rev Dis Primers* 2018; 4:18024.

Dubé C.M., McClelland S., Choy M., Brewster A.L., Noam Y., Baram T.Z. Fever, febrile seizures and epileptogenesis. In: Noebels J.L., Avoli M., Rogawski M.A., Olsen R.W., Delgado-Escueta A.V., editors. *Jasper's Basic Mechanisms of the Epilepsies [Internet]*. 4th edition. Bethesda (MD): National Center for Biotechnology Information (US); 2012.

Fisher R.S., Acevedo C., Arzimanoglou A., Bogacz A., Cross J.H., Elger C.E., Engel Jr. J., Forsgren L., French J.A., Glynn M., Hesdorffer D.C., Lee B.I., Mathern G.W., Moshé S.L., Perucca E., Scheffer I.E., Tomson T., Watanabe M., Wiebe S. ILAE official report: A practical clinical definition of epilepsy. *Epilepsia* 2014; 55(4):475–82.

Fisher R.S., Cross J.H., French J.A., Higurashi N., Hirsch E., Jansen F.E., Lagae L., Moshé S.L., Peltola J., Roulet Perez E., Scheffer I.E., Zuberi S.M. Operational classification of seizure types by the International League Against Epilepsy: Position paper of the ILAE Commission for Classification and Terminology. *Epilepsia* 2017; 58:522–30.

Frank N.A., Greuter L., Guzman R., Soleman J. Early surgical approaches in pediatric epilepsy - a systematic review and meta-analysis. *Childs Nerv Syst* 2022. doi: 10.1007/s00381-022-05699-x.

Galanopoulou A. Developmental patterns in the regulation of chloride homeostasis and GABAA receptor signaling by seizures. *Epilepsia* 2007; 48(Suppl 5):14–8.

Hauser W., Annegers J., Kurland L. Incidence of epilepsy and unprovoked seizures in Rochester, Minnesota: 1935–1984. *Epilepsia* 1993; 34:453–68.

Kho L., Lawn N., Dunne J., Linto J. First seizure presentation: Do multiple seizures within 24 hours predict recurrence? *Neurology* 2006; 67:1047–9.

Gedzelman E.R., Meador K.J. Neurological and psychiatric sequelae of developmental exposure to antiepileptic drugs. *Front Neurol* 2012; 3:182.

Guerrini R., Conti V., Mantegazza M., Balestrini S., Galanopoulou A.S., Benfenati F. Developmental and epileptic encephalopathies: From genetic heterogeneity to phenotypic continuum. *Physiol Rev* 2023; 103(1):433–513.

Kriegstein A., Noctor S. Patterns of neuronal migration in the embryonic cortex. *Trends Neurosci* 2004; 27:392–9.

Kwan P., Brodie M. Early identification of refractory epilepsy. *N Engl J Med* 2000; 342:314–9.

Lizana J., Garcia E., Marina L., Lopez M., Gonzalez M., Hoyos A. Seizure recurrence alter a first unprovoked seizure in childhood: A prospective study. *Epilepsia* 2000; 41:1005–13.

Pohlmann-Eden B., Beghi E., Camfield C., Camfield P. The first seizure and its management in adults and children. *BMJ* 2006; 332:339–42.

Rogawski M.A., Löscher W., Rho J.M. Mechanisms of action of antiseizure drugs and the ketogenic diet. *Cold Spring Harb Perspect Med* 2016; 6(5):a022780.

Sankar R., Rho J. Do seizures affect the developing brain? Lessons from the laboratory. *J Child Neurol* 2007; 22 (Suppl):21S–29S.

Scheffer I.E., Berkovic S., Capovilla G., Connolly M.B., French J., Guilhoto L., Hirsch E., Jain S., Mathern G.W., Moshé S.L., Nordli D.R., Perucca E., Tomson T., Wiebe S., Zhang Y.H., Zuberi S.M. ILAE classification of the epilepsies: Position paper of the ILAE commission for classification and terminology. *Epilepsia* 2017; 58:512–21.

Tellez-Zenteno J., Dhar R., Wiebe S. Long-term seizure outcomes following epilepsy surgery: A systematic review and meta-analysis. *Brain* 2005; 128:1188–98.

Tsou A.Y., Kessler S.K., Wu M., Abend N.S., Massey S., Treadwell J.R. Surgical treatments for epilepsies in children aged 1–36 Months: A systematic review. *Neurology* 2022 Oct 21. doi: 10.1212/WNL.0000000000201012.

Velísková J., Claudio O.I., Galanopoulou A.S., Lado F.A., Ravizza T., Velísek L., Moshé S.L. Seizures in the developing brain. *Epilepsia* 2004; 45(Suppl 8):6–12.

2 Epilepsy Genetics Primer

Kimberly Wiltrout
Boston Children's Hospital

Annapurna Poduri
Boston Children's Hospital

CONTENTS

Genetics has long been recognized as having an important causal role in epilepsy. From the first gene discoveries of familial epilepsies in the 1990s to now, there has been rapid growth in the identification of monogenic causes of epilepsy as well as in the delineation of the principles underlying the genetics of epilepsy. In this chapter, we will highlight the advances in clinical practice that have come from the growth of epilepsy genetics and will review the principles that guide a rational approach to genetic testing in epilepsy.

EPILEPSY GENETICS PRINCIPLES

Genetic epilepsies are defined as epilepsies with a known or presumed genetic etiology. Generally, people with presumed genetic epilepsy lack an acquired cause, such as trauma or infection, although newer studies are beginning to examine the role of genetic susceptibility to developing epilepsy after events such as traumatic brain injury and stroke.

In the past 30 years, there has been a veritable boom in the identification of genetic causes of epilepsy (Figure 2.1). Like other diseases, the genetic variants associated with epilepsy include single nucleotide variants (one base pair), small insertions and deletions that may or may not lead to a shift in the reading frame of the gene, copy number abnormalities ranging from microdeletions/microduplications to larger structural variation in the form of monosomies and trisomies, and genomic rearrangements that include inversions, translocations, and ring chromosomes. Copy number variants (CNVs) are a type of genomic rearrangement that have 1 Kb or larger

DOI: 10.1201/9781003296478-3

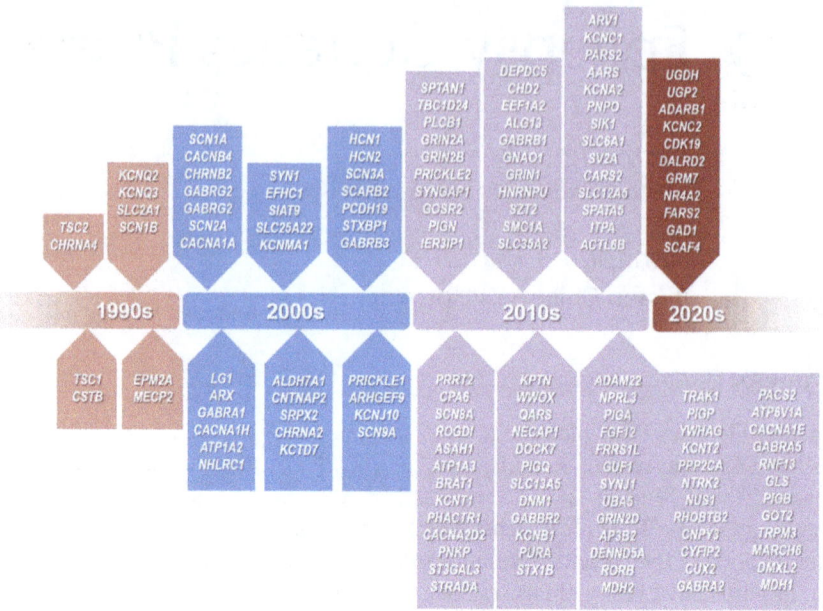

FIGURE 2.1 Timeline of epilepsy gene discoveries during the past 25 years. (Created by Alfred George and reprinted with permission from Poduri et al., 2021, *How We Got to Where We're Going, Elements in Genetics of Epilepsy.*)

differences in copy number compared to the reference genome. CNVs mainly consist of microdeletions and microduplications. Other less common types of genetic variation associated with epilepsy include trinucleotide repeat expansions and genomic imprinting, which is an epigenetic phenomenon.

Familial segregation and twin studies provided the first evidence for genetic causes of familial epilepsy. *De novo* variants are variants that are considered new in an individual and are detectable in the individual but not detected in their parents when DNA is assayed, typically from peripheral blood leukocytes or buccal samples. *De novo* variants have been demonstrated to play an important role in causing epilepsy, particularly in the case of developmental and epileptic encephalopathies (DEEs).

De novo variants most often arise during meiosis during the formation of the oocyte or spermatocyte, and so are present starting from the individual's zygote stage and should be detectable in a blood sample. A *de novo* variant may also occur in the postzygotic stage, with the implication that it is present in only a fraction of cells and may potentially be restricted to only the brain or only certain neuron populations in the brain. These mosaic variants may not be detectable with the routine DNA analysis of blood leukocytes. This phenomenon of somatic mosaicism has been demonstrated to be a mechanism for focal cortical dysplasia, hemimegalencephaly, and other brain malformations that have an association with epilepsy. Genetic testing may only be successful at identifying the causative variant if performed on the brain tissue removed during epilepsy surgery. Rarely, mosaicism has occurred in a parent's oocytes or spermatocytes, meaning that multiple eggs or sperm may have the variant but the rest of the parent's cells do not, resulting in "negative" testing from DNA assayed in leukocytes and an apparently *de novo* testing result but a slightly higher (1%–10%) risk of recurrence in offspring compared to a truly *de novo* variant in which only one oocyte or spermatocyte had the variant DNA.

For most familial epilepsies and *de novo* epilepsies identified during the initial periods of gene discovery, the genetic causes have been monogenic, meaning the causal variant is in a single gene and follows basic inheritance patterns of autosomal dominant, autosomal recessive, X-linked, etc. However, for many of the common, more drug-responsive forms of epilepsy, such as genetic generalized epilepsies (GGEs), efforts to identify monogenic causes have not been as successful, and there is likely a multifactorial etiology that involves risk incurred from multiple gene variants, called "polygenic risk," and possibly epigenetic factors. The understanding of these polygenic and epigenetic risk factors is still in its infancy, and their clinical applicability has not yet been established.

UTILITY OF GENETIC TESTING

Identification of the genetic cause of epilepsy has a multitude of benefits, including both clinical and personal benefits for the patient/family. From a clinical standpoint, identification of a genetic etiology ends the diagnostic odyssey, providing clarity of the diagnosis and stopping the cycle of invasive tests. A diagnostic genetic test may also provide prognostic value and lead to targeted diagnostics to screen for known comorbidities, such as with *TSC1/TSC2*-, *MECP2*-, and *WDR45*-related disorders, to name a few. Identification of the genetic etiology of epilepsy may also guide antiseizure medication (ASM) or other treatment choices and may affect clinical trial eligibility (Table 2.1). For those with drug-resistant epilepsy, growing evidence supporting genetic testing may also inform predictions of surgical candidacy and surgical outcomes, particularly in focal epilepsy without MRI-identified lesions.

Beyond the clinical utility, genetic testing is also of personal utility. Although a more formal assessment of the psychosocial impact of genetic testing is needed, there is general agreement about the importance of psychosocial factors. Several papers have described that a positive genetic result may alleviate parental guilt, provide a sense of closure, and facilitate processing of the diagnosis and prognosis. It may increase the family's understanding of the diagnosis and enable communication of the diagnosis to family members, schools, other healthcare providers, and other caretakers to increase understanding and potentially improve access to services. It also opens doors to family support networks. Lastly, it provides important information for recurrence risk determination and family planning.

GENETIC TESTING METHODS

Multiple techniques are used in the genetic evaluation of epilepsy, although not all techniques have the same clinical utility. The range of tests available continues to evolve and improve diagnostic yield. No single technology currently available can screen for all possible genetic mechanisms of epilepsy. The ordering clinician must

TABLE 2.1

Genetic Epilepsies and Syndromes with Epilepsy as a Prominent Feature in Which Genetic Etiology Influences Treatment and Trial Eligibility

Gene	Treatment
ALDH7A1	Pyridoxine
CAD	Uridine
CHRNA4, *CHRNB2*, and *CHRNA2*	Potential precision therapy: transdermal nicotine
CLN2	Cerliponase alfa to delay motor impairment
DEPDC5, *NPRL2*, and *NPRL3*	Potential precision therapy: mTOR inhibitors
GRIN1, *GRIN2A*, *GRIN2B*, and *GRIN2D*	Potential precision therapy: memantine, dextromethorphan for gain-of-function variants
KCNQ2	Sodium channel-blocking ASMs generally helpful. Potential precision therapy: ezogabine (in trial currently)
KCNT1 and *KCNT2*	Potential precision therapy: quinidine for gain-of-function variants
MECP2	Symptomatic treatments and trials ongoing
PNPO	Pyridoxal 5-phosphate
PRRT2	Carbamazepine helpful
SCN1A	Avoid sodium channel-blocking ASMs (generally) Potential precision therapy: fenfluramine and stiripentol
SCN2A	Sodium channel blocking ASM for gain-of-function variants. Generally, avoid sodium channel blocking ASM for loss-of-function variants
SCN8A	Sodium channel blocking ASM for gain-of-function variants Potential precision therapy: Trials ongoing
SLC2A1	Ketogenic diet
TSC1 and *TSC2*	Vigabatrin for infantile spasms Precision therapy: mTOR inhibitors
CDKL5	Ganaxolone
UBE3A	Potential precision therapy: trials ongoing

consider the phenotype of the individual and decide the test most likely to target the genes associated with the phenotype:

- Karyotype

  Karyotypes are images of a person's chromosomes isolated from an individual cell and arranged in pairs in numerical order based on size and banding patterns to look for abnormalities in chromosome number or structure. Historically, karyotypes have been used for identification of chromosomal aberrations in those with dysmorphic features or congenital anomalies (e.g., trisomy 21). However, chromosomal microarray analysis (CMA) has largely replaced the karyotype as the preferred modality in these situations due to greater resolution. Karyotype remains useful in epilepsy genetics evaluation if there is suspicion of a complex chromosomal rearrangement, such as a ring chromosome.

- Chromosomal Microarray Analysis

  CMA evaluates for CNVs (i.e., deletions and duplications). Laboratory technologies vary in the size of deletions and duplications that they can detect, to a minimum reporting threshold of 25 Kb. CMA is also able to detect regions of homozygosity, which may be due to parental consanguinity or uniparental disomy. The yield of testing with CMA is higher in individuals with epilepsy cooccurring with dysmorphic features or neurodevelopmental disorders (NDDs) such as developmental delay and autism spectrum disorder. CNVs are also more prevalent in the GGEs.

- Single Gene Testing with Sanger Sequencing

  Targeted testing for a variant in a single gene can be performed by polymerase chain reaction (PCR) and Sanger sequencing. Although, historically, this has been a mainstay of genetic testing, particularly for disorders such as Dravet syndrome, in which variants in a single gene are predominantly the explanation for the disorder, and more recently, gene panels have replaced single gene testing. Even in Dravet syndrome, where *SCN1A* variants are the predominant cause of the phenotype, there remains some genetic heterogeneity, in which other genes may cause a similar phenotype, particularly early in the course of the disorder. This genetic heterogeneity contributes to the higher yield of gene panels and exome sequencing over single gene testing. There are also reports of missed identification of variants due to errors in the Sanger sequencing technique. Single gene testing with Sanger sequencing remains useful to validate previously identified single nucleotide variants and for family segregation analysis.

- Next Generation Sequencing (NGS)

  NGS technologies allow for sequencing of the DNA and RNA at a faster and more cost-effective rate than Sanger sequencing. NGS includes three testing techniques: multigene panels, whole exome sequencing, and whole genome sequencing.

- Gene Panels

  Multigene panels (MGP) feature sequencing of the coding regions and surrounding splice sites, and depending on the panel, CNV analysis for targeted genes specific to a group of disorders, such as infantile-onset epilepsy. The panels may include several to hundreds of known epilepsy genes. The obvious limitation of MGP is that only genes in the panel will be tested. Several studies have found that the more genes included in the panel, the higher the diagnostic yield of the panel.

- Exome Sequencing

  Exome sequencing (ES) evaluates for sequence changes within the entire coding regions of approximately 20,000 genes and intronic regions near the exons. With the exception of splice sites immediately flanking an exon, intra- and intergenic noncoding regions are not included in the analysis. More recently, some laboratories are also able to detect CNV within the exons. ES may be analyzed for the patient alone or the patient and parent data may be analyzed together as a "duo" or "trio." Analysis of trio-based exome increases the diagnostic yield, as it improves the ability to classify any variants identified during testing. Exome sequencing allows for the option of reanalysis in the future if negative.

• Genome Sequencing

  Genome sequencing (GS) includes sequencing of the entire human genome, including the coding sequences, as well as the noncoding regions, and can detect SNVs, insertions/deletions, CNVs, and structural variants. GS has the potential to yield more variants of uncertain significance (VUS) than other methods, making a trio-based approach a key component of variant interpretation. GS is a more expensive testing method that is not often covered by insurance, but, as has been experienced with the other testing methods, the costs are expected to decline over time. As analysis methods develop, we anticipate more detection of noncoding variants in the regions of known genes and novel genes.

• Other

  In specific cases, additional targeted genetic testing may be required, guided by epilepsy-related phenotypes that suggest specific syndromes or genes.

Detection of Repeat Expansion Disorders. If disorders with tandem repeats as a causative mechanism of disease are suspected, targeted testing for the expansion triplet repeat within the gene should be considered. Examples of these disorders include Fragile X Syndrome (CGG repeats in the *FMR1* gene), *ARX*-related infantile epileptic-dyskinetic encephalopathy, Unverricht Lundborg Disease, and Familial Adult Myoclonic Epilepsy (FAME). Technologies utilizing long-read NGS platforms may improve the yield for identifying tandem repeat disorders using GS in the future.

Methylation Studies. If Angelman syndrome or Prader–Willi syndrome is suspected, methylation studies of 15q11.2-q13 chromosome region via methylation-sensitive multiplex ligation-dependent probe amplification (MS-MLPA) should be considered to detect deletions, uniparental disomy, and imprinting defects.

CHOOSING GENETIC TESTS FOR PATIENTS WITH EPILEPSIES

Just as there is not one test that will screen for all possible mechanisms of genetic variation in epilepsy, there is not a single algorithm for genetic testing in epilepsy. Similar to other diagnostic tests in medicine, there are pros and cons for each testing strategy that must be considered. The first step in genetic testing is to determine the phenotype of the individual, as this both inform the expected diagnostic yield of the genetic test and will also play a role in the interpretation of any results (Table 2.2). Detailed phenotype information should be provided to the testing lab to aid in their interpretation of any variants identified.

In general, for epilepsy, diagnostic yields for ES and GS are higher than those of MGP and CMA. As such, ES or epilepsy-focused MGP is generally considered the initial methodology of choice for most epilepsies. DEE and the presence of epilepsy with other neurodevelopmental comorbidities, such as intellectual disability or autism, increases the diagnostic yield for all of the testing techniques, and supports the continued testing with an alternative technique if the first test is negative. ES and

TABLE 2.2
Diagnostic Yield of Genetic Testing Techniques in Epilepsy

	Diagnostic Yield			
	Total Epilepsy		**Epilepsy + Other**	
Test	**Cohort (%)**	**DEEs (%)**	**NDDs (%)**	**Focal Epilepsy (%)**
CMA	9		9	
Multigene Panel	19	24		7
Exome Sequencing	24	29	27	8
Genome Sequencing	48			

Source: Percentages obtained from Sheidley et al. (2022).

GS provide the additional benefit of opportunity for reanalysis after an initial negative test. The yield of CMA is higher in those with epilepsy and dysmorphic features or other systemic abnormalities, supporting the use of CMA earlier in the diagnostic testing algorithm for these individuals.

INTERPRETATION OF THE GENETIC TESTING RESULTS

The work of epilepsy genetics does not end with receiving a genetic testing result. Any identified variant must be interpreted in the context of the patient's phenotype and what is known (or not known) about the structure and function of the gene, as well as previously identified variants in the gene. The interpretation of variants is guided by the American College of Medical Genetics and Genomics (ACMG) standard terminology, which includes five categories: pathogenic, likely pathogenic, uncertain significance, likely benign, and benign.

When receiving a genetic test result from the laboratory, the first step is determining if the clinical features are fully explained by the detected genetic variant. For some genes, the associated disorder, prognosis, and therapeutic implications depend on the functional consequence of the variant. This requires obtaining data on whether the variant has loss-of-function or gain-of-function properties, which may be reported in the literature or may require contacting a research group studying the gene and inquiring about the possibility of performing functional testing.

If the detected variant is of uncertain significance, there are several steps that may be taken to aid in interpretation. First, if parents have not been tested for the variant, parental testing may be helpful, as an unaffected parent with the same variant is often, although not always, a hint that it is not the cause of the epilepsy. If other family members are affected and available for testing, performing a familial segregation analysis of the variant and disorder can also be helpful. In addition, gaining a deeper understanding of the phenotype may aid interpretation of the variant. The clinician may reach out to the laboratory or use GeneMatcher to identify other clinicians and researchers to combine individuals with variants in the gene and evaluate for any potential gene–disease relationships.

If no genetic cause is identified, there may still be a genetic cause, but it has not yet been identified by the methods used in testing. If one is still suspicious of a genetic cause, a new technique may be employed to detect different types of variants, or if some time has passed, a benefit from improvement in technology. Reanalysis of ES or GS data after an appropriate time interval has also been shown to be successful at identifying causative genetic variants, as the scientific knowledge of gene variants continues to grow.

THE IMPORTANCE OF PRE- AND POSTTEST GENETIC COUNSELING

Prior to sending genetic testing, genetic counseling should be provided to individuals and families to review the reasons for testing, any anticipated results, and limitations of the tests. A discussion of potential results, including the meaning of ACMG variant interpretation classifications (pathogenic, likely pathogenic, variant of uncertain significance), and additional testing that may be undertaken for negative or uncertain results. It is also important to review the possible outcomes from positive results, including the impact (or potential lack of impact) on therapies and candidacy for trials.

For ES and GS, counseling must be provided on the possibility of identification of actionable secondary findings, which mostly include variants in cancer predisposition genes and cardiac arrhythmia genes. Individuals and parents may opt not to receive these secondary findings and should be counseled regarding this decision prior to testing. Nonclinical implications for genetic testing also need to be weighed by families prior to testing, and these include costs of the test, the effect on insurance, and potential implications for family dynamics.

CONCLUSIONS

Genetic testing has an established role in the evaluation of familial epilepsy and drug-resistant and early-onset epilepsy, and the understanding of the role of genetics in more common, non-drug-resistant epilepsy continues to grow. The pace of new discoveries in the genomics of epilepsy continues to be rapid. Genetic testing is becoming routine in the care of patients with epilepsy, presenting a challenge even to the well-informed neurologist, who must triage individuals who might benefit from testing, determine the appropriate and available tests, partner with genetic counselors or geneticists to consent patients and families, and interpret and explain findings, as well as implement the findings into a treatment plan that includes expanding prognostic and therapeutic implications.

SUGGESTED REFERENCES

Benke T.A., Park K., Krey I., Camp C.R., Sojng R., Ramsey A.J., Yuan H., Traynelis S.F., Lemke J. Clinical and therapeutic significance of genetic variation in the GRIN gene family encoding NMDARs. *Neuropharmacology* 2021;199: 108805.

Beygo J., Buiting K., Ramsden S.C., Ellis R., Clayton-Smith J., Kanber D. Update of the EMQN/ACGS best practice guidelines for molecular analysis of Prader-Willi and Angelman syndromes. *Eur J Hum Genet* 2019;27: 1326–40.

Borlot F., Abushama A., Morrison-Levy N., Jain P., Puthenveettil Vinayan K., Abukhalid M., Aldhalaan H.M., Almuzaini H.S., Gulati S., Hershkovitz T., Konanki R., Lingappa L., Luat A.F., Shafi S., Tabarki B., Thomas M., Yoganathan S., Alfadhel M., Arya R., Donner E.J., Ehaideb S.N., Gowda V.K., Jain V., Madaan P., Myers K.A., Otsubo H., Panda P., Sahu J.K., Sampaio L.P.B., Sharma S., Simard-Tremblay E., Zak M., Whitney R. KCNT1-related epilepsy: An international multicenter cohort of 27 pediatric cases. *Epilepsia* 2020;61: 679–92.

Chandrasekar I., Tourney A., Loo K., Carmichael J., James K., Ellsworth K.A., Dimmock D., Joseph M. Hemimegalencephaly and intractable seizures associated with the NPRL3 gene variant in a newborn: A case report. *Am J Med Genet A* 2021;185: 2126–30.

Chintalaphani S.R., Pineda S.S., Deveson I.W., Kumar K.R. An update on the neurological short tandem repeat expansion disorders and the emergence of long-read sequencing diagnostics. *Acta Neuropathol Commun* 2021;9: 98.

Chou I.C., Lin S.S., Lin W.D., Wang C.H., Chang Y.T., Tsai F.J., Tsai C.H. Successful control with carbamazepine of family with paroxysmal kinesigenic dyskinesia of PRRT2 mutation. *Biomedicine (Taipei)* 2014;4: 15.

Claes L., Del-Favero J., Ceulemans B., Lagae L., Van Broeckhoven C., De Jonghe P. De novo mutations in the sodium-channel gene SCN1A cause severe myoclonic epilepsy of infancy. *Am J Hum Genet* 2001;68: 1327–32.

Coughlin 2nd C.R., Tseng L.A., Abdenur J.E., Ashmore C., Boemer F., Bok L.A., Boyer M., Buhas D., Clayton P.T., Das A., Dekker H., Evangeliou A., Feillet F., Footitt E.J., Gospe Jr. S.M., Hartmann H., Kara M., Kristensen E., Lee J., Lilje R., Longo N., Lunsing R.J., Mills P., Papadopoulou M.T., Pearl P.L., Piazzon F., Plecko B., Saini A.G., Santra S., Sjarif D.R., Stockler-Ipsiroglu S., Striano P., Van Hove J.L.K., Verhoeven-Duif N.M., Wijburg F.A., Zuberi S.M., van Karnebeek C.D.M. Consensus guidelines for the diagnosis and management of pyridoxine-dependent epilepsy due to α-aminoadipic semialdehyde dehydrogenase deficiency. *J Inherit Metab Dis* 2021;44: 178–92.

Cowley M.J., Liu Y.C., Oliver K.L., Carvill G., Myers C.T., Gayevskiy V., Delatycki M., Vlaskamp D.R.M., Zhu Y., Mefford H., Buckley M.F., Bahlo M., Scheffer I.E., Dinger M.E., Roscioli T. Reanalysis and optimisation of bioinformatic pipelines is critical for mutation detection. *Hum Mutat* 2019;40: 374–9.

Djémié T., Weckhuysen S., von Spiczak S., Carvill G.L., Jaehn J., Anttonen A.K., Brilstra E., Caglayan H.S., de Kovel C.G., Depienne C., Gaily E., Gennaro E., Giraldez B.G., Gormley P., Guerrero-López R., Guerrini R., Hämäläinen E., Hartmann C., Hernandez-Hernandez L., Hjalgrim H., Koeleman B.P., Leguern E., Lehesjoki A.E., Lemke J.R., Leu C., Marini C., McMahon J.M., Mei D., Møller R.S., Muhle H., Myers C.T., Nava C., Serratosa J.M., Sisodiya S.M., Stephani U., Striano P., van Kempen M.J., Verbeek N.E., Usluer S., Zara F., Palotie A., Mefford H.C., Scheffer I.E., De Jonghe P., Helbig I., Suls A., EuroEPINOMICS-RES Dravet working group. Pitfalls in genetic testing: The story of missed SCN1A mutations. *Mol Genet Genomic Med* 2016;4: 457–64.

Epilepsy Genetics Initiative. The epilepsy genetics initiative: Systematic reanalysis of diagnostic exomes increases yield. *Epilepsia* 2019;60: 797–806.

Epilepsy Phenome/Genome Project EiKC. Diverse genetic causes of polymicrogyria with epilepsy. *Epilepsia* 2021;62: 973–83.

Franz D.N., Lawson J.A., Yapici Z., Ikeda H., Polster T., Nabbout R., Curatolo P., de Vries P.J., Dlugos D.J., Herbst F., Peyrard S., Pelov D., French J.A. Adjunctive everolimus therapy for tuberous sclerosis complex-associated refractory seizures: Results from the postextension phase of EXIST-3. *Epilepsia* 2021;62: 3029–41.

French J.A., Lawson J.A., Yapici Z., Ikeda H., Polster T., Nabbout R., Curatolo P., de Vries P.J., Dlugos D.J., Berkowitz N., Voi M., Peyrard S., Pelov D., Franz D.N. Adjunctive everolimus therapy for treatment-resistant focal-onset seizures associated with tuberous sclerosis (EXIST-3): A phase 3, randomised, double-blind, placebo-controlled study. *Lancet* 2016;388: 2153–63.

Fu C., Armstrong D., Marsh E., Lieberman D., Motil K., Witt R., Standridge S., Nues P., Lane J., Dinkel T., Coenraads M., von Hehn J., Jones M., Hale K., Suter B., Glaze D., Neul J., Percy A., Benke T. Consensus guidelines on managing Rett syndrome across the lifespan. *BMJ Paediatr Open* 2020;4: e000717.

Guerrini R., Dravet C., Genton P., Belmonte A., Kaminska A., Dulac O. Lamotrigine and seizure aggravation in severe myoclonic epilepsy. *Epilepsia* 1998;39: 508–12.

Helbig I., Ellis C.A. Personalized medicine in genetic epilepsies - Possibilities, challenges, and new frontiers. *Neuropharmacology* 2020;172: 107970.

Hong W., Haviland I., Pestana-Knight E., Weisenberg J.L., Demarest S., Marsh E.D., Olson H.E. CDKL5 deficiency disorder-related epilepsy: A review of current and emerging treatment. *CNS Drugs* 2022;36: 591–604.

Ibañez K., Polke J., Hagelstrom R.T., Dolzhenko E., Pasko D., Thomas E.R.A., Daugherty L.C., Kasperaviciute D., Smith K.R.; WGS for Neurological Diseases Group, Deans Z.C., Hill S., Fowler T., Scott R.H., Hardy J., Chinnery P.F., Houlden H., Rendon A., Caulfield M.J., Eberle M.A., Taft R.J., Tucci A.; Genomics England Research Consortium. Whole genome sequencing for the diagnosis of neurological repeat expansion disorders in the UK: A retrospective diagnostic accuracy and prospective clinical validation study. *Lancet Neurol* 2022;21: 234–45.

Ivy A.S., Standridge S.M. Rett syndrome: A timely review from recognition to current clinical approaches and clinical study updates. *Semin Pediatr Neurol* 2021;37: 100881.

Johannesen K.M., Liu Y., Koko M., Gjerulfsen C.E., Sonnenberg L., Schubert J., Fenger C.D., Eltokhi A., Rannap M., Koch N.A., Lauxmann S., Krüger J., Kegele J., Canafoglia L., Franceschetti S., Mayer T., Rebstock J., Zacher P., Ruf S., Alber M., Sterbova K., Lassuthová P., Vlckova M., Lemke J.R., Platzer K., Krey I., Heine C., Wieczorek D., Kroell-Seger J., Lund C., Klein K.M., Au P.Y.B., Rho J.M., Ho A.W., Masnada S., Veggiotti P., Giordano L., Accorsi P., Hoei-Hansen C.E., Striano P., Zara F., Verhelst H., Verhoeven J.S., Braakman H.M.H., van der Zwaag B., Harder A.V.E., Brilstra E., Pendziwiat M., Lebon S., Vaccarezza M., Le N.M., Christensen J., Grønborg S., Scherer S.W., Howe J., Fazeli W., Howell K.B., Leventer R., Stutterd C., Walsh S., Gerard M., Gerard B., Matricardi S., Bonardi C.M., Sartori S., Berger A., Hoffman-Zacharska D., Mastrangelo M., Darra F., Vøllo A., Motazacker M.M., Lakeman P., Nizon M., Betzler C., Altuzarra C., Caume R., Roubertie A., Gélisse P., Marini C., Guerrini R., Bilan F., Tibussek D., Koch-Hogrebe M., Perry M.S., Ichikawa S., Dadali E., Sharkov A., Mishina I., Abramov M., Kanivets I., Korostelev S., Kutsev S., Wain K.E., Eisenhauer N., Wagner M., Savatt J.M., Müller-Schlüter K., Bassan H., Borovikov A., Nassogne M.C., Destrée A., Schoonjans A.S., Meuwissen M., Buzatu M., Jansen A., Scalais E., Srivastava S., Tan W.H., Olson H.E., Loddenkemper T., Poduri A., Helbig K.L., Helbig I., Fitzgerald M.P., Goldberg E.M., Roser T., Borggraefe I., Brünger T., May P., Lal D., Lederer D., Rubboli G., Heyne H.O., Lesca G., Hedrich U.B.S., Benda J., Gardella E., Lerche H., Møller R.S. Genotype-phenotype correlations in SCN8A-related disorders reveal prognostic and therapeutic implications. *Brain* 2021;145: 2991–3009.

Kalachikov S., Evgrafov O., Ross B., Winawer M., Barker-Cummings C., Martinelli Boneschi F., Choi C., Morozov P., Das K., Teplitskaya E., Yu A., Cayanis E., Penchaszadeh G., Kottmann A.H., Pedley T.A., Hauser W.A., Ottman R., Gilliam T.C. Mutations in LGI1 cause autosomal-dominant partial epilepsy with auditory features. *Nat Genet* 2002;30: 335–41.

Klepper J., Akman C., Armeno M., Auvin S., Cervenka M., Cross H.J., De Giorgis V., Della Marina A., Engelstad K., Heussinger N., Kossoff E.H., Leen W.G., Leiendecker B., Monani U.R., Oguni H., Neal E., Pascual J.M., Pearson T.S., Pons R., Scheffer I.E., Veggiotti P., Willemsen M., Zuberi S.M., De Vivo D.C. Glut1 Deficiency Syndrome (Glut1DS): State of the art in 2020 and recommendations of the international Glut1DS study group. *Epilepsia Open* 2020;5: 354–65.

Kobow K., Reid C.A., van Vliet E.A., Becker A.J., Carvill G.L., Goldman A.M., Hirose S., Lopes-Cendes I., Khiari H.M., Poduri A., Johnson M.R., Henshall D.C. Epigenetics explained: A topic "primer" for the epilepsy community by the ILAE Genetics/Epigenetics Task Force. *Epileptic Disord* 2020;22: 127–41.

Koch J., Mayr J.A., Alhaddad B., Rauscher C., Bierau J., Kovacs-Nagy R., Coene K.L., Bader I., Holzhacker M., Prokisch H., Venselaar H., Wevers R.A., Distelmaier F., Polster T., Leiz S., Betzler C., Strom T.M., Sperl W., Meitinger T., Wortmann S.B., Haack T.B. CAD mutations and uridine-responsive epileptic encephalopathy. *Brain* 2017;140: 279–286.

Lai D., Gade M., Yang E., Koh H.Y., Lu J., Walley N.M., Buckley A.F., Sands T.T., Akman C.I., Mikati M.A., McKhann G.M., Goldman J.E., Canoll P., Alexander A.L., Park K.L., Von Allmen G.K., Rodziyevska O., Bhattacharjee M.B., Lidov H.G.W., Vogel H., Grant G.A., Porter B.E., Poduri A.H., Crino P.B., Heinzen E.L. Somatic variants in diverse genes leads to a spectrum of focal cortical malformations. *Brain* 2022;145(8): 2704–2720.

Leu C., Stevelink R., Smith A.W., Goleva S.B., Kanai M., Ferguson L., Campbell C., Kamatani Y., Okada Y., Sisodiya S.M., Cavalleri G.L., Koeleman B.P.C., Lerche H., Jehi L., Davis L.K., Najm I.M., Palotie A., Daly M.J., Busch R.M.; Epi25 Consortium, Lal D. Polygenic burden in focal and generalized epilepsies. *Brain* 2019;142: 3473–81.

Lossius K., de Saint Martin A., Myren-Svelstad S., Bjørnvold M., Minken G., Seegmuller C., Valenti Hirsch M.P., Chelly J., Steinlein O., Picard F., Brodtkorb E. Remarkable effect of transdermal nicotine in children with CHRNA4-related autosomal dominant sleep-related hypermotor epilepsy. *Epilepsy Behav* 2020;105: 106944.

Millichap J.J., Park K.L., Tsuchida T., Ben-Zeev B., Carmant L., Flamini R., Joshi N., Levisohn P.M., Marsh E., Nangia S., Narayanan V., Ortiz-Gonzalez X.R., Patterson M.C., Pearl P.L., Porter B., Ramsey K., McGinnis E.L., Taglialatela M., Tracy M., Tran B., Venkatesan C., Weckhuysen S., Cooper E.C. KCNQ2 encephalopathy: Features, mutational hot spots, and ezogabine treatment of 11 patients. *Neurol Genet* 2016;2: e96.

Mills P.B., Camuzeaux S.S., Footitt E.J., Mills K.A., Gissen P., Fisher L., Das K.B., Varadkar S.M., Zuberi S., McWilliam R., Stödberg T., Plecko B., Baumgartner M.R., Maier O., Calvert S., Riney K., Wolf N.I., Livingston J.H., Bala P., Morel C.F., Feillet F., Raimondi F., Del Giudice E., Chong W.K., Pitt M., Clayton P.T. Epilepsy due to PNPO mutations: Genotype, environment and treatment affect presentation and outcome. *Brain* 2014;137: 1350–60.

Mole S.E., Schulz A., Badoe E., Berkovic S.F., de Los Reyes E.C., Dulz S., Gissen P., Guelbert N., Lourenco C.M., Mason H.L., Mink J.W., Murphy N., Nickel M., Olaya J.E., Scarpa M., Scheffer I.E., Simonati A., Specchio N., Von Löbbecke I., Wang R.Y., Williams R.E. Guidelines on the diagnosis, clinical assessments, treatment and management for CLN2 disease patients. *Orphanet J Rare Dis* 2021;16: 185.

Møller R.S., Liebmann N., Larsen L.H.G., Stiller M., Hentschel J., Kako N., Abdin D., Di Donato N., Pal D.K., Zacher P., Syrbe S., Dahl H.A., Lemke J.R. Parental mosaicism in epilepsies due to alleged de novo variants. *Epilepsia* 2019;60: e63–e66.

Moloney P.B., Dugan P., Widdess-Walsh P., Devinsky O., Delanty N. Genomics in the presurgical epilepsy evaluation. *Epilepsy Res* 2022;184: 106951.

Northrup H., Aronow M.E., Bebin E.M., Bissler J., Darling T.N., de Vries P.J., Frost M.D., Fuchs Z., Gosnell E.S., Gupta N., Jansen A.C., Jóźwiak S., Kingswood J.C., Knilans T.K., McCormack F.X., Pounders A., Roberds S.L., Rodriguez-Buritica D.F., Roth J.,

Sampson J.R., Sparagana S., Thiele E.A., Weiner H.L., Wheless J.W., Towbin A.J., Krueger D.A.; International Tuberous Sclerosis Complex Consensus Group. Updated international tuberous sclerosis complex diagnostic criteria and surveillance and management recommendations. *Pediatr Neurol* 2021;123: 50–66.

Oliver K.L., Ellis C.A., Scheffer I.E., Ganesan S., Leu C., Sadleir L.G., Heinzen E.L., Mefford H.C., Bass A.J., Curtis S.W., Harris R.V.; Epi4K Consortium, Whiteman D.C., Helbig I., Ottman R., Epstein M.P., Bahlo M., Berkovic S.F. Common risk variants for epilepsy are enriched in families previously targeted for rare monogenic variant discovery. *EBioMedicine* 2022;81: 104079.

Perucca P., Scheffer I.E. Genetic contributions to acquired epilepsies. *Epilepsy Curr* 2021;21: 5–13.

Peters L., Depienne C., Klebe S. Familial adult myoclonic epilepsy (FAME): Clinical features, molecular characteristics, pathophysiological aspects and diagnostic work-up. *Medizinische Genetik* 2021;33: 311–8.

Poduri A.H., George J., Alfred L., Heinzen E.L., Lowenstein D., James S. (editors). *How We Got to Where We're Going.* Cambridge: Cambridge University Press, 2021.

Retterer K., Scuffins J., Schmidt D., Lewis R., Pineda-Alvarez D., Stafford A., Schmidt L., Warren S., Gibellini F., Kondakova A., Blair A., Bale S., Matyakhina L., Meck J., Aradhya S., Haverfield E. Assessing copy number from exome sequencing and exome array CGH based on CNV spectrum in a large clinical cohort. *Genet Med* 2015;17: 623–629.

Richards S., Aziz N., Bale S., Bick D., Das S., Gastier-Foster J., Grody W.W., Hegde M., Lyon E., Spector E., Voelkerding K., Rehm H.L.; ACMG Laboratory Quality Assurance Committee. Standards and guidelines for the interpretation of sequence variants: A joint consensus recommendation of the American College of Medical Genetics and Genomics and the Association for Molecular Pathology. *Genet Med* 2015;17: 405–24.

Riggs E.R., Andersen E.F., Cherry A.M., Kantarci S., Kearney H., Patel A., Raca G., Ritter D.I., South S.T., Thorland E.C., Pineda-Alvarez D., Aradhya S., Martin C.L. Technical standards for the interpretation and reporting of constitutional copy-number variants: A joint consensus 11recommendation of the American College of Medical Genetics and Genomics (ACMG) and the Clinical Genome Resource (ClinGen). *Genet Med* 2020;22: 245–57.

Rochtus A., Olson H.E., Smith L., Keith L.G., El Achkar C., Taylor A., Mahida S., Park M., Kelly M., Shain C., Rockowitz S., Rosen Sheidley B., Poduri A. Genetic diagnoses in epilepsy: The impact of dynamic exome analysis in a pediatric cohort. *Epilepsia* 2020;61: 249–58.

Sánchez Fernández I., Loddenkemper T., Gaínza-Lein M., Sheidley B.R., Poduri A. Diagnostic yield of genetic tests in epilepsy: A meta-analysis and cost-effectiveness study. *Neurology* 2019;92: e418–e428.

Sheidley B.R., Malinowski J., Bergner A.L., Bier L., Gloss D.S., Mu W., Mulhern M.M., Partack EJ, Poduri A. Genetic testing for the epilepsies: A systematic review. *Epilepsia* 2022;63: 375–87.

Shoubridge C., Fullston T., Gécz J. ARX spectrum disorders: Making inroads into the molecular pathology. *Hum Mutat* 2010;31: 889–900.

Spector E., Behlmann A., Kronquist K., Rose N.C., Lyon E., Reddi H.V.; ACMG Laboratory Quality Assurance Committee. Laboratory testing for fragile X, 2021 revision: A technical standard of the American College of Medical Genetics and Genomics (ACMG). *Genet Med* 2021;23: 799–812.

Steinlein O.K., Mulley J.C., Propping P., Wallace R.H., Phillips H.A., Sutherland G.R., Scheffer I.E., Berkovic S.F. A missense mutation in the neuronal nicotinic acetylcholine receptor alpha 4 subunit is associated with autosomal dominant nocturnal frontal lobe epilepsy. *Nat Genet* 1995;11: 201–3.

Vanoye C.G., Desai R.R., Ji Z., Adusumilli S., Jairam N., Ghabra N., Joshi N., Fitch E., Helbig K.L., McKnight D., Lindy A.S., Zou F., Helbig I., Cooper E.C., George Jr. A.L. High-throughput evaluation of epilepsy-associated KCNQ2 variants reveals functional and pharmacological heterogeneity. *JCI Insight*. 2022; 7: e156314.

Vawter-Lee M., Franz D.N., Fuller C.E., Greiner H.M. Clinical Letter: A case report of targeted therapy with sirolimus for NPRL3 epilepsy. *Seizure* 2019;73: 43–45.

Virtaneva K., D'Amato E., Miao J., Koskiniemi M., Norio R., Avanzini G., Franceschetti S., Michelucci R., Tassinari C.A., Omer S., Pennacchio L.A., Myers R.M., Dieguez-Lucena J.L., Krahe R., de la Chapelle A., Lehesjoki A.E. Unstable minisatellite expansion causing recessively inherited myoclonus epilepsy, EPM1. *Nat Genet* 1997;15: 393–6.

Wallace R.H., Scheffer I.E., Barnett S., Richards M., Dibbens L., Desai R.R., Lerman-Sagie T., Lev D., Mazarib A., Brand N., Ben-Zeev B., Goikhman I., Singh R., Kremmidiotis G., Gardner A., Sutherland G.R., George Jr. A.L., Mulley J.C., Berkovic S.F. Neuronal sodium-channel alpha1-subunit mutations in generalized epilepsy with febrile seizures plus. *Am J Hum Genet* 2001;68: 859–65.

Wilson J.L., Gregory A., Kurian M.A., Bushlin I., Mochel F., Emrick L., Adang L.; BPAN Guideline Contributing Author Group, Hogarth P., Hayflick S.J. Consensus clinical management guideline for beta-propeller protein-associated neurodegeneration. *Dev Med Child Neurol* 2021;63: 1402–9.

Wolff M., Johannesen K.M., Hedrich U.B.S., Masnada S., Rubboli G., Gardella E., Lesca G., Ville D., Milh M., Villard L., Afenjar A., Chantot-Bastaraud S., Mignot C., Lardennois C., Nava C., Schwarz N., Gérard M., Perrin L., Doummar D., Auvin S., Miranda M.J., Hempel M., Brilstra E., Knoers N., Verbeek N., van Kempen M., Braun K.P., Mancini G., Biskup S., Hörtnagel K., Döcker M., Bast T., Loddenkemper T., Wong-Kisiel L., Baumeister F.M., Fazeli W., Striano P., Dilena R., Fontana E., Zara F., Kurlemann G., Klepper J., Thoene J.G., Arndt D.H., Deconinck N., Schmitt-Mechelke T., Maier O., Muhle H., Wical B., Finetti C., Brückner R., Pietz J., Golla G., Jillella D., Linnet K.M., Charles P., Moog U., Õiglane-Shlik E., Mantovani J.F., Park K., Deprez M., Lederer D., Mary S., Scalais E., Selim L., Van Coster R., Lagae L., Nikanorova M., Hjalgrim H., Korenke G.C., Trivisano M., Specchio N., Ceulemans B., Dorn T., Helbig K.L., Hardies K., Stamberger H., de Jonghe P., Weckhuysen S., Lemke J.R., Krägeloh-Mann I., Helbig I., Kluger G., Lerche H., Møller R.S. Genetic and phenotypic heterogeneity suggest therapeutic implications in SCN2A-related disorders. *Brain* 2017;140: 1316–36.

Xu Y., Song R., Chen W., Strong K., Shrey D., Gedela S., Traynelis S.F., Zhang G., Yuan H. Recurrent seizure-related GRIN1 variant: Molecular mechanism and targeted therapy. *Ann Clin Transl Neurol* 2021;8: 1480–94.

Yuskaitis C.J., Ruzhnikov M.R.Z., Howell K.B., Allen I.E., Kapur K., Dlugos D.J., Scheffer I.E., Poduri A., Sherr E.H. Infantile spasms of unknown cause: Predictors of outcome and genotype-phenotype correlation. *Pediatr Neurol* 2018;87: 48–56.

3 Developmental Pharmacokinetics
Principles and Practice

Melissa Barker-Haliski
University of Washington

CONTENTS

Many age-related variables influence the pharmacokinetic properties of drugs. Absorption of drugs delivered by the oral route is age dependent but can occur in the stomach, small intestine, and colon. Maturation of the gastrointestinal tract is a major driver of age-related differences in pharmacokinetics of orally administered drugs used in children and infants.

With respect to absorption, gastric pH is increased in neonates, infants, and young children but decreases to adult levels after age 2. Gastric emptying time does not markedly differ in neonates relative to older children or adults and largely approximates that of human milk or formula (~48–78 minutes). Many factors can influence the *a*bsorption, *d*istribution, *m*etabolism, and *e*xcretion (ADME) of an orally administered drug in neonates and infants, including, but not limited to, gastric acid production, residence time, absorptive surface area, intestinal transit time, and biotransformation reactions. Importantly, neonates are unique relative to older children or adults in that the colon plays an outsized role in drug absorption, allowing for more frequent colonic administration in this age range.

Once absorbed, a drug is distributed to various body compartments in a manner that is dependent on its unique physiochemical properties, such as molecular size, ionization constant, and relative aqueous and lipid solubility. In neonates and infants, the increased total-body-water to body-fat ratio contributes to an increase in the volume of distribution (V_d) of drugs. The direction of the change will also depend on the drug's physiochemical characteristics. The plasma concentration that results from a

DOI: 10.1201/9781003296478-4

loading dose of a drug is inversely proportional to the V_d. Therefore, determination of loading doses for a given drug should account for age-related changes in V_d.

Protein binding is another important variable that affects V_d. Albumin and α_1-acid-glycoprotein concentrations are decreased in the neonate and infant and only reach adult levels after the first year of life. The decreased protein binding alters the ratio of unbound to total plasma concentrations of antiseizure medications (ASMs). For highly protein-bound ASMs (Table 3.1), total concentrations are not reliable for therapeutic drug monitoring and will underestimate the unbound or active concentration of ASMs in neonates. Assessments of unbound plasma concentrations are required to avoid dose-dependent adverse events.

Elimination of ASMs occurs through either renal excretion of unchanged parent drug, hepatic biotransformation to metabolites (both active and inactive), or a combination of both. At birth, renal blood flow, glomerular filtration rates, and tubular secretion and reabsorption are at approximately 25%–30% of adult values but increase steadily to 50%–75% of adult values by 6 months of age. Full maturation of renal function is generally attained in approximately 1 year. In preterm neonates, renal function is not only immature at birth, but it also remains significantly delayed from achieving its full capacity. As with the gastrointestinal tract, transporter proteins participate in active renal excretion of many drugs. In general, weight-normalized doses of ASMs, excreted predominately unchanged by the kidneys, need to be reduced only for neonates and infants. Drug interactions occur less frequently with drugs metabolized by non-CYP or UGT pathway, or if eliminated unchanged.

The influence of developmental maturation on hepatic metabolism is dependent on the enzymes involved. The cytochrome P450 (CYP) and uridine diphosphate (UDP) glucuronosyltransferase (UGT) family of enzymes catalyze biotransformation of most of the older (first and second generation) ASMs, whereas newer ASMs are eliminated by a variety of pathways (Table 3.1). CYP-dependent metabolism is low at birth – approximately 50%–70% of adult levels.

However, by 3 years of age, CYP enzymatic activity actually surpasses adult values. Therefore, infants aged <1 year generally have decreased ability to eliminate drugs, while young children have an increased ability (relative to adults) to eliminate drugs metabolized by the CYP isozymes. By puberty, the CYP activity decreases to adult levels. The one exception is CYP2C19, which appears to have similar activity in children versus adults. UGT activity in neonates is deficient at birth and reaches adult levels by 4 years of age.

Children have slightly increased UGT activity relative to adults; however, this difference is significantly less than with the CYP isozymes. The effect of age on drugs that are eliminated by a combination of pathways (i.e., renal and hepatic) will depend both on the relative maturation of these pathways as well as the relative fraction of each drug eliminated through them.

The pharmacokinetic properties of the ASMs are summarized in Table 3.1. The remainder of this chapter will thus define the critical ADME properties relevant to ASM administration in infants and children.

TABLE 3.1

Pharmacokinetic Properties of the Antiseizure Medications (ASMs)

Drug	ASD Generation	Absorption		Protein Bound	Children Require Larger mg/kg Doses?[a]	Effect of Enzyme Inducers?	Major Metabolic Pathway
		F	T_{max} (hr)				
Renal Elimination							
Gabapentin	3rd	<60%	2–3	0	Yes, 30%–50%	No	N/A
Pregabalin	3rd	>90%	3	0	Yes, 40%	No	N/A
Vigabatrin	3rd	60%–80%	0.5–2	0	No	No	N/A
Metabolic Elimination							
Carbamazepine	2nd	>80%	4–8	75	Yes, 50%–100%	Yes	CYP3A4, 1A2, 2C8
Clobazam	2nd	>85%	0.5–2	90	No	Yes	Multiple
Clonazepam	2nd	>80%	1–4	85	No	Yes	Multiple
Diazepam	2nd	>95%	0.5–1.5	94–99	Yes, 50%–100%	Yes	CYP3A4 and CYP2C19
Lamotrigine	3rd	>95%	2–4	50	No	Yes	Glucuronidation
Lorazepam	3rd	>90%	1–2	85–91	No	Yes	Multiple
Phenytoin	1st	>90%	Varied	90	Yes, 50%–100%	Yes	UDP-glucuronyl-transferase and CYP2C9
Tiagabine	3rd	>95%	1	96	Yes, 50%	Yes	UGT and CYP3A4
Valproate	2nd	>95%	Varied	7–15	Yes, 50%–100%	Yes	β-oxidation & glucuronidation
Cannabidiol	3rd	Varied	2–5	94	No	Yes	CYP3A4

(Continued)

TABLE 3.1 (*Continued*)
Pharmacokinetic Properties of the Antiseizure Medications (ASMs)

Drug	ASD Generation	Absorption F	Absorption T$_{max}$ (hr)	Protein Bound	Children Require Larger mg/kg Doses?[a]	Effect of Enzyme Inducers?	Major Metabolic Pathway
Stiripentol	3rd	Varied	2–3	99	No	Yes	Multiple
Brivaracetam	3rd	>99%	1	<20	No	Yes	CYP2C19
Perampanel	3rd	>99%	0.5–2.5	95–96	No	Yes	CYP3A4
Eslicarbazepine acetate	3rd	>90%	1–4	40	No	Yes	Unchanged once active metabolite
Metabolic and Renal Elimination							
Ethosuximide	1st	100%	3–7	0	Yes, 50%–100%	Yes	CYP3A4
Felbamate	3rd	>95%	2–4	30	Yes, 40%	Yes	Glucuronidation & CYP3A4
Levetiracetam	3rd	>95%	1	0	Yes, 30%–50%	No	N/A
Oxcarbazepine	3rd	>95%	7 (MHD)	40	Yes, 30%–80%	Yes	Ketoreductase
Phenobarbital	1st	>95%	1–4	50	Yes, 50%–100%	Yes	CYP2C9, 2C19, and 2E1
Topiramate	3rd	~80%	3–4	20	Yes, 30%–50%	Yes	N/A
Zonisamide	3rd	>90%	2–4	50	Yes, 50%–100%	Yes	Mixed, CYP3A4
Lacosamide	3rd	>99%	1–4	15	No	Yes	Demethylation
Fenfluramine	3rd	68%–74%	4–5	50	No	Yes	Multiple CYPs
Rufinamide	3rd	>85%	4–6	34	No	Yes	Hydrolysis

[a] Approximately estimated based on available data.

ASMs ELIMINATED RENALLY

For ASMs eliminated by renal excretion of unchanged drug, neonates and infants require significantly lower doses than children and adults due to immature renal function. Weight-corrected doses should be approximately the same in children and adults if there are no age-related effects on absorption.

Gabapentin is less than completely absorbed (<60%) and is highly variable due to saturation of active L-neutral amino acid transporters in the gastrointestinal tract. Children less than 5 years of age have significantly higher and more variable oral gabapentin clearance than older children. Infants and young children (<5 years) require greater weight-normalized doses to attain similar concentrations. The weight-normalized oral clearance in children aged >5 years is comparable to adults. Further, children older than >5 years may also need higher weight-normalized doses than adults.

Pregabalin is approved as adjunctive therapy for focal-onset seizures in individuals older than 1 month. It has linear pharmacokinetics and does not bind plasma proteins. In patients aged 1 month to 16 years, body weight-normalized pregabalin clearance is ~40% higher in individuals weighing <30 kg compared with patients weighing ≥ 30 kg. Use of pregabalin in children (4–16 years) weighing <30 kg should be adjusted to a 40% higher dose (per kg of body weight) than in patients weighing ≥30 kg to achieve similar exposure.

Vigabatrin is renally eliminated almost completely unchanged. Children aged <5 years have lower concentration-to-dose ratios than adults; however, there is no clear relationship between vigabatrin plasma concentrations and clinical effect. Vigabatrin is titrated slowly to clinical effect and not to therapeutic plasma concentrations.

ASMs ELIMINATED BY CYP-DEPENDENT METABOLISM

For the older generation ASMs (Table 3.1) that are eliminated predominantly by CYP-dependent metabolism, neonates and infants require lower doses than young children. Young children will need approximately 50% higher mg/kg doses than older children, and older children will need approximately 50% higher mg/kg doses than adults.

Carbamazepine (CBZ) is extensively metabolized. CBZ-epoxide is the predominant pharmacologically active metabolite, accounting for approximately 25% of the dose in monotherapy and 50% in polytherapy with other enzyme-inducing ASMs. There is a higher weight-adjusted total body clearance and higher CBZ-epoxide to carbamazepine ratio in children versus adults. Carbamazepine has a significantly shorter $t_{1/2}$ in children versus adults, which may require more frequent dosing. Controlled-release formulations significantly reduce fluctuations in plasma concentrations and toxicity associated with high peak concentrations. Children generally need 50%–100% higher weight-normalized maintenance doses than adults to achieve comparable serum levels.

Cannabidiol was first approved for Dravet syndrome, a rare pediatric genetic epilepsy in 2018. It has rapid uptake following oral administration. It is extensively metabolized by first-pass metabolism via CYP3A4 and has relatively low oral bioavailability (6%–10%). Bioavailability is further limited by the hydropho-bic nature of cannabidiol, which also exhibits limited solubility in the gut. While bioavailability decreases in adults that receive high doses of cannabidiol, the lower doses needed for children results in a linear increase in systemic exposure between 10 and 40 mg/kg/day. However, there is wide variability in cannabidiol disposition between adults and children, and even between infants and older pediatric patients, primarily due to developmental maturation differences.

Diazepam is extensively metabolized to several active metabolites, including desmethyldiazepam, temazepam, and oxazepam, through reactions catalyzed by CYP2C19 and CYP3A4. Notably, the mean $t_{1/2}$ of diazepam and desmethyldiazepam is significantly prolonged in poor metabolizers by CYP2C19.

Fenfluramine was approved for use in Dravet syndrome in 2020. It is lipid soluble and has good oral bioavailability that is unaffected by food intake. Fenfluramine is partially metabolized to d(+)- (6)- and l(−)-(1)-norfenfluramine by a diversity of CYP enzymes, including CYP1A2, CYP2B6, CYP2D6, CYP2C9, CYP2C19, and CYP3A4, before undergoing renal elimination. While metabolism by several CYP enzymes largely minimizes potential drug–drug interactions, reduction in fenflura-mine dose in combination with stiripentol is recommended to avoid adverse effects.

Perampanel is metabolized extensively in the liver, primarily by CYP3A4. Perampanel is rapidly absorbed after oral administration and pharmacokinetics are independent of age, weight, or liver function. There is no need for age- or weight-based adjustments to achieve effective exposures in patients ≥2 years of age. Due to CYP3A4 metabolism, enzyme-inducing ASMs dose-dependently reduce perampanel concentrations in adults, although studies have not yet been extended to children.

Phenytoin is eliminated predominately by saturable CYP2C9 and CYP2C19-dependent hepatic metabolism. Individuals with CYP2C9 or CYP2C19 poor metab-olizer variants will exhibit significantly increased concentration-to-dose ratios. Neonates have decreased weight-normalized unbound clearance. In neonates, decreased albumin results in decreased protein binding and, as such, total phenytoin concentrations will not reflect the unbound or active phenytoin.

ASMs ELIMINATED BY UGT-DEPENDENT HEPATIC METABOLISM

For drugs eliminated predominately by UGT, neonates and infants will require lower doses; however, weight-corrected doses should be approximately the same for chil-dren and adults.

Lamotrigine is predominately eliminated by hepatic metabolism by UGT1A4 and then renally eliminated. Weight-normalized oral clearance in neonates under 1 month of age is approximately 50% lower than in infants aged 2–12 months. However, compared with adults, young children (<2 years) have higher weight-corrected clearance. Therefore, lamotrigine monotherapy should be adjusted for age; however, enzyme-inducing ASM comedication in children may require higher weight-normalized doses.

Lorazepam is extensively metabolized to a glucuronide conjugate. Neonates have significantly decreased oral clearance versus children and adults. The pharmacokinet-ics of lorazepam in young children does not significantly differ from values obtained in adults. Age-related dosing is not necessary. Glucuronidation reaches adult levels by age 3 years, thus weight-corrected doses in children >3 years of age should be the same as adults. Infants and children <3 years old should receive reduced doses.

ASMs ELIMINATED BY MIXED CYP, UGT, AND OTHER METABOLIC PATHWAYS

Several ASMs are extensively metabolized by multiple metabolic pathways, with minimal excretion of unchanged drug in the urine. Predicting age-related effects is more difficult due to the larger intersubject variability in the fraction eliminated by each pathway, and lack of data on the effect of age on the non-CYP and UGT enzymes.

Clobazam is eliminated predominately by hepatic metabolism to multiple metabolites. The primary metabolite, N-desmethylclobazam, is active and accumulates to approximately eight-fold higher serum concentrations than clobazam after multiple doses. It is unclear if children require higher doses of clobazam than adults. Doses of clobazam should be initiated and titrated to effect and tolerability in both children and adults.

Clonazepam is approved as an adjunctive treatment for seizures associated with Lennox–Gastaut syndrome in patients > 2 years old. It is extensively metabolized. Neonates receiving clonazepam require lower weight-normalized doses than older children and adults. The $t_{1/2}$ of clonazepam is prolonged in neonates, with a significantly lower clearance than found in older children and adults.

Tiagabine is extensively metabolized via CYP3A4 and UGT-predominant pathways. The weight-corrected clearance of tiagabine is two-fold higher in children than adults not receiving enzyme-inducing ASMs. The weight-corrected clearance is similar to older children and adults receiving enzyme-inducing drugs.

Valproate undergoes extensive hepatic metabolism by UGT-catalyzed glucuronide conjugation and β-oxidation. Neonates with intractable seizures have highly variable but similar total clearances as compared to adults. Due to low albumin concentrations in neonates, total valproate concentrations underestimate the unbound or pharmacologically active valproate concentration. During the first 2 months of life, clearance increases significantly due to maturation of hepatic enzymes. Older infants – aged 3–36 months – exhibit significantly higher weight-normalized clearance than adults. School-age children have clearances intermediate to those found in infants and adults. Infants and young children thus need weight-adjusted doses 50%–100% higher than adults to attain similar plasma concentrations.

Stiripentol is approved as adjunctive therapy with clobazam in patients with Dravet syndrome. Stiripentol is a potent inhibitor of several CYP450 enzymes, including CYP3A4, 2C9, 2C19, and 2D6, thus having a high potential for drug–drug interactions. Clobazam levels are particularly susceptible to fluctuations. Therefore, therapeutic drug monitoring is advised to avoid toxicity. Stiripentol administration in children is associated with nonlinear dose-related clearance. Stiripentol exposures increase by up to 300% in children weighing >30 kg; therefore, the dose of stiripentol should be adjusted as children enter adolescence.

Eslicarbazepine acetate is the prodrug of eslicarbazepine, the major pharmacologically active metabolite, and is structurally related to carbamazepine and oxcarbazepine. Eslicarbazepine acetate is rapidly and extensively hydrolyzed in both children and adolescents, consistent with metabolism in adults. It shows dose-proportional exposures in children and adolescents, but the relative exposure is age limited. Older children with epilepsy (aged 12–17) will have higher relative exposure than younger children (aged <12 years).

ASMs ELIMINATED BY HEPATIC METABOLISM AND RENAL EXCRETION

Many ASMs are eliminated by a combination of hepatic metabolism and renal excretion.

Ethosuximide is eliminated primarily by CYP3A4-dependent metabolism, with approximately 20% renally excreted unchanged. The weight-adjusted oral clearance of ethosuximide is higher in children than adults, and the concentration-to-dose ratio is 50% higher in children aged 2.5–10 years versus older children (≥15 years). Children also need approximately 50%–100% higher mg/kg maintenance doses than adults to attain similar concentrations.

Felbamate is approved for adjunctive use in individuals of all ages with Lennox–Gastaut syndrome. It is eliminated via renal excretion of unchanged drug (50%), glucuronidation (20%), and is a substrate for CYP3A4 (20%) and CYP2E1. It can also induce CYP3A4; therefore, the use of felbamate in combination with other enzyme-inducing ASMs or ASMs that are metabolized by these enzymes can increase the risk for adverse effects. The weight-adjusted clearance of felbamate is approximately 40% higher in children aged 2–12 years than adults. There is also higher clearance in very young children that decreases to adult values by age 12.

Lacosamide demonstrates near complete oral bioavailability. It is largely metabolized by CYP2C19, but roughly 40% is renally excreted unchanged. Concomitant use of enzyme-inducing ASMs can substantially decrease average plasma concentration.

Levetiracetam and brivaracetam are structurally related, highly bioavailable, and rapidly absorbed. Levetiracetam is eliminated predominantly by renal excretion of unchanged drug. Weight-normalized oral clearance of levetiracetam in children ages 6 months to 4 years and 6–12 years is approximately 30%–40% higher in children than adults. Lower clearance rates occur in infants and neonates due to immature renal function. Children aged >6 months require 30%–50% higher weight-normalized dose than adults to achieve similar concentrations whereas neonates have lower clearance, higher volume of distribution, and a longer half-life as compared with older children and adults. Notably, levetiracetam and brivaracetam have a low potential for drug–drug interactions.

Oxcarbazepine is a prodrug that is rapidly converted to 10,11-dihydro, 10-hydroxycarbazepine (MHD; monohydroxy-derivative) upon oral administration. MHD is predominantly renally excreted unchanged or conjugated by UGT and then excreted. Children aged 6–12 years exhibit higher weight-normalized clearance of MHD. Children <6 years and between 6 and 11 years of age will require 80% higher and 30% higher weight-normalized doses, respectively, than adults to achieve similar concentrations.

Phenobarbital is eliminated by both renal excretion of unchanged drug and hepatic metabolism by CYP2C9 and CYP2C19 and glucosidation. Newborns receiving phenobarbital have a decreased clearance relative to young infants and children. During the first year of life, young children have a two- three-fold greater weight-normalized clearance than adults. Therefore, weight-normalized maintenance doses of phenobarbital in children should generally be 50%–100% higher than in adults.

Topiramate is eliminated as a combination of hepatic metabolism and renal excretion of unchanged drug. Weight-adjusted clearance of topiramate is ~50% higher in children aged 4–11 years than in adults, resulting in approximately 33% lower concentrations. The weight-adjusted clearance is slightly higher in infants than in children and significantly higher than in adults, resulting in an increased dose requirement.

Zonisamide is rapidly absorbed after oral administration and food intake can delay the extent of absorption. It is eliminated by a combination of renal excretion of unchanged drug (~15%–30%) and hepatic metabolism via CYP3A4-mediated reduction to 2-sulfamoyolacetylphenol (SMAP). As a result, zonisamide $t_{1/2}$ can be substantially reduced in patients taking enzyme-inducing ASMs. Clearance is also significantly higher in young children (aged <4 years) versus older children, requiring dose adjustment.

Rufinamide is structurally unrelated to other available ASMs and is approved for adjunctive use in patients with Lennox–Gastaut syndrome ≥1 year of age. Rufinamide is extensively metabolized by enzymatic hydrolysis. In Lennox–Gastaut syndrome patients aged 1–4 years, the pharmacokinetic profile of rufinamide was independent of dose. Further, there is evidence of mild-to-moderate interindividual variability in clearance, which increases with body weight. Rufinamide is not highly protein bound (~30%) but can be subject to drug-to-drug interactions with adjunctive use.

CONCLUSION

Neonates, young infants, and children undergo significant (and nonlinear) maturational changes in organ systems that prominently affect ADME properties of ASMs. Dosing therefore needs to be carefully adjusted if therapeutic serum concentrations are to be achieved to enable seizure freedom (Table 3.2).

Young infants and children generally need increases in weight-normalized dosages of ASMs, as these patients have a greater capacity for drug disposition than adolescents and adults. Of course, clinical judgment, combined with judicious use of serum levels and rational selection to avoid drug–drug interactions will maximize clinical efficacy and tolerability.

Age-related pharmacokinetic properties of ASMs are increasingly being investigated as more orphan drug indications are pursued for pediatric developmental epileptic encephalopathies. Future efforts to enhance treatment for these patients will improve understanding of developmental pharmacokinetics, pharmacogenomics, and the drug-to-drug interaction potential for existing and new ASMs.

TABLE 3.2
Age-Specific Maintenance Dosing of Antiseizure Drugs Used in Monotherapy[a]

Drug	Neonates	Infants	Children	Adults
			Average Dose	
Phenobarbital	3–4 mg/kg qd	2.5–3.0 mg/kg q12h	2–4 mg/kg q12h	0.5–1.0 mg/kg q12h
Phenytoin	2.5–4.0 mg/kg q12h	2–3 mg/kg q8h	2.3–2.6 mg/kg q8h	2 mg/kg q12h
Carbamazepine	NE	3–10 mg/kg q8h	3–10 mg/kg q8h	5–8 mg/kg q12h
Valproate	NE	5–10 mg/kg q8h	5–10 mg/kg q8h	5–10 mg/kg q12h
Ethosuximide	NE	NE	10–20 mg/kg q12h	250–500 mg q12h
Felbamate	NE	NE	5–15 mg/kg q8h	900–1800 mg q12h
Gabapentin	NE	NE	5–15 mg/kg q8h	600–1200 mg q8h
Pregabalin	NE	NE	2.5–3.5 mg/kg/day (divided into 2–3 doses)	75–300 mg q12h
Topiramate	NE	NE	2–5 mg/kg q12h	100–200 mg q12h
Lamotrigine	NE	NE	2–5 mg/kg q12h	75–150 mg q12h
Tiagabine	NE	NE	0.5–2 mg/kg qd	32–56 mg qd
Oxcarbazepine	NE	NE	5–15 mg/kg q8h	300–1,200 mg q12h
Levetiracetam	NE	NE	5–20 mg/kg q12h	500–1,500 mg q12h
Zonisamide	NE	NE	2–6 mg/kg q12h	100–200 mg q12h
Vigabatrin	NE	50–100 mg/kg q12h	25–75 mg/kg q12h	1,000–1,500 mg q12h
Cannabidiol	NE	NE	2.5–5 mg/kg q12h	5–10 mg/kg q12h
Stiripentol	NE	NE	16.67 mg/kg q8h or 25 mg/kg q12h	16.67 mg/kg q8h or 25 mg/kg q12h
Brivaracetam	NE	NE	25–50 mg q12h	50 mg q12h
Cenobamate	NE	NE	NE	12.5–200 mg once daily (titration required)
Lacosamide	NE	NE	Initial: 50 mg q12h Maintenance: 150–200 mg q12h	Initial: 100 mg q12h Maintenance: 150–200 mg q12h
Fenfluramine	NE	NE	0.1 mg/kg-0.35 mg/kg q12h	0.1–0.35 mg/kg q12h
Perampanel	NE	NE	Initial: 2 mg qhs Maintenance: 8–12 mg qhs	Initial: 2 mg qhs Maintenance: 8–12 mg qhs
Eslicarbazepine acetate	NE	NE	Initial: 200–400 mg once daily Maintenance: 800–1,200 mg once daily (weight based)	Initial: 400 mg once daily Maintenance: 800–1,600 mg once daily

(Continued)

TABLE 3.2 (*Continued*)
Age-Specific Maintenance Dosing of Antiseizure Drugs Used in Monotherapy[a]

Drug	Average Dose			
	Neonates	Infants	Children	Adults
Rufinamide	NE	5 mg/kg q12h (titrate up to target of 22.5 mg/kg q12h)	5 mg/kg q12h (titrate up to target of 22.5 mg/kg q12h)	200–400 mg q12h (may titrate to maximum TDD of 1,600 mg q12h)

NE, not established.

[a] Not all antiseizure medications (ASMs) have FDA-approved indications for monotherapy. When used in conjunction with other ASMs, or drugs that affect hepatic metabolism and/or renal function, doses should be adjusted according to clinical judgment.

SUGGESTED REFERENCES

Brown T.R., Leduc B. Phenytoin: Chemistry and biotransformation. In: Levy R.H., Mattson R.H., Meldrum B.S., et al., editors. *Antiepileptic Drugs.* 5th ed. Philadelphia, PA: Lippincott Williams & Wilkins; 2002, pp. 565–80.

Kearns G.L., Abdel-Rahman S.M., Alander S.W., Blowey D.L., Leeder J.S., Kauffman R.E. Developmental pharmacology–drug disposition, action, and therapy in infants and children. *N Engl J Med* 2003;349: 1157–67.

Neal-Kluever A., Fisher J., Grylack L., Kakiuchi-Kiyota S., Halpern W. Physiology of the neonatal gastrointestinal system relevant to the disposition of orally administered medications. *Drug Metab Dispos* 2019;47: 296–313.

Sulemanji M., Vakili K. Neonatal renal physiology. *Semin Pediatr Surg* 2013;22: 195–8.

4 Dietary Therapies for Epilepsy

Eric H. Kossoff
The Johns Hopkins Hospital

CONTENTS

WHAT IS THE KETOGENIC DIET?

The ketogenic diet (KD) is a high-fat, adequate protein, very low-carbohydrate diet that is both calorie and fluid calculated (not restricted) and carefully designed by a ketogenic diet-trained dietitian. Typical foods eaten include butter, eggs, cheese, heavy whipping cream, avocado, nuts, coconut, canola and olive oils, mayonnaise, green vegetables, chicken, hot dogs, fish, and ground beef. Sugar-free and carbohydrate-free snacks can be incorporated to help make the KD more palatable. Infants and children with gastrostomy tubes can be relatively easily started on the KD by substituting their current formula for one of several that are ketogenic.

The mechanism of KD action is undoubtedly multifactorial and still subject to active investigation, including recent studies suggesting a role of the gut microbiota. In nearly 200 retrospective and prospective studies, since its introduction in 1921, it has been clearly demonstrated as effective. The KD causes a >50% reduction in seizures in approximately 55%–60% of the children who begin it by 6 months, and seizure reduction is often maintained long term. Approximately 10% of children become seizure free. The onset of KD action is usually rapid, with studies suggesting seizure reduction within 1–2 weeks (and this has led to recent interest in "emergency" use of KD including for status epilepticus). Many epileptologists believe the KD is more likely to be effective than additional medications after two antiseizure medications (ASMs) have been unsuccessful, especially for generalized epilepsies, and will recommend its use at that time.

DOI: 10.1201/9781003296478-5

39

The KD is started gradually as an inpatient in approximately 80% of ketogenic diet centers. Although originally designed to mimic fasting and starvation, the 24-hour fasting period (with carbohydrate-free fluids) is now deemed optional. The fast has been demonstrated in several retrospective and prospective studies to be unnecessary for long-term control; however, it appears to lead to a more rapid seizure improvement in many children. The KD is provided as a typically 4:1 or 3:1 ratio (by weight of fat to protein and carbohydrate grams combined). During the 3–4-day admission period, families and children are educated for several hours per day regarding the KD attributes and its outpatient management. Following the admission, children are seen back at 1, 3, 6, and 12 months for follow-up in outpatient clinics.

ARE THERE INDICATIONS FOR THE DIET?

Although, prior to the 1990s, there did not appear to be any specific epilepsy etiologies or syndromes more (or less) likely to respond to the KD, this does not currently appear to be the case. The typical child started on the diet is 3–10 years old, with a mixed epilepsy syndrome such as Lennox–Gastaut syndrome, who is not a candidate for epilepsy surgery. However, evidence exists that the KD is effective in infants, adolescents, and even adults. Several studies have even suggested infants may be the age group most likely to respond.

Over the past few decades, there has been a significant increase in case series describing seizure reductions higher than usually seen with the KD (e.g., >70% responder rates) for conditions such as severe myoclonic epilepsy of infancy (i.e., Dravet syndrome), tuberous sclerosis complex, mitochondrial disorders, febrile infection-related epilepsy syndrome (or FIRES), Angelman syndrome, and epilepsy with myoclonic-atonic seizures (i.e., Doose syndrome). Children with GLUT-1 deficiency syndrome and pyruvate dehydrogenase deficiency should be empirically placed on the KD as soon as the diagnosis is made given that it is the treatment of choice. In addition, patients with infantile spasms respond well to the KD, especially if the KD is used earlier in the course of their disorder. Two studies have demonstrated efficacy of the KD as a first-line therapy for infantile spasms. Children receiving formula-only diets (e.g., infants on formulas and children with gastrostomy tubes) also do extremely well, with one study reporting a two-fold increase in the likelihood of a >90% seizure reduction.

It is also important to recognize that there are metabolic disorders that are contraindications to the KD. Such disorders involve difficulties with the metabolism of a high-fat diet and include pyruvate carboxylase deficiency, carnitine deficiencies, and fatty acid oxidation defects. Although it is not a true contraindication, children who are candidates for surgery (e.g., a focal dysplasia or stroke) do not appear to be likely to be seizure free with the KD when compared to resective surgery. In addition, if the nutritional status of the child cannot be assured (e.g., failure to thrive), then the KD should be postponed until proper dietary intake and compliance are confirmed.

ANTISEIZURE MEDICATIONS AND THE DIET

Considering the intractable nature of the epilepsy in most children starting the KD, it is not surprising that over 80% of children remain on ASMs during their time on the KD. Medications can be changed from liquid to tablet formulations to ensure an absence of carbohydrates, although studies have shown that a small increase in the ketogenic ratio can compensate well for the small amount of daily carbohydrates ingested from liquid formulations of ASMs. It is important for the physician to realize that the second most common reason for starting the KD following seizure reduction is ASM reduction. Although our center generally discourages making two changes at once by immediately reducing medications, evidence suggests that it is safe to do if parents request and physicians believe it is prudent, even in the first month of KD use.

Most ASMs do not exhibit significant fluctuations in blood levels when the KD is started in children. Carbonic anhydrase inhibitors such as topiramate and zonisamide have inherently increased risks of acidosis and kidney stones. When used in combination with the KD, the risks are not clearly higher; therefore, they do not need to be discontinued automatically. Valproic acid, which has been reported to lower both serum carnitine levels and serum ketosis, does not lead to increased side effects or lower efficacy when used in combination.

ADVERSE EFFECTS OF THE KETOGENIC DIET

The KD is neither all natural nor holistic; side effects can and do occur. Fortunately, they tend to be transient and treatable, and only very rarely lead to KD discontinuation. They are traditionally divided into "common" (>50%), "occasional" (5%), and "rare" (<1%) when evaluated in the literature and are listed in Table 4.1. The most common adverse effects are a lack of weight gain (or rarely weight loss), constipation, low-grade acidosis, and hypoglycemia during the fasting period. All these side effects can be easily treated with additional calories, oral fiber products (Miralax™),

TABLE 4.1
Reported Side Effects of the Ketogenic Diet

Common:
- Lack of weight gain
- Constipation
- Hypoglycemia (with fasting)

Occasional:
- Gastrointestinal upset or gastroesophageal reflux
- Dehydration or acidosis (more frequent with illness)
- Dyslipidemia
- Growth retardation
- Bone density changes (more common with long-term use)

Rare (case reports):
- Kidney stones
- Pancreatitis
- Cardiomyopathy
- Prolonged QT syndrome
- Basal ganglia changes
- Vitamin and/or mineral deficiencies (if not supplemented)
- Carnitine deficiency (symptomatic)

extra fluids, oral alkalinization with citrate products, and extra glucose in the form of orange juice if symptomatic, respectively.

Less common side effects include kidney stones, dyslipidemia, and diminished growth. Early studies suggested that the risk of either uric acid or calcium carbonate kidney stones was 6% and was associated with hypercalciuria (urine calcium/creatinine ratio higher than 0.2). A retrospective study demonstrated that the use of oral alkalinization (Polycitra K™, 2 mEq/kg/day divided twice daily), historically started in the setting of hypercalciuria, is associated with a three-fold decrease in kidney stone risk when used. As a result of this study, since January 2006, our center now empirically starts all children on Polycitra K™ at diet onset. Cholesterol increases by approximately 30% after 6 months on the KD, then plateaus by 9–12 months, and returns frequently to baseline values. Growth and bone density can be adversely affected by the KD, more so in young infants and after several years on the diet. Gastrointestinal upset has also been described in large series. Again, none of the above-mentioned side effects typically necessitate KD discontinuation and all can be treated with either KD modifications (usually to the ketogenic ratio) or supplemental medications. Rare side effects reported include vitamin and mineral deficiencies (prevented with typical supplementation), selenium deficiency, pancreatitis, cardiomyopathy, bruising, basal ganglia change, and prolonged QT intervals.

"ALTERNATIVE" KETOGENIC DIETS

Modified Atkins Diet

First reported in 2003, the modified Atkins diet (MAD) has emerged as a viable dietary treatment for seizures. This diet is less restrictive, but perhaps equally effective as the traditional KD, based on clinical studies that have directly compared the two diets. The term "modified" describes the lower carbohydrate limit compared to published Atkins diet recommendations for their "induction phase" (20 g/day indefinitely) and the emphasis on high-fat intake (Table 4.2). The MAD can induce ketosis

---

TABLE 4.2

Modified Atkins diet (MAD) protocol

- Copy of a carbohydrate counting guide (paperback) provided.
- Carbohydrates described in detail and restricted to 20 g/day. Carbohydrates can be increased after 2 months in patients if desired.
- Fats (e.g., 36% heavy whipping cream, oils, butter, mayonnaise) encouraged.
- Clear, carbohydrate-free, fluids not restricted.
- Daily low-carbohydrate multivitamin and calcium supplementation.
- Urine ketones checked weekly for the first 2 months and weight checked weekly throughout dietary therapy.
- Antiseizure medications left unchanged for at least the initial month, but reformulated if necessary to tablet or sprinkle preparations.
- Complete blood count, liver and kidney functions, and fasting lipid profile at baseline, 3, and 6 months.
- Discontinue the MAD if ineffective after 3 months.

---

without any protein, fluid, or calorie restriction. In addition, this diet does not require an admission or a fast. In reviewing food records of children on this diet, it approximates a 1:1 ratio of fat:carbohydrate and protein, compared to a typical 3:1 or 4:1 ketogenic diet. Low-carbohydrate foods and meals can also be eaten in restaurants. It is commonly used in adolescents and adults today. A study is underway evaluating the MAD vs. ethosuximide for new-onset childhood absence epilepsy. Side effects of the MAD seem slightly better to that seen with the KD.

LOW-GLYCEMIC INDEX TREATMENT

There is also evidence that a low-glycemic index treatment (LGIT), similar in many ways to the South Beach diet, can be helpful for seizure control. This diet is perhaps even less restrictive than the MAD and does not induce similar levels of ketosis, possibly acting by stabilizing serum glucose. Foods implemented during the LGIT are still relatively high in fat and protein but allow 40–60 g of low-glycemic (glycemic index < 50) carbohydrates, and calories are only roughly monitored as well. In a study of 20 patients aged 5–34 years, 50% had a >90% reduction in seizures and 25% had a 50%–90% improvement.

CONCLUSIONS

Dietary therapies are a useful treatment option for children with medically intractable epilepsy and have been used for over 100 years. While diets can improve seizure control in many patients with epilepsy, certain specific epilepsy syndromes may respond better to the KD than others. While often seen as a more "natural" treatment, side effects from the various diets do occur and their complexity sometimes makes it difficult for some families. The recent emergence of "alternative" ketogenic diets such as the MAD and the LGIT has also led to additional options for patients, especially adolescents and adults. Understanding the many advantages of dietary treatments for epilepsy is very important in the care of children with medically refractory epilepsy, even in the current era of plentiful new and old ASMs.

SUGGESTED REFERENCES

Bergqvist A.G., Schall J.I., Gallagher P.R., Cnaan A., Stallings V.A. Fasting versus gradual initiation of the ketogenic diet: A prospective, randomized clinical trial of efficacy. *Epilepsia* 2005;46: 1810–9.

Groesbeck, D.K., Bluml R.M., Kossoff E.H. Long-term use of the ketogenic diet. *Dev Med Child Neurol* 2006;48: 978–81.

Kossoff E.H., Turner Z., Cervenka M.C., Barron B.H. *Ketogenic Diet Therapies for Epilepsy and Other Conditions.* 7th ed. New York: Springer, 2021.

Kossoff E.H., Zupec-Kania B.A., Auvin S., Ballaban-Gil K.R., Bergqvist A.G.C., Blackford R., Buchhalter J.R., Caraballo R.H., Cross J.H., Dahlin M.G., Donner E.J., Guzel O., Jehle R.S., Klepper J., Kang H.C., Lambrechts D.A., Liu Y.M.C., Nathan J.K., Nordli Jr. D.R., Pfeifer H.H., Rho J.M., Scheffer I.E., Sharma S., Stafstrom C.E., Thiele E.A., Turner Z., Vaccarezza M.M., van der Louw E.J.T.M., Veggiotti P., Wheless J.W., Wirrell

E.C. Optimal clinical management of children receiving dietary therapies for epilepsy: Updated recommendations of the International Ketogenic Diet Study Group. *Epilepsia Open* 2018;3: 175–92.

Nickels K., Kossoff E.H., Eschbach K., Joshi C. Epilepsy with myoclonic-atonic seizures (Doose syndrome): Clarification of diagnosis and treatment options through a large retrospective multicenter cohort. *Epilepsia* 2021;62: 120–7.

Wheless J.W. The ketogenic diet: An effective medical therapy with side effects. *J Child Neurol* 2001;16: 633–5.

5 Vagus Nerve Stimulation Therapy

James W. Wheless, Nitish Chourasia,
and Andrew J. Gienapp
Le Bonheur Children's Hospital & The University
of Tennessee Health Science Center

CONTENTS

THE VAGUS NERVE STIMULATION THERAPY SYSTEM

Vagus nerve stimulation (VNS), which attenuates seizure frequency, severity, and duration by chronic intermittent stimulation of the vagus nerve, is intended for use as an adjunctive treatment with antiseizure medication (ASM) therapies (see Figure 5.1 for device history). As of 2022, more than 135,000 patients with epilepsy have been implanted with the VNS therapy system worldwide, with approximately 30% of those patients being younger than 18 years of age at the time of first implant. Approximately 50%–60% of patients receiving VNS therapy experienced at least a 50% reduction in seizure frequency with no adverse cognitive or systemic effects. Moreover, clinical findings have indicated that the effectiveness of VNS therapy continues to improve over time, independent of changes in ASMs or stimulation parameters. Tolerance does not appear to be a factor with VNS therapy, even after extended periods of time. The long-term safety and effectiveness seen with this treatment have made VNS therapy a mainstream treatment option for a broad range of epilepsy patients, including children and adolescents.

DOI: 10.1201/9781003296478-6

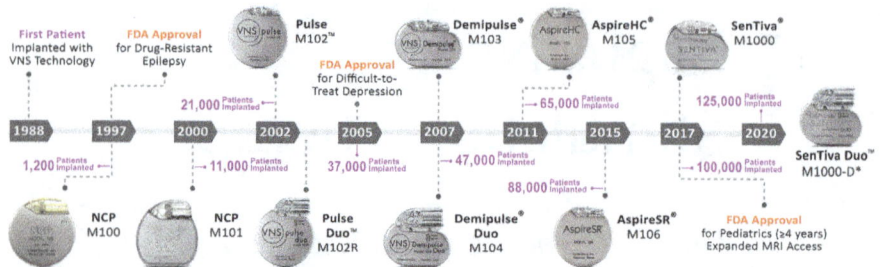

FIGURE 5.1 Timeline of the clinical studies that analyzed the safety and effectiveness of VNS therapy.

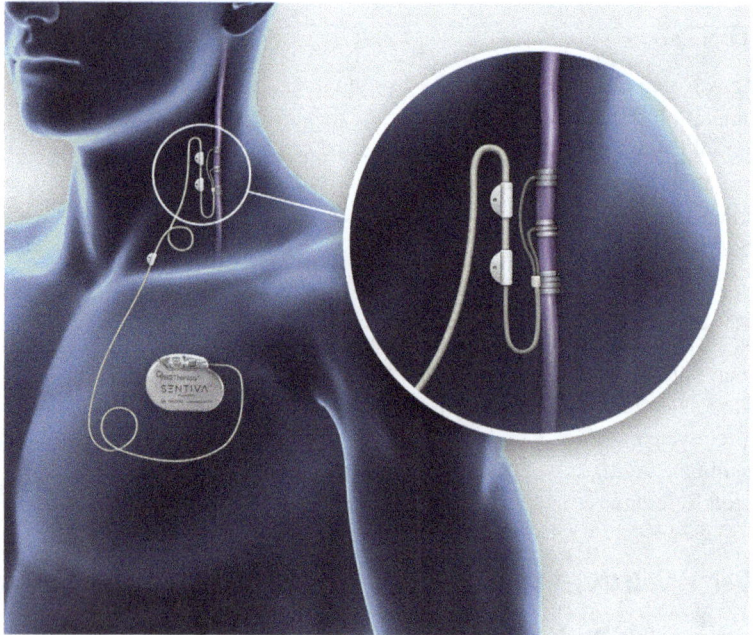

FIGURE 5.2 Implantable components of the VNS therapy system.

The VNS therapy system consists of the implantable pulse generator and bipolar VNS therapy lead, a programming wand with software, a tunneling tool, and a handheld magnet (Figures 5.2 and 5.3). The software allows placement of the programming wand over the generator for reading and altering stimulation parameters (Figure 5.4). There are many possible parameter options available; guidance is provided to allow clinicians to start with the most common and effective settings for each generator model available (Table 5.1).

Four models of the VNS therapy generators are currently available: the Demipulse Model 103, the Demipulse Duo Model 104 (this is the only model available as a dual-pin), the AspireSR Model 106, and the SenTiva Model 1000 (the AspireSR and

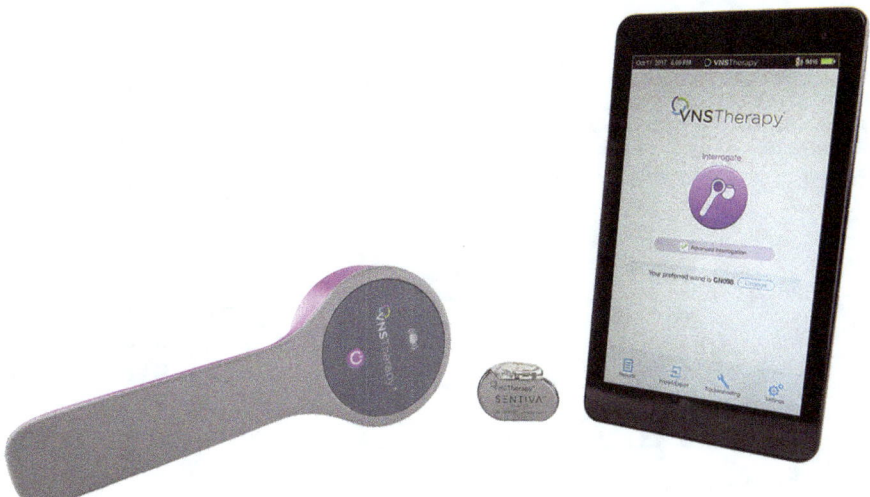

FIGURE 5.3   SenTiva (Model 1000) wireless programming wand, tablet, and device.

TABLE 5.1
Vagus Nerve Stimulation Variables Ranges

Parameter	Units	Range	Suggested
Output current	Milliamps	0–3.5	>1.50–2.25
Signal frequency	Hertz	1–30	20
Pulse width	Microseconds	130–1000	250
On time[a]	Seconds	7–60	30 (7)
Off time[a]	Minutes	0.2–180	1.8, 3, 5 (0.3)
Magnet Settings			
Output current	Milliamps	0–3.5	>1.75–2.25
Pulse width	Microseconds	130–1000	250
On time	Seconds	7–60	14

[a] If using an On time of 30 seconds, use an Off time of 1.8, 3, or 5 minutes. If using an On time of 7 seconds, use an Off time of 0.3 minutes and turn off AutoStim Program (for Models 106 & 1000).

SenTiva are only available as a single-pin model) (Figure 5.5). The average battery life for the generator is approximately 6–8 years with normal use but depends on stimulation parameters (i.e., frequency and intensity), as well as model type.

The magnet allows for on-demand stimulation, which has the potential to abort seizures, either consistently or occasionally, and is provided to patients as part of the VNS therapy system. The added ability of on-demand stimulation provides a greater sense of control for patients and their caregivers over their disorder, which can help improve how they perceive their quality of life. The magnet also allows temporary interruption of stimulation if needed, particularly when singing or playing woodwind

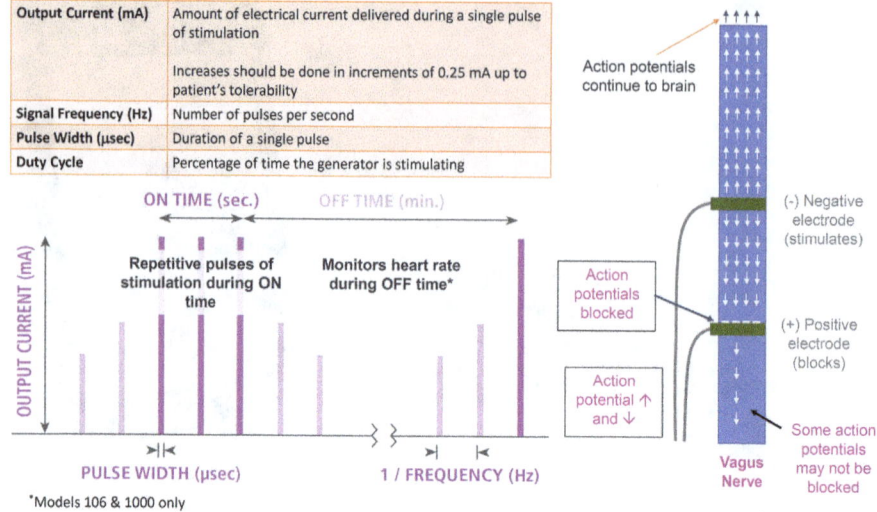

FIGURE 5.4   VNS therapy dosing terminology and stimulation parameters.

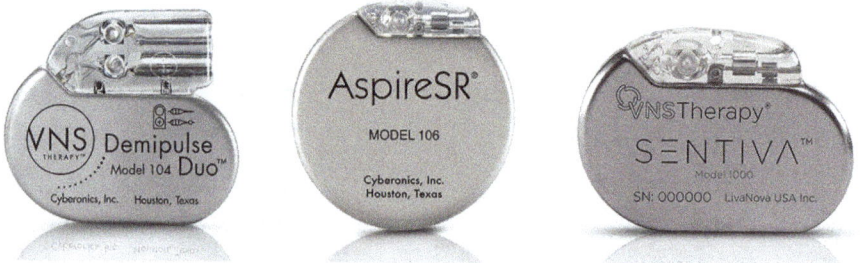

FIGURE 5.5   VNS therapy generators: models 104, 106, and 1000.

instruments or during speaking engagements. However, stopping the stimulus should be done sparingly, and with care, as doing so creates the potential risk of seizures.

Advances in VNS technology have provided seizure detection based on heart rate changes (AutoStim). As the vast majority of refractory epilepsies are associated with ictal tachycardia, rapid changes in heart rate can be used as a surrogate marker for seizure onset, which converts standard VNS therapy from an open-loop form of stimulation to a closed-loop responsive stimulation based on ictal tachycardia detection. This observation has led to changes in VNS technology with the newest models (106 and 1000) incorporating these and other features into the device software. The AspireSR (Model 106) and SenTiva (Model 1000) devices detect ictal tachycardia and then deliver a timed therapy dose to attempt prevention of seizure progression and abort the seizure (AutoStim feature). Long-term outcomes in patients (children, adolescents, and adults with focal seizures and generalized epilepsies) using the newer model generators that incorporate cardiac-based seizure detection documented additional improvement in seizure control with the AutoStim feature compared with traditional open-loop VNS. Additional data collected by the Model 1000 device included detections that occurred in the prone position and/or were associated with bradycardia, potentially allowing individual patient strategies to be put in place to lower sudden unexpected death in epilepsy (SUDEP) risk. Other advanced features of the Model 1000 device have streamlined dosing and patient management, even allowing incremental preprogrammed dosing out-of-office or differential dosing for different time periods during the day.

IMPLANTATION PROCEDURE

The implant surgery is most often performed as a day surgery under general anesthesia and typically lasts approximately 1 hour. The pacemaker-like generator device is generally implanted in the subcutaneous tissues of the upper left pectoral region, with a lead running from the generator device to the left vagus nerve in the neck (Figure 5.6). Two incisions are made during the procedure—one in the chest to create the generator pocket, and the other along a fold in the neck to expose the vagus nerve for placement of the electrode (Figure 5.7). The device is often turned on in the operating room or in the office immediately after surgery, generally with a low initial setting of 0.25 mA. The programming wand is used at follow-up visits to check and fine-tune the stimulation settings according to patient comfort and level of seizure control (see Table 5.1 for suggested parameter settings).

Once a generator reaches its end of service, another surgery is required to replace the generator. Oftentimes, an increase in seizure frequency or intensity suggests the clinical end of service. The entire generator is replaced rather than just the battery to prevent opening the hermetically sealed titanium case of the generator, which could

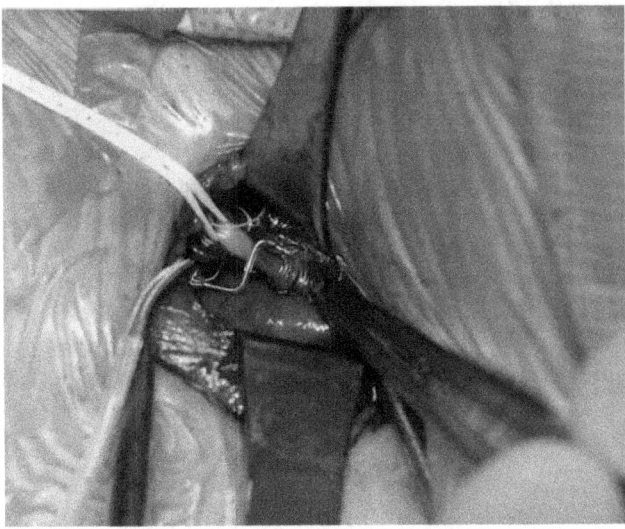

FIGURE 5.6 VNS lead wire prior to placement on the left vagus nerve. Cathode electrode (green suture) placed proximal (right side of picture), then anode electrode (white suture), and then anchor tether (green suture; caudal; left side of picture).

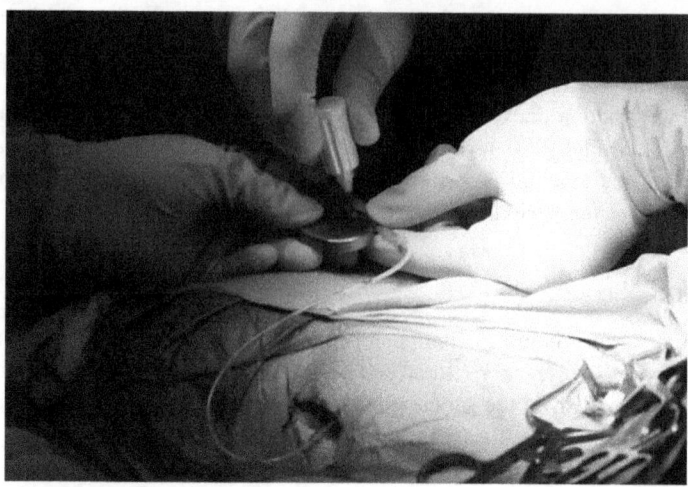

FIGURE 5.7 Implantation of the VNS generator and lead wire (chest incision middle of figure, neck incision on bottom right).

lead to a rejection reaction. Generator-replacement surgery typically lasts 10–15 minutes and is performed as a day surgery. Because the leads remain untouched during a generator replacement, only one chest incision is needed. Generator replacement is recommended before the battery is completely depleted to prevent an interruption in treatment and worsening of seizure control.

POTENTIAL COMPLICATIONS

One possible risk resulting from the implantation surgery is infection at the implant site. This risk may be increased in the pediatric population because young children or patients with neurocognitive disorders may tamper with the wound before the incision has had time to heal properly. Such infections can be treated with antibiotics, but typically lead to explantation of the device, if antibiotic treatment is not effective.

The routine lead test performed during surgery also has resulted in reports of bradycardia and asystole in a small number of patients (~0.1%). Neither of these cardiac events, however, has occurred after surgery during day-to-day treatment with VNS therapy or in children. Usually, they are self-limited and rarely of clinical significance. Vocal cord paresis, although rare, can be caused by manipulation of the vagus nerve during the implant procedure, but such paresis is most often transient.

STIMULATION PARAMETERS

VNS therapy "dosing" is defined by five inter-related stimulation parameters (Figure 5.4): output current (measured in mA), signal frequency (Hz), pulse width (µs), signal "On" time (s), and signal "Off" time (s/min). The output current, signal frequency, and pulse width define how much energy is delivered to the patient, with the combination of settings for these three parameters being analogous to the size or dose of a pill. The signal "On" and "Off" times constitute the duty cycle (i.e., how often the energy is delivered) and are analogous to the dosing schedule for drug therapy. An optimal dose–response relationship for VNS therapy, however, is due to the intraindividual variability between patients and to the number of parameters involved in regulating the dose.

Standard parameter settings as determined from clinical trials are 20 Hz, pulse width of 250 µs, and an output current of 1.5–2.25 mA for 30 seconds of "On" time and 5 minutes of "Off" time (Table 5.1). Initial stimulation is set at the low end of these ranges and slowly adjusted over time and within the safety limits on the basis of patient tolerance and response. Patients should be closely monitored during the dose-adjustment phase of VNS therapy, typically every 2–4 weeks for the first 8–12 weeks following generator implantation. Once a patient responds to a tolerated dose, further parameter adjustments are performed only as clinically necessary. However, routine assessment of lead-wire integrity and generator function should be performed.

MECHANISMS OF ACTION

The mechanisms of action of VNS therapy are not fully understood but are believed to be manifold, due to the diffuse distribution of vagal afferents throughout the central nervous system, and unique from those of traditional ASM therapy. Studies suggest that altered vagal afferent activities resulting from VNS are responsible for mediating seizures. Rat studies indicate that VNS activation of the locus coeruleus may be a significant factor for the attenuation of seizures. Human imaging studies also implicate the thalamus in having an important role in regulating seizure activity. The exact antiseizure role of the thalamus is likely complex, however, owing to the diffuse connections of the thalamus throughout the brain.

Imaging findings, coupled with the clinical findings that the effectiveness of VNS therapy continues to improve over time, seem to indicate that rapidly occurring sub-cortical effects rather than rapidly occurring cortical effects may be more important in the VNS antiseizure mechanism. It is believed that rapidly altered intrathalamic synaptic activities, as well as other mechanisms likely occurring independently of thalamic activation, comprise the therapeutic mechanisms of VNS.

More recently, resting-state fMRI and phase-based and amplitude-based studies of connectivity have provided insights into the interrelations among key nodes of the vagus afferent network. The emergence of functional connectomics has helped to elucidate the underlying circuitry within the vagus afferent network that may be involved in VNS treatment effect and responsiveness.

Seizure Efficacy: Clinical Trials

Results from two randomized, placebo-controlled, double-blind trials (E03 and E05) were pivotal in demonstrating the antiseizure effect of VNS therapy (Table 5.2). In addition, studies have indicated that response to VNS therapy is independent of age, seizure type, or epilepsy syndrome. In a large consecutive series of 141 children 18 years of age and younger with treatment-resistant epilepsy and at least 1 year of follow-up, seizure frequency significantly improved with VNS therapy (mean

TABLE 5.2

Efficacy of VNS Therapy in Regulatory Clinical Studies

Study	Design	Seizure Type	No. of Patients	Age of Patients (years)	First Implant	No. of Patients with >50% Response (%)	Mean Reduction in Seizures/Day (%)
E01	Pilot, longitudinal	Focal	11	20–58	1998	30	24[a]
E02	Pilot, longitudinal	Focal	5	18–42	1990	50	40
E04	Open, longitudinal	All types	124	3–63	1990	29	7[a]
E03	Randomized, parallel, high/low	Focal	115	13–57	1991	31/14	24[a]/6
E05	Randomized, parallel, high/low	Focal	198	13–60	1995	23/16	28[b]/15[b]

[a] Student t-test, $p \leq 0.05$.
[b] Analysis of Variance, $p < 0.0001$.

reduction, 58.9%; $p < 0.0001$). The mean age at initiation of VNS therapy was 11.1 years (range, 1–18); 86 (61%) patients were under the age of 12 years when they received VNS therapy. The mean duration of VNS therapy was 5.2 years (range, 25 days–11.4 years). The overall responder rate for this population was 65% with 41% of the patients experiencing a reduction in seizure frequency of 75% or greater. Comparisons between patients older than 12 years of age and patients younger than 12 years of age showed no differences in efficacy or safety between the groups. Additional pediatric studies have reported similar findings, in addition to showing increasing response rates over time like those seen in the real-world outcome data for adults with VNS.

A recent retrospective European multicenter study investigated the efficacy of VNS over an extended follow-up period (up to 24 months) in 347 children (ages 6 months to 17.9 years) with drug-resistant epilepsy. At 6-, 12-, and 24-month postimplant, 32.5%, 37.6%, and 43.8%, respectively, of children were responders (a 50% or greater seizure reduction). Higher responder rates were seen in children who had no changes in ASMs during the study. A dose–response correlation for VNS was identified with increasing response correlating with total VNS charge delivered per day. Additional improvement was seen in other measures: seizure duration, ictal severity, postictal severity, quality of life, and safety. Vagus nerve stimulation in the first 3 years of life was retrospectively evaluated in 17 children Of these patients, 33% had improvement in seizure frequency at 1 year of treatment, and all who had a prior history of status epilepticus ($n = 6$) had none during this period of time. Fifty-six children were followed for at least 5 years after VNS implant and at the last follow-up, 62.5% were responders with 11 being seizure-free.

Special Patient Populations

Although few prospective or controlled trials have been performed among pediatric epilepsy patients, the number of young patients receiving VNS therapy across the United States and Europe is growing. Observations of pediatric patients with age-related or specialized syndromes receiving VNS therapy have indicated that this treatment is safe and effective across a broad range of seizure types and syndromes, independent of age. Table 5.3 lists the epilepsy syndromes, seizure types, and associated conditions where VNS therapy may be helpful. Additionally, VNS therapy also seems to be a palliative treatment option for patients who have failed cranial surgery (Figures 5.8 and 5.9).

Particularly favorable results, including reduced seizure frequency and severity and improved quality of life, have been reported among patients in open-label studies of Lennox–Gastaut syndrome and other refractory childhood epilepsies, such as hypothalamic hamartomas, epileptic encephalopathies, Rett syndrome, Dravet syndrome, and tuberous sclerosis complex.

The lowest response rate (13% at 2-year postimplantation of VNS) was seen in children with epileptic spasms and tonic spasms. Case reports have described improvement in generalized tonic-clonic seizures and myoclonus in progressive myoclonic epilepsies. A retrospective study showed that improved quality of life—particularly in the area of alertness—was associated with VNS therapy in patients with autism ($n = 59$) or Landau–Kleffner syndrome (LKS; $n = 6$) with more than half of the patients in each group also experiencing a 50% or more reduction in seizure frequency at follow-up (12 months of follow-up for autism and 6 months for LKS patients). Studies have also shown both seizure frequency reductions and improved

---

TABLE 5.3
Epilepsy Syndromes, Seizure Types, and Associated Patient Conditions Where VNS Therapy May Be of Benefit

- Focal seizures with awareness; focal seizures with awareness progressing to impaired awareness or bilateral tonic-clonic seizures; and focal seizures with impaired awareness with or without progression to bilateral tonic-clonic seizures
- Symptomatic generalized tonic-clonic seizures
- Drop attacks and other seizures associated with Lennox–Gastaut syndrome
- Refractory primary genetic generalized epilepsy (i.e., Juvenile Myoclonic Epilepsy, Juvenile Absence Epilepsy)
- Seizures associated with Tuberous Sclerosis Complex or Dravet Syndrome
- Seizures associated with frequent emergency department (ED) visits
- Autism with symptomatic epilepsy
- Sensitive to antiseizure medication side effects (does not tolerate medium to high medication doses)
- Comorbid mood disorder/depression
- Poor adherence with antiseizure medication regimen

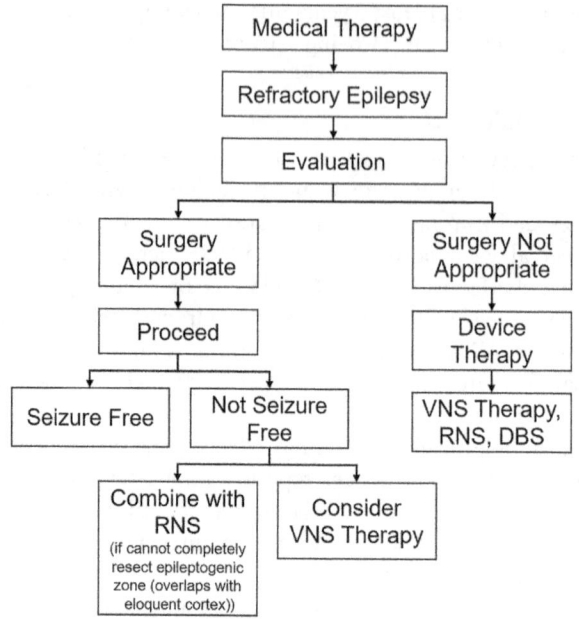

FIGURE 5.8   Epilepsy: treatment sequence for epilepsy surgery and devices. DBS, deep brain stimulation for epilepsy; RNS, responsive neurostimulation.

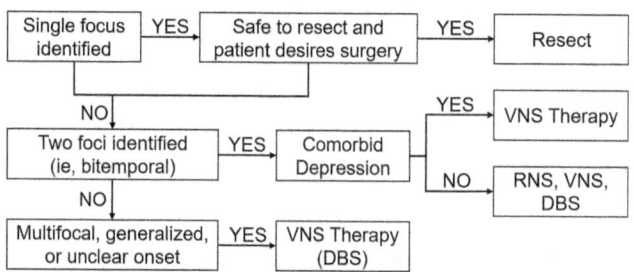

FIGURE 5.9   Device therapy options. Comorbidities, invasiveness of device, and seizure focus determine which device may be used initially (some patients may benefit from more than 1 device). DBS, deep brain stimulation for epilepsy; RNS, responsive neurostimulation.

quality of life among both institutionalized and noninstitutionalized children and adults with mental impairment/developmental delay.

VNS therapy was first reported in 2001 as a possible treatment for refractory generalized convulsive status epilepticus in an adolescent at 13 years of age, and since has been reported in adults and children as a treatment option to help control refractory status epilepticus. VNS therapy also dramatically resolved electroencephalogram findings and achieved seizure freedom in a 12-year-old girl with electrographic status epilepticus in slow-wave sleep. Another report of three children admitted to the intensive care unit (ICU) after developing status epilepticus showed that VNS therapy allowed early cessation of status and discharge from the ICU.

A recent meta-analysis of VNS therapy efficacy showed that children and patients with generalized epilepsy benefited significantly from VNS therapy. Eleven children with genetic epilepsy (absence or juvenile myoclonic epilepsy) at 1-year follow-up reported improved seizure frequency in 64%.

SAFETY

Adverse Events

Adverse events reported with VNS therapy are generally transient and mild and are often related to the duration and intensity of stimulation. Serious adverse events have not been reported with standard therapy and no patients have died or have had a higher mortality risk as a result of VNS therapy. The most common adverse events reported during the clinical trials were mild hoarseness or voice alterations, coughing, and paresthesia (primarily at the implant site), which decreased over time and were not considered clinically significant. Other side effects reported less frequently during these studies included dyspnea, pain, headache, pharyngitis, dyspepsia, nausea, vomiting, fever, infection, depression, and accidental injury. Not all of these side effects were related to VNS therapy. Outside of the clinical trials, occasional reports of additional adverse events, such as shortness of breath and vocal cord paresis, have been reported but did not result in discontinuation of therapy. Moreover, many of the side effects tend to diminish or disappear altogether, as patients adjust to the stimulation therapy. If side effects persist or are bothersome to the patient, reductions in stimulation intensity or frequency oftentimes alleviate the side effects, most of which occur only during active stimulation. Pediatric patients seem to have a higher tolerance for VNS therapy. Rare reports of increased salivation, increased hyperactivity, and swallowing difficulties occur in children. Overall, the side effects reported for pediatric patients are often mild and transient.

Device Safety

Safety features are built into the VNS therapy system to protect patients from stimulation-related nerve injury. The primary safety feature is the "Off" switch effect of the magnet. If a patient begins to experience continuous stimulation or uncomfortable side effects as a result of VNS therapy, the magnet can be held or taped over the generator to stop stimulation until the patient can visit the physician. A watchdog timer also is programmed into the device to monitor the number of pulses a patient receives. If a certain number of pulses are delivered without an "Off" time, the device will turn itself off in order to prevent excess stimulation from potentially causing nerve injury.

Diathermy, which could heat the system above safe levels and thereby cause either temporary or permanent tissue or nerve damage, should be avoided in patients receiving VNS therapy. According to the manufacturer of the device, a (1) transmit-and-receive head coil MRI or extremity coil (excluding the C7–T8 region) or (2) whole body coil (excluding the C7–L3 region) can be used for head and extremity scans by MRI with the generator programmed to 0 mA for the procedure and returned to the original settings thereafter. MRI scans following these procedures are safe in 1.5T and 3T scanners for model 103, 104, 106, and 1000 generators. However, successful head coil MRIs have been performed among patients with both devices turned on and off. If the device does remain on during the MRI, the device should be interrogated post-procedure to ensure that the magnetic field did not deactivate the device or change pre-MRI settings. Advances in device safety during MRI imaging will allow more patients to have routine MRI scans performed without concern for device-related side effects or malfunction.

CANDIDATE SELECTION

Although optimal use parameters continue to be defined, candidates should meet the following criteria: (1) presence of medically refractory seizures, (2) adequately completed trials of at least two ASMs, (3) exclusion of nonepileptic events, and (4) ineligibility for epilepsy surgery (Figures 5.8 and 5.9). Focal resective surgery (temporal lobectomy or lesional neocortical epilepsy) is preferred in appropriate patients because of its superior seizure-freedom rate. Recent open studies suggest that VNS therapy may be used among patients considered for corpus callosotomy, producing lower rates of morbidity, and among those who have previously undergone epilepsy surgery.

In October 2013, the American Academy of Neurology updated its evidence-based VNS therapy guidelines for the treatment of epilepsy, which provided an update on data regarding the efficacy and safety of VNS therapy for epilepsy since the publication of the original guidelines in 1999. Previous guidelines did not provide guidance on many of the epilepsy patient populations in which VNS therapy is actively being used. The literature review for the new guidelines found 1274 manuscripts for VNS therapy since the last review. Of these, 216 articles were reviewed to answer eight clinical questions, which are summarized in Table 5.4. The clinical evidence supported the use of VNS therapy across a range of refractory epilepsy populations, and the impact of the reviewed studies (with a specific focus on the intensity and magnitude of the responses) continued to be quite supportive.

Patients of any age should be considered for VNS therapy if they experience seizures refractory to other therapies, including ASMs, the ketogenic diet, and epilepsy surgery. Preliminary data suggested that patients treated with VNS therapy earlier in the course of their epilepsy (i.e., when seizures fail to respond to treatment with two or three ASMs within 2 years of epilepsy onset) may have a higher response rate to treatment.

Patients with a history of partial adherence to their ASM regimens, particularly those on polypharmacy, may also be good candidates for VNS therapy because of the assured compliance and lack of further drug-drug interactions with VNS therapy. Additional considerations that would positively impact the decision to use VNS would include patients who have a comorbid mood disorder, or frequent emergency room visits or hospitalizations secondary to poorly controlled seizures (Figure 5.9).

Precautions should be taken with patients predisposed to cardiac dysfunction and obstructive sleep apnea (OSA) as stimulation may increase apneic events, and chronic obstructive pulmonary disease may increase the risk of dyspnea. Lowering

TABLE 5.4
Summary of AAN Updated Evidence-Based Guidelines for VNS Therapy

Clinical Question	Recommendation/Clinical Context
Is VNS therapy beneficial in children with epilepsy?	VNS therapy may be considered as adjunctive treatment for children with partial or generalized epilepsy (C)
Is VNS therapy beneficial in patients with LGS?	VNS therapy may be considered in patients with LGS (C)
Is VNS therapy associated with mood improvement in patients with epilepsy?	In adult patients receiving VNS therapy for epilepsy, improvement in mood may be an additional benefit (C)
Is VNS therapy associated with reduced seizure frequency over time?	VNS therapy may be considered progressively effective in patients over multiple years of exposure (C)
Does rapid cycling[a] improve seizure frequency more often than do standard stimulation settings?	Optimal VNS therapy settings are still unknown. The evidence is insufficient to support a recommendation for the use of standard stimulation vs. rapid stimulation
Does using additional magnet-activated stimulation trains for auras or at seizure onset interrupt seizures?	VNS therapy magnet activation may be associated with seizure abortion when used at the time of seizure auras (C) Seizure abortion with the magnet use may be associated with overall response to VNS treatment (C)
Have new safety concerns emerged since the last VNS therapy assessment?	No new safety concerns were identified The rates of SUDEP dropped in the first 2 years of VNS therapy
Do adverse effects differ among children and adults?	Children may have greater risk for wound infection than adults due to behaviors more common in children. Extra vigilance in monitoring for occurrence of site infection in children should be undertaken

[a] Rapid cycling is shorter On and Off times, typically 7 seconds On and 18 seconds Off compared with standard settings, typically 30 seconds On and 5 minutes Off.

C, based on data from class III studies; LGS, Lennox–Gastaut Syndrome; SUDEP, sudden unexpected death in epilepsy; U, unproven, or data inadequate or conflicting.

the stimulus frequency or increasing the "Off" time may prevent exacerbation. It is not known whether the effects of VNS on sleep-related breathing diminish over time.

Patients who have undergone a bilateral or left cervical vagotomy are not considered candidates for VNS therapy. Evaluation by a cardiologist is recommended for patients with a personal or family history of cardiac dysfunction. If clinically indicated, Holter monitor tests and electrocardiograms also should be done before implant. The impact of VNS on mortality and SUDEP remains unsettled with some data suggesting that it might reduce the risk of SUDEP.

COST-EFFECTIVENESS

Previous fiscal analyses for VNS therapy indicate that the initial costs of VNS are offset over time by reductions in health care costs and hospital admissions following implantation. The reductions in the economic burden for both patients and society were seen even among patients with less than a 25% reduction in seizures, indicating that even those without a substantial improvement in seizure frequency receive some benefit from the device. Therefore, the decision to proceed with VNS therapy for a patient population with few options should be made on the basis of clinical judgment rather than short-term costs.

CONCLUSION

VNS is emerging at the forefront of epilepsy treatments as a well-tolerated adjunctive therapy. With its minimal adverse side effects, lack of pharmacokinetic interactions with drug therapies, negligible compliance issues, improvements in quality of life, and cumulative efficacy over time, VNS therapy may be particularly effective among pediatric patients and patients with comorbid conditions.

VNS therapy has raised interest in the role of neurostimulation as a treatment for refractory epilepsy. Since the first device implantation more than 34 years ago, the number of ASMs has increased, yet uncontrolled seizures continue. The codification of refractory epilepsy by the International League Against Epilepsy (ILAE) in 2010 increased visibility around the need for nonpharmacologic treatment options earlier in the course of the disease rather than waiting until multiple medications have failed, and surgery is not an option. The use of VNS therapy, however, must be balanced against the necessity of surgery, although VNS therapy surgery is well tolerated. As our understanding of what characterizes refractory epilepsy continues to evolve, adjunctive treatments like VNS therapy will play an increasingly larger role in improving the lives of patients with epilepsy.

SUGGESTED REFERENCES

Benbadis S.R., Geller E., Ryvlin P., Schachter S., Wheless J., Doyle W., Vale F.L. Putting it all together: Options for intractable epilepsy: An updated algorithm on the use of epilepsy surgery and neurostimulation. *Epilepsy Behav* 2018;88S: 33–8.

Morris 3rd G.L., Gloss D., Buchhalter J., Mack K.J., Nickels K., Harden C. Evidence-based guideline update: Vagus nerve stimulation for the treatment of epilepsy: Report of the Guideline Development Subcommittee of the American Academy of Neurology. *Neurology* 2013;81: 1453–9.

Orosz I., McCormick D., Zamponi N., Varadkar S., Feucht M., Parain D., Griens R., Vallee L., Boon P., Rittey C., Jayewardene A.K., Bunker M., Arzimanoglou A., Lagae L. Vagus nerve stimulation for drug-resistant epilepsy: A European long-term study up to 24 months in 347 children. *Epilepsia* 2014;55: 1576–84.

Wheless J.W., Baumgartner J. Vagus nerve stimulation therapy. *Drugs Today (Barc)* 2004;40: 501–15.

Wheless J.W., Gienapp A.J., Ryvlin P. Vagus nerve stimulation (VNS) therapy update. *Epilepsy Behav* 2018;88S: 2–10.

6 Neuromodulation Devices

Responsive Neurostimulation and Deep Brain Stimulation

Shifteh S. Sattar
UC San Diego School of Medicine

CONTENTS

Approximately 30% of patients with epilepsy have drug-resistant epilepsy. The first neuromodulatory therapy for epilepsy was the Vagus Nerve Stimulator (VNS) which was approved by the Food and Drug Administration (FDA) in 1997. Brain responsive neurostimulation (RNS) and deep brain stimulation (DBS) are recent neuromodulatory devices approved in patients with medically refractory epilepsy that are over the age of 18 years and have been demonstrated to be safe and effective treatments to reduce seizure frequency.

Although the RNS and DBS devices have no formal approval to be used in the pediatric population, they have great potential for the treatment of medically refractory epilepsy in patients that are deemed to be poor surgical candidates due to the lack of clear localization of the epileptogenic focus, multiple epileptogenic foci or owing to demonstration that the area of epileptogenicity is within or adjacent to eloquent cortex.

RESPONSIVE NEUROSTIMULATION (NEUROPACE)

The RNS system has been approved by the FDA as an adjunctive treatment for adults with medical refractory focal-onset seizures that arise from one or two epileptogenic

DOI: 10.1201/9781003296478-7

foci in 2013. The RNS device allows for continuous electrocorticography (ECoG) of one or two seizure foci with the use of intracranial electrodes, either with four-contact strips or four-contact depths. These electrodes are placed over (strip electrode) or within (depth electrode) the epileptogenic zone, which is often identified by the use of invasive electroencephalography (EEG) using stereotactic EEG or subdural grid implantation.

Once the RNS electrodes are implanted, the device is programmed to detect and respond to specific ECoG patterns, electrographic seizures, or interictal discharges. Although the device continuously senses the ECoG, a limited quantity of ECoG recordings is stored per day as a sample of the events being treated.

IMPLANTATION AND PROGRAMMING OF THE RNS DEVICE

The neurostimulator is placed under the scalp and within the skull and connected to two electrodes placed either on the surface of the brain, into the brain, or a combination of both. Initially, the neurosurgeon makes a window in the skull to fit a titanium tray that is secured in the skull. The neurostimulator is then secured in the tray. The neurostimulator is as thick as the skull and has a curved design to be even with the skull surface; and since it is implanted underneath the scalp, the device is not visible or palpable. The surgical procedure generally takes 3–5 hours, and most patients stay 1–2 nights in the hospital after device implantation.

The external components of the RNS system are comprised of the RNS tablet for programming by the physician, a remote monitor for patient use which includes a wand that can be placed over the neurostimulator device on the scalp and connected to an RNS laptop. The information from the neurostimulator is transferred to the laptop computer which then can be transferred to a secure database called the patient data management system (PDMS) where they are available for physician review. In addition, a magnet is provided to the patient that can be used to mark a clinical seizure and store the ECoG data.

The neurostimulator is a battery-powered device that stores and records electrographic pattern from the electrodes with a battery life of 6–12.4 years for the RNS-320 model. The device allows for the connection of four electrodes; however, ECoG information can only be obtained only from two electrodes. Intraoperative ECoG and impedance check is performed once the device and electrodes are implanted. The device is enabled to detect and record abnormal activity in the operating room. Information can be downloaded from the neurostimulator. Generally, treatment with electrical stimulation is not immediately enabled in order to capture electrographic seizures and tailor programming of the device based on the abnormal ECoG activity.

The RNS system takes a closed-loop approach in contrast to open-loop approaches to neuromodulation in which therapy is delivered continuously or on a fixed schedule (VNS and DBS). The most common stimulation therapy settings are two bursts of stimulation at 100–200 Hz, 160 μs pulse width, and 100 milliseconds burst duration with initial current current-controlled stimulation treatments of 0.5–1 mA. Titration of the treatment or modification of detection settings is usually made every 3–4 months to allow time for modulatory effects to occur (Figure 6.1).

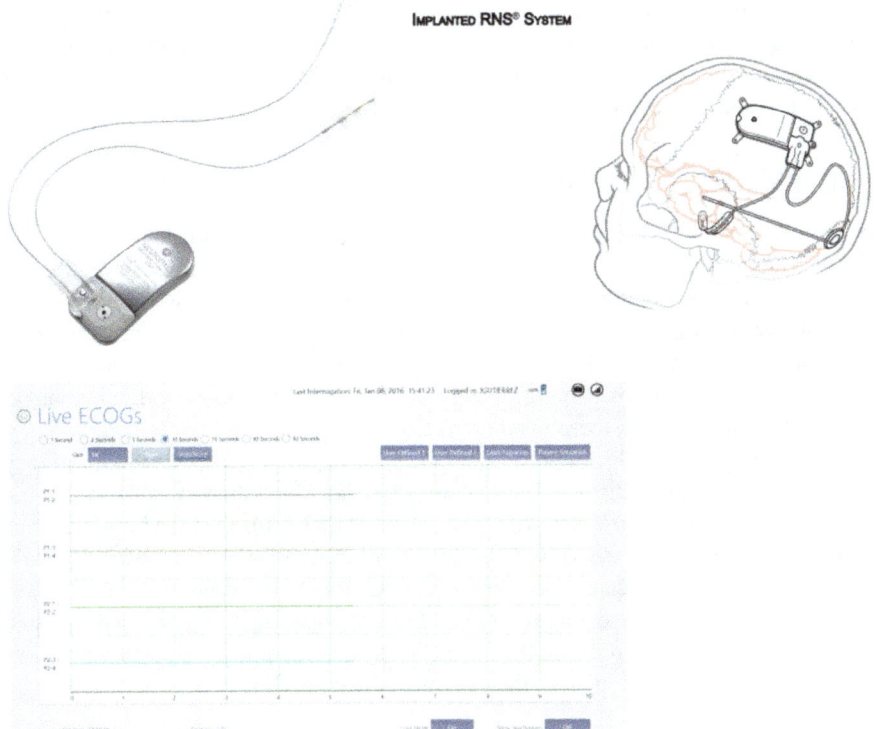

IMPLANTED RNS® SYSTEM

FIGURE 6.1 Live ECoG screen on RNS tablet.

CLINICAL TRIALS VALIDATING THE SAFETY AND EFFECTIVENESS

The key study was a multicenter, randomized, controlled, and double-blinded trial of responsive neurostimulation in 191 patients with drug-resistant epilepsy. The initial portion of the study consisted of a 12-week blinded period followed by an 84-week open-label period. This study showed an overall reduction in disabling seizures over the 4-month blinded period in the treatment group (37.9%), which was significantly larger than the sham-treated patients (17.3% with $p = 0.012$).

Disabling seizures were defined as focal motor, focal impaired awareness, and/or focal to bilateral tonic-clonic seizures. In addition to these findings, the seizure frequency reduction increased to 41.5% after 5 months of stimulation treatment, compared to the sham-stimulated patients that had 9.4% seizure frequency reduction ($p = 0.008$). The open-label long-term treatment trial, where all patients received responsive stimulation, had a median seizure frequency reduction of 44% in the first year, 53% in the second year, 60%–66% in years 3–6, and 75% reduction at 9 years.

In the initial randomized controlled pivotal study, 3.7% infection rate was noted with the initial implantation or replacement of the neurostimulator, 2.6% of lead damage, and 3.7% of lead revisions. Stimulation was well tolerated, and there was no difference in the type of serious adverse events between the treated and sham groups over the blinded period. RNS did not identify any significant adverse issues in mood, suicidality, or cognition. In patients that were implanted in a neocortical area, a significant improvement in naming was seen ($p < 0.0001$). In patients with mesial temporal lobe seizures, significant improvements in verbal learning, delayed free recall, and recognition were seen.

DEEP BRAIN STIMULATION

Although DBS has been used for movement disorders such as Parkinson's disease and DYT1 dystonia in the pediatric population, it received FDA approval in December 2018 for adjunctive treatment of medically refractory focal-onset seizures in adults over the age of 18 years old who have been unresponsive to three or more antiseizure medications (ASMs). DBS is the third neuromodulatory approach for epilepsy treatment. Although the mechanism of action for DBS is poorly understood, it is thought to alter the Papez circuit, thereby reducing seizure frequency.

The Papez circuit links hippocampal output through the fornix and mammillary nuclei to the anterior nucleus of the thalamus (ANT) which then travels through the cingulate gyrus to the parahippocampal cortex and then returns to the hippocampus. Alterations in the Papez circuit with placement of electrodes within the subthalamic nucleus (STN) and the centromedian nucleus (CMN) as opposed to the ANT have also been performed for seizure reduction. DBS provides an open-loop therapy with placement of depth electrodes in the ANT. Open-loop therapy provides a continuous electrical stimulation throughout the day, in contrast to RNS.

IMPLANTATION AND PROGRAMMING OF THE DBS DEVICE

The DBS surgery is typically a two-step procedure in adult patients. The initial step consists of stereotactic targeting techniques using specific MRI brain sequence imaging for placement of two electrodes into the ANT bilaterally through a small hole created in the skull. The lead extensions are tunneled behind the ear. This is followed by placing the neurostimulator under the skin, typically in the upper chest. The leads that are implanted in the ANT will be connected to the neurostimulator under the skin and usually behind the ears. In most pediatric centers offering DBS, both procedures are done on the same day. Unlike DBS implantation for Parkinson's disease and essential tremor where the patient is awake during the lead-implant surgery, the patient remains under general anesthesia for the complete duration of the procedure.

The programmer is a hand-held device that allows the physician to adjust the neurostimulation settings. An additional hand-held device is provided to the patient and provides battery status with the ability to turn the device on and off. The DBS patient programmer also has a seizure log to document when a seizure has occurred (Figure 6.2).

As for all neuromodulatory devices, initial programming is done within 2–4 weeks of implantation and optimized every 3–4 months. Program optimization can take several months and response to therapy is not immediate as is the case with all neuromodulatory devices. The programming is tailored to each individual. The most common therapy settings are as follows: stimulation at 5 V, 145 Hz, 90 μs, cycling on interval of 1 minute and cycling off interval of 5 minutes (Figure 6.3).

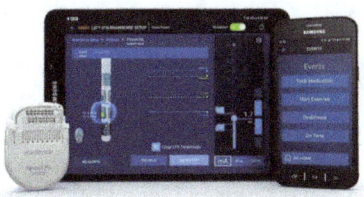

FIGURE 6.2   DBS tablet, programmer, and neurostimulator.

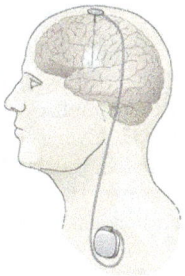

FIGURE 6.3   DBS-implanted location.

CLINICAL TRIALS VALIDATING SAFETY AND EFFECTIVENESS

The Stimulation of the Anterior Nucleus of the Thalamus for Epilepsy (SANTE) trial, was a randomized, double-blind multicenter study involving 110 adults with medically refractory epilepsy who underwent DBS implantation in the ANT. The blinded randomized phase of the study lasted 4 months in which the treatment group received stimulation at 5 V, 145 Hz, 90 μs, cycling 1 minute on and 5 minutes off. The sham or control group was programmed to 0 V, 145 Hz, 90 μs, cycling on 1 minute and cycling off 5 minutes.

Once the blinded phase was completed, the control group had the stimulation programmed to 5 V and the treatment group continued stimulation. The long-term, follow-up open-label study lasted 7 years. The blinded phase of the study showed that the treatment group had 8% fewer seizures compared to the sham group which was not statistically significant. However, the median percent seizure reduction from baseline in year 1 was 41% and in year 5 was 69%, with 16% of patients being seizure-free for at least 6 months. At 7 years, the median percent seizure reduction was 75% ($p < 0.001$).

The Electrical Stimulation of Thalamus for Epilepsy of Lennox–Gastaut phenotype (ESTEL) trial was a prospective double-blind randomized study with electrode implantation in the centromedian nucleus of the thalamus in 20 patients with Lennox–Gastaut Syndrome (LGS). The blinded phase of the study was for 3 months, followed by an unblinded phase of 3 months where all patients received treatment. Half of the stimulation group had a >50% seizure reduction compared to 22% in the control group ($p = 0.25$). The statistically significant finding was in the reduction of electrographic seizures with a >50% seizure reduction in 59% of the treatment group compared to none in the control group ($p = 0.05$).

CONCLUSION

Currently, there are no long-term studies supporting the efficacy and safety of neuromodulatory devices in the pediatric population. However, neuromodulatory strategies offer an adjunctive treatment option for all patients with drug-resistant epilepsy. Due to continued brain growth and development, it remains unclear whether electrode migration could occur and result in complications and/or compromise of the treatment effect in children.

SUGGESTED REFERENCES

Bergey G.K., Morrell M.J., Mizrahi E.M., Goldman A., King-Stephens D., Nair D., Srinivasan S., Jobst B., Gross R.E., Shields D.C., Barkley G., Salanova V., Olejniczak P., Cole A., Cash S.S., Noe K., Wharen R., Worrell G., Murro A.M., Edwards J., Duchowny M., Spencer D., Smith M., Geller E., Gwinn R., Skidmore C., Eisenschenk S., Berg M., Heck C., Van Ness P., Fountain N., Rutecki P., Massey A., O'Donovan C., Labar D., Duckrow R.B., Hirsch L.J., Courtney T., Sun F.T., Seale C.G. Long-term treatment with responsive brain stimulation in adults with refractory partial seizures. *Neurology* 2015;84: 810–7.

Dalic L.J., Warren A.E.L., Bulluss K.J., Thevathasan W., Roten A., Churilov L., Archer J.S. DBS of thalamic centromedian nucleus for Lennox-Gastaut Syndrome (ESTEL Trial). *Ann Neurol* 2022;91: 253–67. Retraction in: *Ann Neurol.* 2022; *Erratum* in: *Ann Neurol* 2022.

Fisher R., Salanova V., Witt T., Worth R., Henry T., Gross R., Oommen K., Osorio I., Nazzaro J., Labar D., Kaplitt M., Sperling M., Sandok E., Neal J., Handforth A., Stern J., DeSalles A., Chung S., Shetter A., Bergen D., Bakay R., Henderson J., French J., Baltuch G., Rosenfeld W., Youkilis A., Marks W., Garcia P., Barbaro N., Fountain N., Bazil C., Goodman R., McKhann G., Babu Krishnamurthy K., Papavassiliou S., Epstein C., Pollard J., Tonder L., Grebin J., Coffey R., Graves N.; SANTE Study Group. Electrical stimulation of the anterior nucleus of thalamus for treatment of refractory epilepsy. *Epilepsia* 2010;51: 899–908.

Heck C.N., King-Stephens D., Massey A.D., Nair D.R., Jobst B.C., Barkley G.L., Salanova V., Cole A.J., Smith M.C., Gwinn R.P., Skidmore C., Van Ness P.C., Bergey G.K., Park Y.D., Miller I., Geller E., Rutecki P.A., Zimmerman R., Spencer D.C., Goldman A., Edwards J.C., Leiphart J.W., Wharen R.E., Fessler J., Fountain N.B., Worrell G.A., Gross R.E., Eisenschenk S., Duckrow R.B., Hirsch L.J., Bazil C., O'Donovan C.A., Sun F.T., Courtney T.A., Seale C.G., Morrell M.J. Two-year seizure reduction in adults with medically intractable partial onset epilepsy treated with responsive neurostimulation: Final results of the RNS system pivotal trial. *Epilepsia* 2014;55: 32–441.

Loring D.W., Kapur R., Meador K.J., Morrell M.J. Differential neuropsychological outcomes following targeted responsive neurostimulation for partial-onset epilepsy. *Epilepsia* 2015;56: 1836–44.

Meador K.J., Kapur R., Loring D.W., Kanner A.M., Morrell M.J. Quality of life and mood in patients with medically intractable epilepsy treated with targeted responsive neurostimulation. *Epilepsy Behav* 2015;45: 242–7.

Morrell M.J. Responsive cortical stimulation for the treatment of medically intractable partial epilepsy. *Neurology* 2011;77: 1295–304.

Nair D.R., Laxer K.D., Weber P.B., Murro A.M., Park Y.D., Barkley G.L., Smith B.J., Gwinn R.P., Doherty M.J., Noe K.H., Zimmerman R.S., Bergey G.K., Anderson W.S., Heck C., Liu C.Y., Lee R.W., Sadler T., Duckrow R.B., Hirsch L.J., Wharen Jr. R.E., Tatum W., Srinivasan S., McKhann G.M., Agostini M.A., Alexopoulos A.V., Jobst B.C., Roberts

D.W., Salanova V., Witt T.C., Cash S.S., Cole A.J., Worrell G.A., Lundstrom B.N., Edwards J.C., Halford J.J., Spencer D.C., Ernst L., Skidmore C.T., Sperling M.R., Miller I., Geller E.B., Berg M.J., Fessler A.J., Rutecki P., Goldman A.M., Mizrahi E.M., Gross R.E., Shields D.C., Schwartz T.H., Labar D.R., Fountain N.B., Elias W.J., Olejniczak P.W., Villemarette-Pittman N.R., Eisenschenk S., Roper S.N., Boggs J.G., Courtney T.A., Sun F.T., Seale C.G., Miller K.L., Skarpaas T.L., Morrell M.J.; RNS System LTT Study. Nine-year prospective safety and effectiveness outcome from the long-term treatment trial of the RNS system. *Neurology* 2020;95: e1244–56.

NeuroPace RNS System Physician Manual - RNS-320, 2018. neuropace-rns-system-manual-320.pdf

Salanova V., Witt T., Worth R., Henry T.R., Gross R.E., Nazzaro J.M., Labar D., Sperling M.R., Sharan A., Sandok E., Handforth A., Stern J.M., Chung S., Henderson J.M., French J., Baltuch G., Rosenfeld W.E., Garcia P., Barbaro N.M., Fountain N.B., Elias W.J., Goodman R.R., Pollard J.R., Tröster A.I., Irwin C.P., Lambrecht K., Graves N., Fisher R.; SANTE Study Group. Long-term efficacy and safety of thalamic stimulation for drug-resistant partial epilepsy. *Neurology* 2015;84: 1017–25.

Skarpaas T.L., Jarosiewicz B., Morrell M.L. Brain-responsive neurostimulation for epilepsy (RNS system). *Epilepsy Res* 2019;153: 68–70.

Velasco F., Velasco A.L., Velasco M., Jiménez F., Carrillo-Ruiz J.D., Castro G. Deep brain stimulation for treatment of the epilepsies: The centromedian thalamic target. *Acta Neurochir* 2007;97: 337–42.

7 Epilepsy Surgery in Children

Ann Hyslop
Stanford University

CONTENTS

INTRODUCTION

Drug-resistant epilepsy is defined as that which does not respond to two appropriately selected and dosed antiseizure medications (ASMs). Approximately one-third of individuals with epilepsy meet criteria for intractability and are unlikely to achieve seizure freedom with medication management alone. Despite the availability of second and third generation ASMs in recent decades, studies have not indicated significantly improved efficacy. Therefore, alternative therapies such as the ketogenic diet, neuromodulation, and epilepsy surgery are important options. Of these, epilepsy surgery, when performed in carefully selected candidates, is the only one that may be curative. A systematic review and metaanalysis of 11 controlled studies found that the odds of obtaining seizure freedom were significantly higher in those undergoing epilepsy surgery compared to those that were medically managed.

DOI: 10.1201/9781003296478-8

UNDERUTILIZATION OF EPILEPSY SURGERY

Despite the clear benefit of epilepsy surgery over medical management in many patients, this approach remains grossly underutilized. It is estimated that of the 10%–50% of patients with drug-resistant epilepsy who are likely surgical candidates, only 1%–11% with this diagnosis undergo surgery in the United States. A systematic review of pediatric epilepsy surgery underutilization found that this stems from many factors, including citing systemic health disparities, patient and family misconceptions about surgery, and low rates of referral to surgical centers due to lack of provider knowledge surrounding criteria for consideration of surgical candidacy.

NONINVASIVE PRESURGICAL EVALUATION

Determining whether a patient is a surgical candidate involves a thorough, carefully designed and personalized presurgical investigation, termed a phase I evaluation. Beyond video-electroencephalography (EEG) and magnetic resonance imaging (MRI), indicated ancillary testing varies based on patient characteristics such as age, patient ability to cooperate with directed tasks, epilepsy etiology, and goals of surgery.

While surgery may offer a path to seizure freedom and discontinuation of ASMs in some, others may be identified as candidates for a palliative surgical intervention. In both populations of patients, three aims exist in the presurgical evaluation: (1) to identify the epileptogenic zones within the cortex, (2) document the child's cognitive and functional baseline, and (3) to delineate regions of eloquent cortex within the child's brain.

The epileptogenic zone, defined as the minimal amount of brain tissue that must be removed to enable seizure freedom, often requires data from multiple testing modalities to be accurately identified. The physical and neurological exams, review of patient history, and detailed neuropsychological testing generate a solid understanding of the baseline functional status of the child while advanced functional imaging techniques yield information on the localization of eloquent functions within the brain, such as speech, motor, and vision.

IDENTIFICATION OF THE EPILEPTOGENIC ZONE

A detailed understanding of the patient's clinical history and seizure semiology in conjunction with assessment of interictal and ictal activity in continuous video-EEG may provide the first lateralizing or localizing information in a child's presurgical evaluation. Corroboration of the semiology during ictal capture on video-EEG with historical descriptions of the seizure behaviors ensures consistency of the seizure appearance over time and aids in the understanding of whether one or more epileptogenic zones exist.

Brain MRI with slice thicknesses of 1 mm performed with a 3-Tesla (3T) magnet allows for the detection of subtle focal cortical dysplasias that may not be detectable in series with thicker slices or obtained on lower Tesla magnets. This, in combination with interpretation by a neuroradiologist with experience in pediatric epilepsy, increases the sensitivity of the MRI significantly.

A method of coregistering electrical dipole data from the EEG onto the patient's anatomic MRI, termed electrical source imaging (ESI), requires postprocessing using specialized software, but adds further localizing information (Figure 7.1). While greater numbers of electrodes increase its localizing power, such as that used in 128- or 256-channel high-density EEG, adding a minimal number of extra scalp electrodes to a phase I video-EEG study can provide helpful information in ESI. EEG-triggered functional MRI, a more technically challenging and resource-intensive procedure, allows for simultaneous acquisition of similar neurophysiologic and anatomic data.

Ancillary testing is often indicated in children undergoing presurgical evaluation and includes positron emission tomography (PET), single photon emission computed tomography (SPECT), and magnetoencephalography (MEG). Use of these modalities depends heavily on their institutional availability and the degree to which they

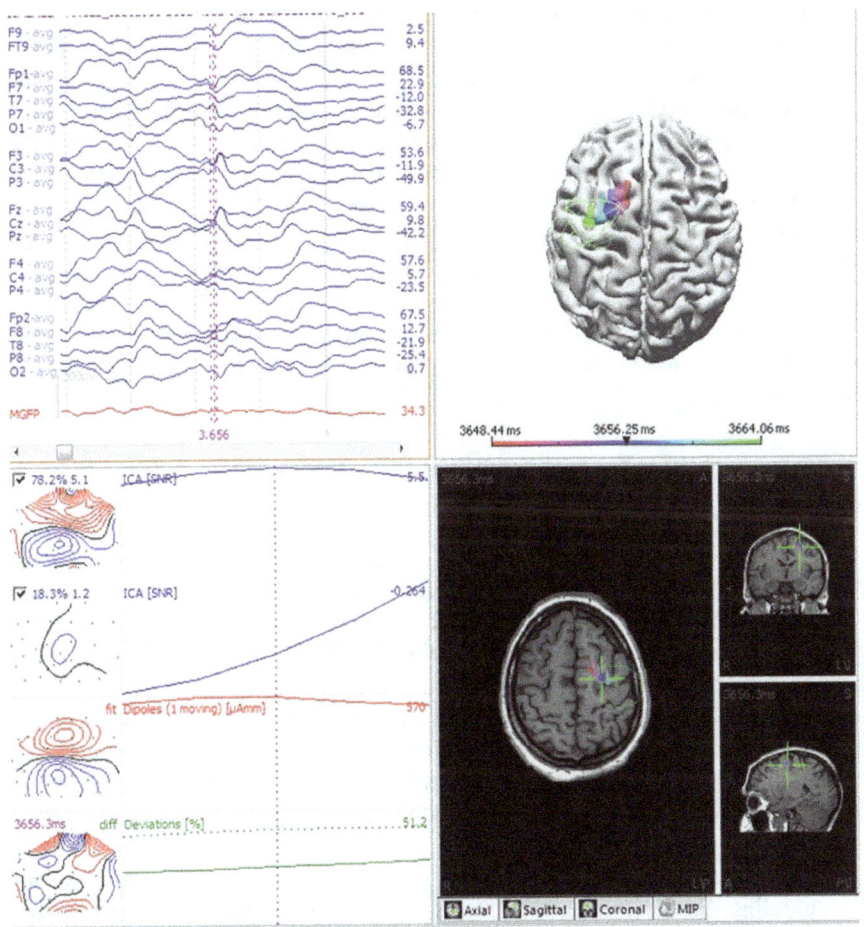

FIGURE 7.1 Electrical source imaging allows the coregistration of electrical dipoles from scalp EEG with the patient's volumetric brain MRI.

offer localizing information is variable and largely based on patient characteristics. FDG (fluorodeoxyglucose)-PET (positon emission tomography) obtained during the interictal state may reveal regions of cortical hypometabolism which indicate focal regions of epileptogenicity.

While removal of the entirety of the lesion has been shown to correlate with improved seizure outcome, the spatial resolution of this technique leads to the possibility of over- or underestimation of the epileptogenic zones. For the same reason, exquisitely focal regions of epileptogenic tissue may not be detectable with this modality. Ictal SPECT scan, which requires injection of a radiotracer through a peripheral intravenous line during a seizure, but ideally within 30 seconds of electrical onset, can be challenging logistically, but offers robust localization in some children.

In this technique, the hyperperfusion of epileptogenic tissue at ictal onset is indicated by increased focal uptake of the radiotracer visible on a scan done within several hours of the injection. Ictal SPECT scans or subtraction of interictal from ictal SPECT sequences (termed subtraction ictal SPECT coregistered to MRI or SISCOM) can offer localizing information when there are regions of encephalomalacia, surgical cavities, or extensive malformations that result in large, potentially non-epileptogenic areas of hypometabolism on PET scan.

MEG is a method by which the magnetic fields generated by electrical activity in the brain are represented as dipoles and superimposed on MRI images. Dipoles generated during interictal states yield localizing data which has been shown to correlate with regions of ictal onset. The dedicated scanners for this technique are costly and therefore not widely available. Overall, PET, SPECT, and MEG offer different types of data, allowing providers to choose the modality, or modalities, most appropriate for a child, yet their complementary nature increases the localizing yield when combined.

DELINEATION OF BASELINE NEURODEVELOPMENTAL FUNCTION AND MAPPING OF ELOQUENT AREAS OF CORTEX

Almost as important as the localization of the epileptogenic zone is the establishment of the overall cognitive function of the child, understanding of the relative strengths and weaknesses of different domains, and mapping of the eloquent functions of language, motor, and vision. Extensive testing performed by a trained neuropsychologist not only provides a comprehensive picture of a child's functional capabilities, but it may also reveal lateralizing or focal areas of dysfunction that support the existence of aberrant networks in specific brain regions.

Interpretation of this testing in the context of localizing data produced by the modalities discussed above allows providers to confirm suspicion of a region of underlying structural or functional abnormality and to better predict the effect of its removal on the child. This is critical not only in surgical decision-making but also in counseling the family about whether epilepsy surgery may benefit, or negatively affect, the trajectory of the child's neurodevelopment.

The more granular process of localizing eloquent functions including expressive and receptive language, motor function, and vision can be achieved in some children with the use of functional MRI, transcranial magnetic stimulation (TMS), and MEG. Task-based functional MRI performed in the awake child requires them to follow commands to envision words for expressive speech mapping or listen to spoken language for receptive speech localization. Motor paradigms require small movements such as finger tapping while vision mapping requires application of visual stimuli. Blood-oxygen-level-dependent (BOLD) signals created during these tasks superimposed on the brain MRI allow for visual representation of these functions. The acquisition of BOLD signals from sedated children produces less optimal results; investigations into the employment of fMRI acquired while in a resting state (termed resting-state fMRI) in this population are promising and concordance of functional localization to task-based fMRI in early studies is high.

TMS requires an awake, cooperative patient as magnetic stimulation is applied with a wand held over the skull of the child to stimulate areas of motor and language (Figure 7.2). Eliciting responses at low intensities can provide very localizing data, but it is not effective on every patient and requires experienced staff to apply and interpret findings. The use of MEG in such mapping is still an area of study but can provide information on language lateralization, even in sedated patients.

MULTIMODAL COREGISTRATION

Coregistration of the data acquired during a phase 1 evaluation is now a reasonable endeavor and can be performed using freeware readily available online.

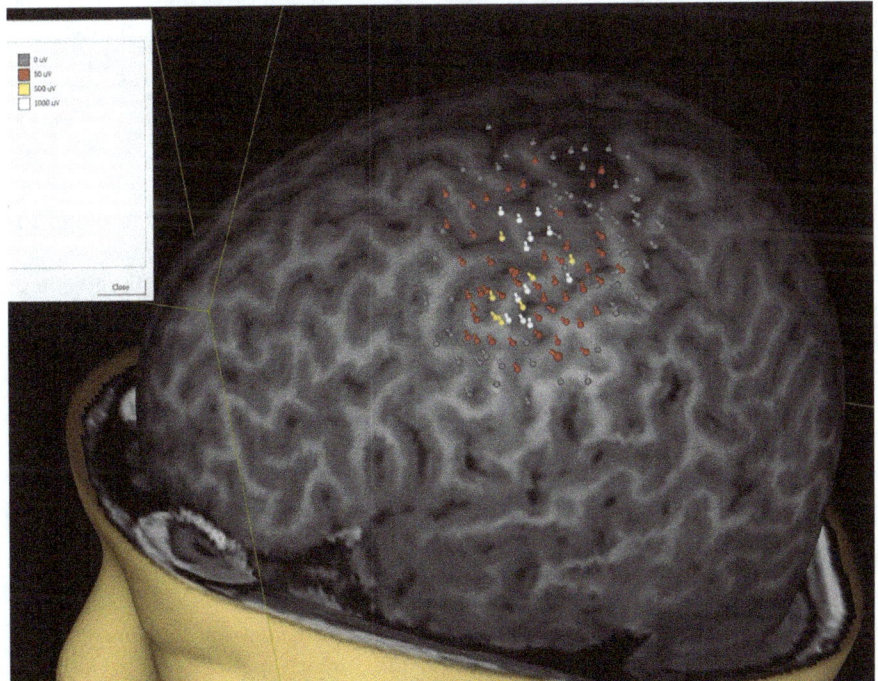

FIGURE 7.2 Successful mapping of the motor cortex in an awake patient with transcranial magnetic stimulation (TMS) offers localizing data of motor function.

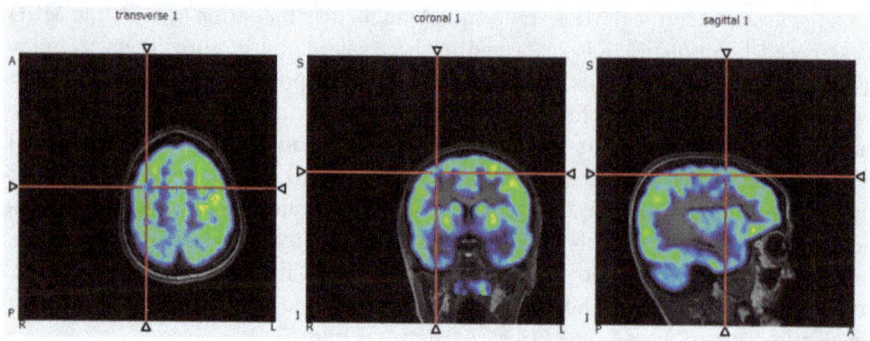

FIGURE 7.3 Coregistration of positron emission tomography (PET) and volumetric brain MRI allows for closer anatomic inspection of hypometabolic cortical regions indicating a potential epileptogenic zone.

Coregistration of the brain MRI, functional neuroimaging data, electrical and magnetic dipoles, as well as data gleaned from the functional mapping of eloquent areas of cortex may be critical to identifying the optimal surgical approach and extent for each child.

A recent study showed that children who had coregistration of their MRI to their PET and/or SPECT were less likely to undergo intracranial EEG monitoring and more likely to achieve postoperative seizure freedom (Figure 7.3). Adding functional data to the coregistration when invasive EEG monitoring is required ensures adequate placement of electrodes and coverage of regions of eloquent cortex in preparation for electrical stimulation mapping.

MULTIDISCIPLINARY MEETING

Discussion of phase I data in the setting of a multidisciplinary meeting of epileptologists, neuroradiologists, neuropsychologists, advanced practice providers, and coordinators is vital for comprehensive analysis of every case. After presentation of the data and through a high-level and detailed discussion, potential benefits as well as the pitfalls and caveats of each case can be realized and discussed. Ideally, each surgical decision is made by consensus, the estimated likelihood of seizure freedom is agreed upon, and points necessary for inclusion in presurgical counseling of the family are determined.

INVASIVE EVALUATION

Ideally, a presurgical evaluation yields enough localizing data to proceed with a successful single-stage surgery with no risk to eloquent tissue. Language and motor mapping can be performed intraoperatively when children are able to cooperate with certain tasks. However, in some cases, epilepsy surgery must involve a two-stage approach in which electrodes placed intracranially provide EEG data and allow for direct cortical stimulation, termed a phase 2 evaluation.

This may be necessary for better epileptogenic zone localization (such as that required when two or more non-adjacent regions are suspected to be involved in seizure onset), determination of the zonal boundaries, or to map the margins of eloquent function using electrical stimulation mapping. This type of mapping is also increasingly utilized as an aid in identifying the primary epileptogenic zone.

SUBDURAL ELECTRODE *VERSUS* STEREO-EEG ELECTRODE PLACEMENT

The two main techniques used in invasive EEG monitoring are placement of subdural grid and/or strip electrodes placed through an open craniotomy (Figure 7.4), stereotactic insertion of depth electrodes through small burr holes in the skull, or a hybrid approach that employs both methodologies. The type of approach and exact electrode placement should be determined by the epilepsy surgery team based on data culled from the presurgical evaluation.

Subdural electrode monitoring has been a mainstay in the United States for several decades while stereo-EEG (sEEG) is increasingly used due to the advent of robot-assistant technology and the need for monitoring of deep-seated regions not

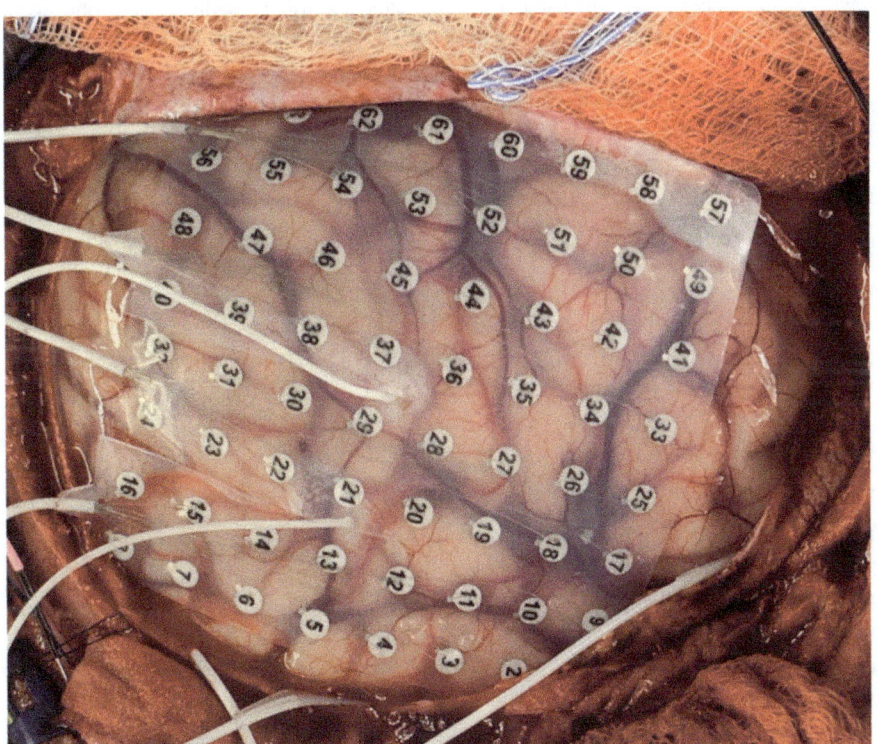

FIGURE 7.4 Placement of subdural grid and strip electrodes through a left-sided craniotomy to allow for mapping of ictal onset, expressive and receptive language function, and the motor cortex.

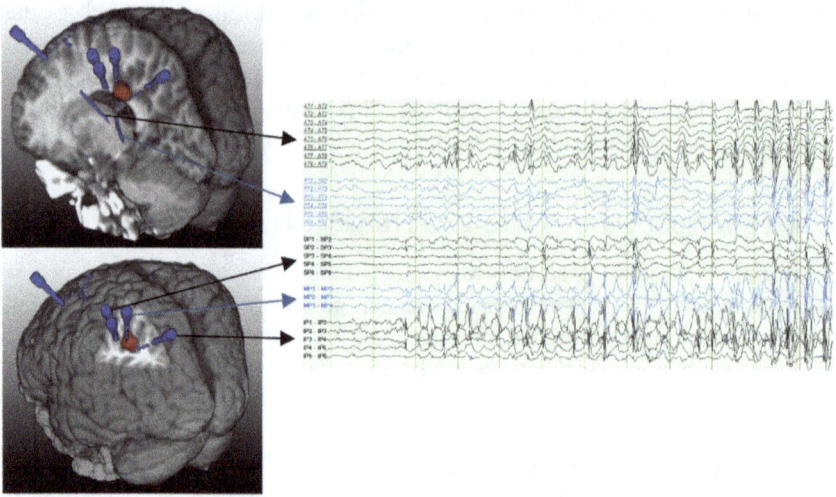

FIGURE 7.5   Invasive exploration of the left parietal cortex and thalamus in a patient with electrical status epilepticus of sleep with stereotactically placed EEG (sEEG). Here, a CT following sEEG placement is coregistered with the patient's MRI and a hypermetabolic signal from PET scan. sEEG signals are shown as recorded from each electrode.

accessible with grid and strip electrodes. In some cases, subdural electrodes provide spatial resolution not achievable with stereotactically placed electrodes (Figure 7.5).

Unfortunately, placement of subdural electrodes has higher rates of complications (15.5% vs. 4.8%), including infection, ischemic injury, and bleeding, as well as higher mortality rates (0.4% vs. 0.2%). Due to institutional preferences in surgical approach and selection bias involved in deciding which technique is most reasonable for each patient, seizure-freedom rates following these procedures are difficult to compare. Regardless, a 2019 metaanalysis found that those undergoing subdural electrode placement had a seizure-freedom rate of 56.4% at 1 year post-operatively, compared to 61% of those who had undergone sEEG.

IDENTIFICATION OF ELOQUENCE AND THE EPILEPTOGENIC ZONE VIA ELECTRICAL STIMULATION MAPPING

Once implanted with any type of the above-mentioned intracranial electrodes, electrical stimulation mapping of the sensory, motor, language, and visual cortices can be performed. Using parameters specific to children, electrical stimulation is typically performed at the bedside while the child is at rest or, for language mapping, engaged in age-appropriate tasks that require either expressive or receptive function. Results often provide confirmation of the functional organization seen on fMRI, but with improved accuracy and clear approximation to eloquent tissue. This procedure is dependent on patient cooperation but can be accomplished even in young children with careful instruction.

Providers with experience in electrical stimulation mapping are assessing the epileptogenic zone using different settings. In this, the goal of stimulation is elicitation of the patent's typical seizure semiology. It has been shown that postoperative outcomes are better when tissue is resected surrounding contacts that, when stimulated, trigger seizures.

SURGICAL PLANNING AND APPROACH

At the conclusion of invasive monitoring and mapping, a discussion between the epileptologist and the neurosurgeon is critical to determine the exact location and extent of a planned resection. In this meeting, the type of surgical procedure as well as the risks to eloquent tissue or potential for incomplete resection are identified. A presurgical discussion with the family and patient then follows.

The intent and type of surgery for each child varies based on presurgical data and, when available, information collected from an invasive evaluation. Palliative surgeries can improve seizure severity or frequency and, therefore, quality of life; it is imperative that these be considered for appropriate patients because of the positive impact seizure reduction can have on a child's quality of life.

These include resections of cortical tissue, lobes, disconnections of multiple lobes, hemispherectomies, corpus callosotomies, or implantation of neurostimulator devices including vagus nerve stimulation, responsive neurostimulation, and deep brain stimulation. Curative surgery may be ideal for carefully chosen patients and also includes focal cortical resections, larger sublobar resections, lobectomies, multilobar disconnections, and hemispherectomies.

The surgical approach for both palliative and curative procedures may require an open craniotomy or a minimally invasive approach such as an endoscopic technique, MRI-guided laser interstitial thermal therapy (MgLITT), radiofrequency thermocoagulation (RFTC), or the noninvasive MRI-guided focused ultrasound (MgFUS).

SURGICAL OUTCOMES

The incidence of seizure freedom varies widely between studies in pediatric epilepsy surgery due to many factors, including whether the intent was curative or palliative. In a systematic review of studies published from centers worldwide, representing a heterogeneous population with wide-ranging follow-up durations, the seizure freedom rate at 1 year was 64.8% and 60.3% at 5 years. This study found that the highest rate of seizure freedom followed hemispheric surgeries (76%) but that similar rates were seen in temporal surgeries (73.4%).

Extratemporal surgery yielded seizure freedom in only 60.2%. In terms of pathology, children with underlying tumors were most likely to be seizure-free postoperatively, followed by those with mesial temporal sclerosis. Lower rates were seen in those with encephalomalacia, malformations of cortical development, tuberous sclerosis, and hemimegalencephaly. Understandably, less favorable outcomes were seen in those with nonlesional epilepsy versus those with lesions appreciable on MRI.

A reduction in or cessation of seizures can result in improvements in the quality of life and/or measures of neuropsychological functioning. Not surprisingly, a recently published systematic review reported that quality of life scores paralleled seizure-freedom rates. Studies analyzed for neuropsychological data were highly variable in measures of neurocognitive function but included reports of stable (70%) or improved (10%–15%) cognition in the majority of the children included.

CONCLUSION

Epilepsy surgery is a highly underutilized approach to improving the quality of life, neurodevelopment, and seizure-freedom rates of children with epilepsy. After a comprehensive presurgical evaluation, a carefully selected candidate can undergo one or more of a variety of surgical procedures that may lead to seizure freedom. Minimally invasive and minimally resective techniques are safe and effective in many children. Palliative options provide a chance of seizure reduction for those with more complex or multifocal epilepsies. Of these, devices employing neuromodulatory stimulation have rapidly advanced and are covered in a separate chapter.

SUGGESTED REFERENCES

Beatty C.W., Lockrow J.P., Gedela S., Gehred A., Ostendorf A.P. The missed value of under-utilizing pediatric epilepsy surgery: A systematic review. *Semin Pediatr Neurol* 2021;39: 100917.

Cuello Oderiz C., von Ellenrieder N., Dubeau F., Eisenberg A., Gotman J., Hall J., Hincapié A.S., Hoffmann D., Job A.S., Khoo H.M., Minotti L., Olivier A., Kahane P., Frauscher B. Association of cortical stimulation-induced seizure with surgical outcome in patients with focal drug-resistant epilepsy. *JAMA Neurol* 2019;76: 1070–8.

Gonzalez L.M., Wrennall J.A. A neuropsychological model for the pre-surgical evaluation of children with focal-onset epilepsy: An integrated approach. *Seizure* 2020;77: 29–39.

Hyslop A., Duchowny M. Electrical stimulation mapping in children. *Seizure* 2020;77: 59–63.

Juhász C., John F. Utility of MRI, PET, and ictal SPECT in presurgical evaluation of non-lesional pediatric epilepsy. *Seizure* 2020;77: 15–28.

Kwan P., Brodie M.J. Early identification of refractory epilepsy. *N Engl J Med* 2000;342: 314–9.

Moosa A.N.V., Wyllie E. Cognitive outcome after epilepsy surgery in children. *Semin Pediatr Neurol* 2017;24: 331–9.

Perry M.S., Bailey L., Freedman D., Donahue D., Malik S., Head H., Keator C., Hernandez A. Coregistration of multimodal imaging is associated with favourable two-year seizure outcome after paediatric epilepsy surgery. *Epileptic Disorders* 2017;19: 40–8.

Romanowski E.F., McNamara N. Surgery for intractable epilepsy in pediatrics, a systematic review of outcomes other than seizure freedom. *Semin Pediatr Neurol* 2021;39: 100928.

Starnes K., Depositario-Cabacar D., Wong-Kisiel L. Presurgical evaluation strategies for intractable epilepsy of childhood. *Semin Pediatr Neurol* 2021;39: 100915.

Widjaja E., Jain P., Demoe L., Guttmann A., Tomlinson G., Sander B. Seizure outcome of pediatric epilepsy surgery: Systematic review and meta-analyses. *Neurology* 2020;94: 311–21.

Yan H., Katz J.S., Anderson M., Mansouri A., Remick M., Ibrahim G.M., Abel T.J. Method of invasive monitoring in epilepsy surgery and seizure freedom and morbidity: A systematic review. *Epilepsia* 2019;60: 1960–72.

8 Status Epilepticus

Sonali Sen and James J. Riviello
Baylor College of Medicine

CONTENTS

Status epilepticus (SE) is defined as a seizure lasting 30 minutes or more of either continuous seizure activity or two or more sequential seizures with persistent altered awareness in-between the seizures. SE is a life-threatening medical emergency requiring prompt recognition and treatment, starting with the basic principles of neuroresuscitation – the A, B, and Cs – followed by a planned treatment protocol. SE is not a specific disease itself and may occur during the course of epilepsy or secondary to a nervous system (CNS) insult. Proper management requires the identification and treatment of the precipitating cause to facilitate seizure control and prevent ongoing neurologic injury.

Status epilepticus (SE) often occurs during an intercurrent illness, and in this scenario, likely represents an exacerbation of the underlying seizure disorder due to inflammation, impaired pharmacokinetics, stress, and other factors. This is a common occurrence, although the differential diagnosis must include encephalitis or meningitis. For epilepsy in general, and especially for SE, it is critical to identify a precipitating cause, even in a patient with an underlying seizure disorder, since a specific precipitant may have caused the exacerbation and require specific treatment.

Blood chemistries should be performed in patients at risk for metabolic abnormalities, such as those with gastroenteritis. While the overall yield is only 6%, it should be considered in at-risk patients. Hyponatremia itself may precipitate seizures and may be caused by carbamazepine, oxcarbazepine, and eslicarbazepine, while metabolic acidosis may occur with topiramate. Neonates often present with hypoglycemic and hypocalcemic seizures, so these should be evaluated for in this age group. A lumbar puncture is diagnostic for a central nervous system (CNS) infection in 12% of patients with SE and should be performed in patients with concerns for intracranial infection, such as those with nuchal rigidity, fever, or unexplained encephalopathy. Other abnormal diagnostic studies included low antiseizure medication (ASM) levels (32%), ingestion of drugs or toxins (3.6%), and inborn errors of metabolism (4.2%). An EEG detects interepileptiform abnormalities in 43% of patients. EEG should be performed in all patients with persistent altered awareness and who do not improve after the control of convulsive movements to exclude NCSE.

DOI: 10.1201/9781003296478-9

In the North London *Status Epilepticus* Surveillance Study (NLSTEPSS), the first prospective pediatric-specific study of only SE, 33% of new-onset SE cases were prolonged febrile seizures and another 16% had an acute CNS insult. In the Richmond study, a mixed adult and child study, the etiology was a medication change in 20%, followed by a metabolic abnormality in 8%, anoxia and CNS infection in 5%, trauma and vascular etiologies in 3.5%, and intoxications in 2.5%.

The most common classification system for SE is done by etiology: symptomatic (acute, remote, progressive, or as defined in a specific electroclinical syndrome) or unknown. In this case, the etiology is remote symptomatic, with an acute precipitant being likely. In a retrospective analysis of SE, the practice parameter from the American Academy of Neurology (AAN) on the diagnostic assessment of the child with SE, an acute precipitant was identified in only 1%. However, the NLSTEPSS identified an acute or remote symptomatic cause in 6%. It is therefore important to identify a precipitant and treat appropriately, since seizure cessation with ASMs does not treat the precipitating cause.

Finally, for SE diagnosis, when is neuroimaging required? Neuroimaging is needed with new-onset SE, or when the baseline neurologic examination has changed, such as with focality, especially if new. In the AAN practice parameter, neuroimaging abnormalities were detected in 8% of the children. These abnormal findings may be related to the cause of the underlying epilepsy, but may not have precipitated the acute episode of SE. In new-onset SE or with a new focal abnormality on the neurologic examination, if there is concern for a CNS infection, neuroimaging should be done prior to a lumbar puncture.

TREATMENT STRATEGY

The strict criterion for SE is 30 minutes of either CSE or serial seizures without recovery of consciousness in between the seizures. However, we do not wait 30 minutes to treat SE, since there is concern about the potential for brain injury. An "operational definition" of SE recommends treatment after 5 minutes for either

- five minutes or more of a continuous tonic-clonic seizure, or
- two or more discrete seizures with incomplete recovery of consciousness in between.

There remains limited information about the long-term consequences from focal or absence SE though it has been suggested that for focal SE, neurologic injury may not occur until 60 minutes of continuous seizure activity. Current recommendations are to treat at 10 minutes for focal seizure activity with impaired awareness or 10–15 minutes for absence seizures.

What are the appropriate ASMs for *status epilepticus*, and is there a specific sequence in which these should be given? Evidence-based guidelines for the treatment of convulsive *status epilepticus* in pediatrics recommend first-line use of benzodiazepines. Intravenous (IV) lorazepam and diazepam are fast and effective. Rectal or intranasal (IN) diazepam, and intramuscular (IM), intranasal, or buccal midazolam are appropriate alternatives, particularly in the out-of-hospital setting. The established *status epilepticus* treatment trial (ESET) showed equal efficacy for

TABLE 8.1

Practice Guideline for the Treatment of Status Epilepticus at Texas Children's Hospital

Lorazepam, 0.1 mg/kg, IV (maximum initial dose 4 mg)

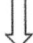 If seizures continue for another 5 minutes, administer

Lorazepam, 0.1 mg/kg, IV,
followed immediately by Fosphenytoin, 30 mg/kg, IV
(maximum dose 1500 mg, given no faster than 150 mg/minute) OR
Levetiracetam, 60 mg/kg (maximum dose 4500 mg).
Note: 30 mg/kg fosphenytoin dose is only for patients with ongoing
status epilepticus

 If seizures continue for another 10
minutes after fosphenytoin infusion
completed:

Admit to Critical Care/anticipate need for intubation
Start midazolam, 0.2 mg/kg (Max 10 mg) and start infusion at
0.1 mg/kg/hr
Consult Neurology (consult neurology sooner if child is
currently on a seizure medication)
In 5 minutes, if seizure continues, repeat 0.2 mg/kg and
increase infusion to 0.2mg/kg/hr
If this does not work, consider another agent (pentobarbital
or ketamine)

levetiracetam, valproic acid, and fosphenytoin in the treatment of benzodiazepine-refractory SE, with similar incidences of adverse events. Phenobarbital can be used but is associated with a higher adverse side-effect profile. Newer ASMs to be considered include lacosamide and brivaracetam, both of which have been shown to be effective for the treatment of SE in adults.

Evidence-based guidelines are important to standardize care, analyze outcomes, and improve treatment. These are extremely important to provide treatment consistency. We have included the current clinical practice guideline for the treatment of SE at Texas Children's Hospital (Table 8.1). Especially in a younger child, consider pyridoxine, 100–200 mg, for the treatment of RSE.

What is the response to treatment of SE? One clinical trial comparing IV lorazepam to IV diazepam demonstrated equivalent efficacy with seizure termination by 10 minutes observed in approximately 72% of patients. The RAMPART showed similar efficacy in seizure termination using IM midazolam and IV lorazepam, but ultimately determined IM midazolam to be superior in the out-of-hospital setting due to a more reliable and rapid route of administration leading to fewer hospital and ICU admissions. Delays in treatment are associated with decreased response to benzodiazepines.

What home or prehospital therapies are available for prolonged or recurrent seizures? When should these be considered? Several preparations are available which can now be given at home. The most used is diazepam rectal gel. There is increasing use of intranasal midazolam or diazepam, which are available as a predosed nasal spray. The intranasal route is likely as effective as IM or IV but more easily administered by a nonmedical caregiver in addition to being more socially appropriate in a public setting. Clonazepam is available as a disintegrating wafer but does not have an immediate effect; it is better to abort seizure clusters.

Why is it important to control SE as soon as possible? Seizures, especially SE, increase cerebral metabolic demands, especially for glucose and oxygen. Initially, CNS compensatory mechanisms are able to meet these demands; however, as the duration of SE increases hypoxemia, hypercarbia, hypotension, and hyperthermia occur. A mismatch develops between the ongoing metabolic needs of the brain and cerebral blood flow with resultant brain depletion of glucose and oxygen. This may result in neuronal injury or death and alteration of neuronal networks, along with other systemic complications. A decreased response to benzodiazepines has been observed with prolonged seizure activity, which is partly the result of internalization of γ-aminobutyric acid type A (GABA$_A$) receptors under conditions of sustained excitability. This results in a progressive impairment of GABA mediated inhibition. Activation of N-methyl-D-aspartate (NMDA) receptors contributes to excitotoxic injury.

LONG-TERM OUTCOME

Neurologic sequelae from SE include cognitive, behavioral, and motor impairments, as well as subsequent epilepsy. The FEBSTAT study demonstrated acute hippocampal injury following febrile *status epilepticus* (FSE). Although still an area of ongoing research, this raises further concern regarding the association between FSE and the development of mesial temporal lobe sclerosis and temporal lobe epilepsy. Risk of epilepsy after unprovoked SE is 25%–40%, though may be higher in acute symptomatic cases.

Delays in treatment are associated with increased morbidity and mortality. In seizures that last greater than 5 minutes, 50% of febrile seizures resolved spontaneously, whereas no acute symptomatic seizures spontaneously resolved. Mortality rates vary from 3% to 11%. In the Richmond study, the overall mortality was 6%, but when age stratified, mortality in the first year was 17.8%, and 24% in the first 6 months. Increased mortality within the first year is associated with a higher incidence of acute symptomatic SE in the youngest children.

SUGGESTED REFERENCES

Chamberlain J.M., Okada P., Holsti M., Mahajan P., Brown K.M., Vance C., Gonzalez V., Lichenstein R., Stanley R., Brousseau D.C., Grubenhoff J., Zemek R., Johnson D.W., Clemons T.E., Baren J.; Pediatric Emergency Care Applied Research Network (PECARN). Lorazepam vs. diazepam for pediatric *status epilepticus*: A randomized clinical trial. *JAMA* 2014;311: 1652–60.

Chin R.F.M., Neville B.G.R., Peckham C., Bedford H., Wade A., Scott R.C. Incidence, cause, and short-term outcome of convulsive *status epilepticus* in children: Prospective, population-based study. *Lancet* 2006;368: 222–9.

DeLorenzo R.J., Towne A.R., Pellock J.M., Ko D. *Status epilepticus* in children, adults, and the elderly. *Epilepsia* 1992;33(Suppl 4): S15–25.

Eriksson E., Metsaranta P., Huhtala H., Auvinen A., Kuusela A.-L., Koivikko M. Treatment delay and the risk of prolonged *status epilepticus*. *Neurology* 2005;65: 1316–8.

Gaínza-Lein M., Sánchez Fernández I., Jackson M., Abend N.S., Arya R., Brenton J.N., Carpenter J.L., Chapman K.E., Gaillard W.D., Glauser T.A., Goldstein J.L., Goodkin H.P., Kapur K., Mikati M.A., Peariso K., Tasker R.C., Tchapyjnikov D., Topjian A.A., Wainwright M.S., Wilfong A., Williams K., Loddenkemper T.; Pediatric Status Epilepticus Research Group. Association of time to treatment with short-term outcomes for pediatric patients with refractory convulsive status epilepticus. *JAMA Neurol* 2018;75: 410–8.

Glauser T., Shinnar S., Gloss D., Alldredge B., Arya R., Bainbridge J., Bare M., Bleck T., Dodson W.E., Garrity L., Jagoda A., Lowenstein D., Pellock J., Riviello J., Sloan E., Treiman D.M. Evidence-based guideline: Treatment of convulsive *Status Epilepticus* in children and adults: Report of the Guideline Committee of the American Epilepsy Society. *Epilepsy Curr* 2016;16: 48–61.

Goodkin H.P., Joshi S., Kozhemyakin M., Kapur J. Impact of receptor changes on treatment of status epilepticus. *Epilepsia* 2007;48(Suppl 8): S14–5.

Harden C.L., Huff J.S., Schwartz T.H., Dubinsky R.M., Zimmerman R.D., Weinstein S., Foltin J.C., Theodore W.H. Therapeutics and technology assessment subcommittee of the American Academy of Neurology. Reassessment: Neuroimaging in the emergency patient presenting with seizure (an evidence-based review): Report of the therapeutics and technology Assessment subcommittee of the American Academy of Neurology. *Neurology* 2007;69: 1772–80.

Kapur J., Elm J., Chamberlain J.M., Barsan W., Cloyd J., Lowenstein D., Shinnar S., Conwit R., Meinzer C., Cock H., Fountain N., Connor J.T., Silbergleit R.; NETT and PECARN Investigators. Randomized trial of three anticonvulsant medications for *status epilepticus*. *N Engl J Med* 2019;318: 2103–13.

Lothman E. The biochemical basis and pathophysiology of *status epilepticus*. *Neurology* 1990;40(Suppl 2): S13–23.

Lowenstein D.H., Bleck T., Macdonald R.L. It's time to revise the definition of *status epilepticus*. *Epilepsia* 1999;40: 120–2.

Riviello J.J., Ashwal Shirtz D., Glauser T., Ballaban-Gil K., Morton L.D., Phillips S., Sloan E., Shinnar S.; American Academy of Neurology Subcommittee; Practice Committee of the Child Neurology Society. Practice parameter: Diagnostic assessment of the child with *status epilepticus* (an evidence-based review): Report of the quality standards subcommittee of the American Academy of Neurology and the practice committee of the Child Neurology Society. *Neurology* 2006;67: 1542–50.

Shinnar S., Bello J.A., Chan S., Hesdorffer D.C., Lewis D.V., Macfall J., Pellock J.M., Nordli D.R., Frank L.M., Moshe S.L., Gomes W., Shinnar R.C., Sun S.; FEBSTAT Study Team. MRI abnormalities following febrile status epilepticus in children: The FEBSTAT study. *Neurology* 2012;79: 871–7.

Silbergleit R., Durkalski V., Lowenstein D., Conwit R., Pancioli A., Palesch Y., Barsan W.; NETT Investigators. Intramuscular versus intravenous therapy for prehospital *status epilepticus*. *N Engl J Med* 2012;366: 591–600.

Status Epilepticus Content Expert Team. (2018) *Initial Management of Status Epilepticus, Evidence Based Guideline*. Evidence-Based Outcomes Center. Texas Children's Hospital, Houston, TX.

Trinka E., Cock H., Hesdorffer D., Rossetti A.O., Scheffer I.E., Shinnar S., Shorvon S., Lowenstein D.H. A definition and classification of status epilepticus-report of the ILAE task force on classification of status epilepticus. *Epilepsia* 2015;56: 1515–23.

9 Focal Cortical Dysplasias

Harvey B. Sarnat
University of Calgary

CONTENTS

INTRODUCTION

Focal cortical dysplasias (FCDs) are circumscribed areas of abnormal architecture and lamination of cerebral cortex. In FCD type I, the neurons are normal in size and form; in FCD type II, many but not all neurons and glial cells are megalocytic and in addition, dysplastic; FCD type III is a zone of FCD I or II associated with another principal lesion of the cortex. All FCDs are congenital lesions and thus developmental malformations. All are highly epileptogenic and seizures often are refractory to medications. The genetic and clinical features are very different in FCD I and II, in addition to distinctive neuropathological findings. Neuropathology also defines subtypes of each FCD type.

The histopathological features that define FCDs were published in 2011 by the International League Against Epilepsy (ILAE) Commission on Neuropathology and a proposal for an update was made in 2018. Proposals for incorporating genetic data and broadening the criteria to include additional distinctive types as well as neuroimaging and clinical data were submitted for consideration. Though neuroimaging features are typical, particularly for FCD II, definitive diagnosis is based upon the histopathology of brain resections for epileptic foci and genetic studies.

Electroencephalography (EEG) and intraoperative electrocorticography (ECoG) and depth electrode recording localize epileptic zones but do not reliably distinguish the types of FCD. Clinical patterns also are not definitive enough alone to establish the diagnosis.

FOCAL CORTICAL DYSPLASIA TYPE I

FCD I is abnormal cortical lamination with normal, not dysplastic, neurons. The lesions usually occur in the parieto-occipital cortex. Onset of epilepsy begins in the neonatal period, in infancy or early childhood. There is a slight female predominance, but all ethnic groups are affected. FCD I is less frequent than FCD II but is not rare. Patients with FCD I are otherwise normal, without neurological, developmental, or cognitive deficits, though some children later exhibit learning disabilities in school or attentional deficits.

Neuropathology. FCD I was divided into three subtypes in the 2011 ILAE scheme: Ia with microcolumnar rather than horizontal laminar cortical architecture (Figure 9.1); Ib with laminar loss of neurons; Ic being a combination of Ia and Ib. But it is now questioned whether subtypes Ib and Ic are true malformations rather than acquired lesions secondary to fetal ischemia or other causes. FCD Ia, by contrast, does appear to be a primary cortical malformation. Layers of synapses also are radial, alternating with the microcolumns of neurons. Radial neuronal columns represent the normal pattern in the first half of gestation, superimposed horizontal lamination beginning at 22 weeks of gestation. It also occurs in a more generalized cortical distribution in certain genetic/metabolic encephalopathies beginning in fetal life.

In the U-fiber layer immediately beneath FCD I, there are excessive heterotopic or displaced neurons, mostly pyramidal cells of layer 6. These neurons of the U-fibers are not demonstrated in the deep subcortical white matter. They form a dense synaptic plexus (Figure 9.2) that also project axons into the cortex to integrate into epileptic networks and likely contribute to propagation but not necessarily initiation of seizures.

Inflammation, vasculitis, and neoplasia are not pathological features of FCD I. Other brain malformations also are not found.

Genetics. A genetic basis for FCD I is poorly established. A consistent genetic mutation has been demonstrated to date only in certain metabolic diseases with generalized microcolumnar cortical architecture. In rodents, the

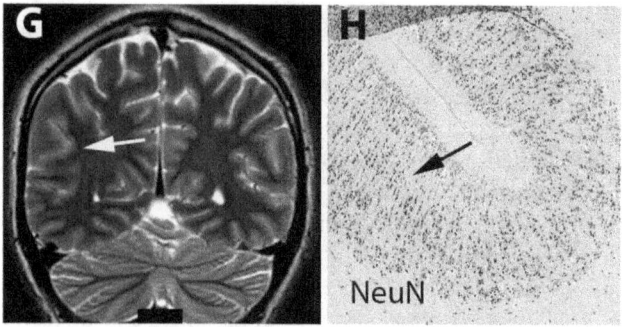

FIGURE 9.1 Nineteen-year-old boy with severe refractory epilepsy with onset at age of 9 months. Right parietal FCD 1a. (G) MRI-T2 of right parietal lobe shows no distinctive changes at the site of electrographic interictal paroxysmal activity and ictal epileptiform discharge (white arrow) (H) Surgical resection of area indicated by the arrow in MRI shows predominant microcolumnar architecture well demonstrated by neuronal nuclear antigen (NeuN) immunocytochemistry (black arrow), diagnostic of FCD Ia. He was free of seizures postoperatively and had no neurological deficits. (From Coras et al. 2021.)

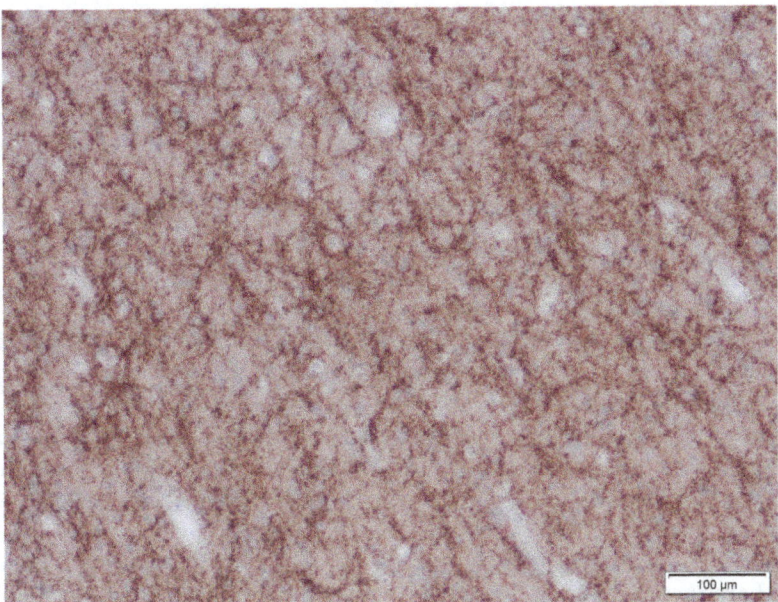

FIGURE 9.2   Subcortical U-fiber layer beneath an FCD Ia, showing heterotopic neurons forming a complex synaptic plexus to interconnect them and to extend into the overlying cortex to join the epileptic network. Synaptophysin reactivity is seen not only surrounding neuronal somata but also within their axons because of the high metabolic rate of heterotopic neurons. A three-year-old girl with refractory focal epilepsy secondary to FCD Ia in the posterior temporal lobe. (From Sarnat et al. 2018.)

Reelin gene is strongly expressed in Cajal–Retzius neurons that are essential to the normal development of the microcolumnar architecture in early fetal life and later fetal cortical laminar organization, but defective *Reelin* or deficiency of Cajal–Retzius neurons has not been demonstrated in human FCD Ia.

Neuroimaging. The abnormal lamination of the cortex does not change neuronal density, and neurons are morphologically normal and vascularization is not altered, so that the cortex at the site of electrographic paroxysmal foci, as seen in routine T1 and T2 images or in FLAIR sequences, does not usually disclose a gray matter lesion. However, there is often blurring of the gray/white matter junction at the site of the FCD due to the heterotopic neurons and their synaptic plexi within the U-fiber layer. Positron emission tomography (PET) scanning may disclose a zone of hypometabolism at the site of FCD I, but this is not diagnostic.

Management and Outcome. The epilepsy arising from FCD Ia often is refractory to medical treatment with antiseizure medications (ASMs) of all types. Surgical resection of the epileptic focus is the most useful approach to seizure control. The prognosis for recurrent seizures is not as good as in FCD II because lesions may be more extensive and their margins more difficult to identify pre- or intraoperatively. Postoperative management should include serial EEGs over several years, even in patients who are free of seizures. Second surgeries to resect residual epileptogenic brain tissue are needed in a minority of cases, months or years after the initial surgery. A ketogenic diet is effective in some, avoiding a second surgery. Vagus nerve stimulation is not effective.

FOCAL CORTICAL DYSPLASIA TYPE II

FCD II is the most frequent congenital focal epileptogenic cortical lesions, is strongly suspected on the basis of MRI, exhibits typical and diagnostic neuropathological findings, and has a well-established genetic basis. FCD II is highly epileptogenic for focal seizures.

Neuropathology. Not only is there disruption of cortical lamination and architecture, with many displaced and disoriented neurons, but many (not all) neurons themselves are megalocytic (enlarged) and dysplastic (altered morphology). Glial cells are similarly involved. In addition, there is an excess of heterotopic neurons in the U-fiber layer that form synaptic plexi similar to FCD I. In FCD II and hemimegalencephaly, there is an upregulation of abnormal phosphorylated tau protein in the cortex, maximal in the superficial layers. FCD II is divided into two subtypes, the difference being that FCD IIb also includes *balloon cells*, which are lacking in FCD IIa. Balloon cells are large, globular cells with eccentric nuclei that express primitive proteins of progenitor cells, such as nestin and vimentin, which help distinguish them from megalocytic, dysplastic neurons (Figure 9.3). Balloon cells also express both glial and neuronal proteins: they are cells of mixed lineage. Though they express synaptophysin, they exhibit infrequent electrophysiological paroxysmal discharges.

Genetics. FCD II, hemimegalencephaly, and tuberous sclerosis complex (TSC) are postzygotic somatic mutations not inherited as a Mendelian trait, though a component of germline mutation also is now recognized in FCD II and hemimegalencephaly and is prominent in TSC. Some but not all neuroepithelial progenitor cell clones are affected at various times during their 33 mitotic cycles; those expressed in early cycles cause more extensive cortical malformations than those expressed in later cycles.

The genetic basis of this postzygotic somatic mutation is a disorder causing upregulation of the *mammalian target of rapamycin* (mTOR) signaling pathway or one of the closely related pathways upstream of mTOR (Figure 9.4). Somatic mutations are expressed after fertilization is complete and affect progenitor cells at various embryonic ages, resulting in mixtures of normal and abnormal clones because not all progenitors are affected. Such mTOR mutations may be confined to one organ, such as the brain in FCD II, or may affect multiple organs, skin, and extremities with overgrowth and tissue architectural abnormalities, as in TSC and epidermal nevus syndromes.

Neuroimaging. MRI findings in FCD II are characteristic and almost diagnostic with good neuropathological correlation. Some findings also can be demonstrated by computed tomography (CT), but prenatal ultrasound examination is less reliable. The T1 and T2 sequences of MRI often show a hyperintense focal lesion within

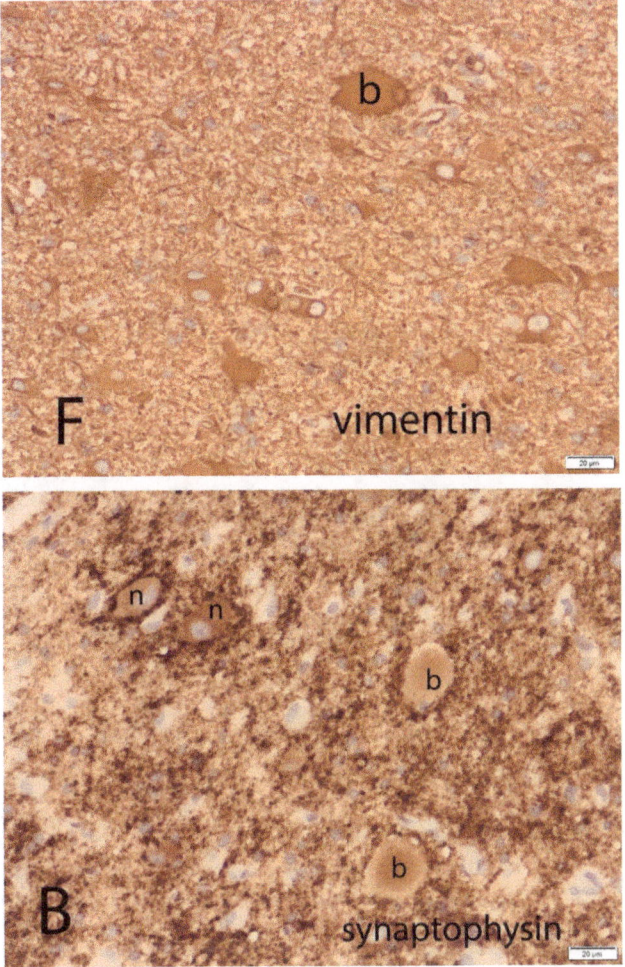

FIGURE 9.3   Surgical resection of focal cortical dysplasia IIb in lateral temporal neocortex of a 13-year-old boy with intractable epilepsy. (F) Vimentin, an intermediate filament protein of early differentiating but not mature neural cells, is strongly reactive in large globular balloon cells (b) and in smaller immature dysplastic or regenerating astrocytes, some of which are abnormally binuclear. Glial fibrillary acidic protein (GFAP) also was reactive (not illustrated). No neurons were reactive to vimentin or GFAP. (B) Balloon cells (b) and dysplastic neurons (n) both exhibit synaptophysin reactivity. Balloon cells are of mixed cellular lineage, expressing both neuronal and glial proteins as well as primitive proteins of differentiating cells. (Reproduced from Sarnat 2021.)

the cortex, usually at the bottom of a sulcus or base of a gyrus. It may also exhibit linear radial continuity of this lesion with a zone at the periventricular wall, called the *transmantle dysplasia sign*. This radial line from ventricular ependyma to the base of a gyrus or of a sulcus between two gyri corresponds neuropathologically to a trail of dysplastic neurons and heterotopia of incompletely migrated neuroblasts and

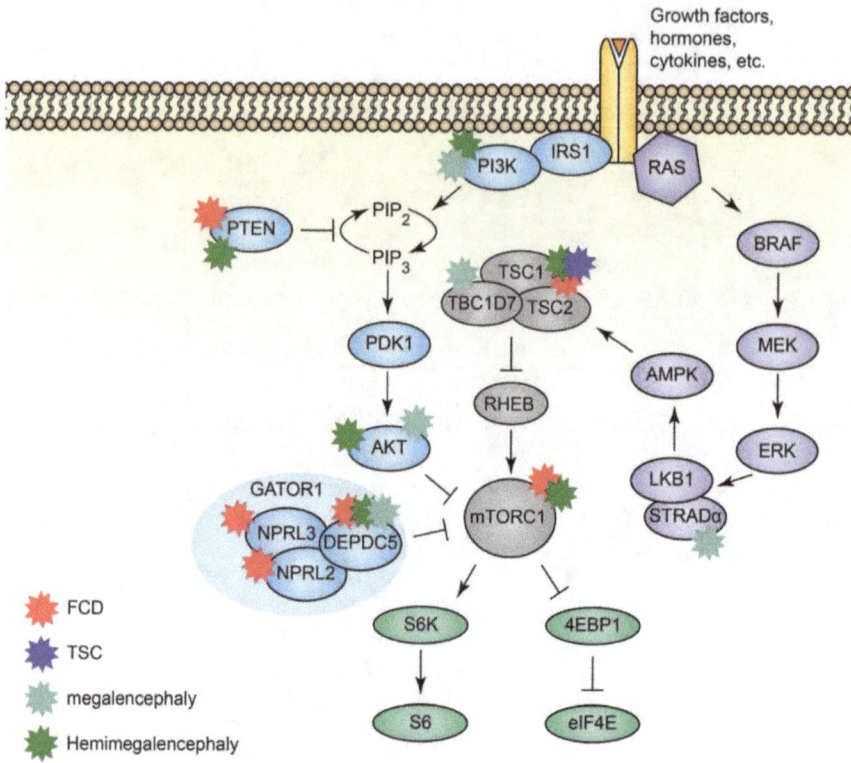

FIGURE 9.4 Diagram of the mTOR (mTORC1) signaling pathway and related upstream pathways that influence it and various epileptogenic cerebral dysplasias that are thus genetically related: FCD, focal cortical dysplasia type II; TSC, tuberous sclerosis complex. Hemimegalencephaly includes epidermal nevus syndromes. (Reproduced from Mühlebner et al. 2019.)

glioblasts within the white matter. It is also frequent in TSC. Other more isolated deep white matter heterotopia also may occur. Focal gray/white matter blurring is common even in the absence of the transmantle sign. The cerebral cortex at the site of FCD II is often thicker than the more normal cortex elsewhere.

Management and Outcome. In isolated FCD II or hemimegalencephaly, control of epilepsy is the most urgent goal. ASMs of all types usually are minimal if at all effective. Currently, surgical resection of the epileptogenic FCD is the most reliable treatment but must be preceded by meticulous history taking and documentation of neurological deficits, intensive preoperative investigations that include extended video-EEG monitoring, MRI with epilepsy surgery protocol, PET and other functional neuroimaging studies, and age-appropriate neuropsychological testing. Intraoperative electrophysiological procedures should be carried out in a medical center where the special resources and experienced epileptologists and neurosurgeons are available. Equally important is the availability of a neuropathologist with expertise in tissue resections for epilepsy requiring specialized workup and immunohistochemical antibodies for modern diagnostic neuropathological studies. Genetic studies of the resected brain tissue also are essential.

Postoperative EEG and MRI are essential. The decision about continued administration of ASMs is made on an individual patient basis. Administration of steroids in the postoperative period may be useful in a minority of patients if significant cerebral edema is present. Serial long-term EEG recordings, even in the absence of clinical seizures, are a useful noninvasive procedure. Some patients with recurrent seizures due to subtotal resection of the FCD may later require additional surgery. In some instances, however, a ketogenic diet may be effective to obviate or delay repeat surgery. Vagus nerve stimulators are not effective.

Promising new approaches for pre- and postoperative management include mTOR-inhibiting medications such as rapamycin (Everolimus; Sirolimus) but these are still under clinical investigation and not yet recommended in routine protocols. In TSC, the cortical tubers are not reduced in size as much as subependymal SEGA tumors, but mTOR inhibitors do suppress epileptic activity associated with cortical tubers. These mTOR inhibitors also may reduce the cerebral overgrowth and epilepsy of hemimegalencephaly.

Prognosis for epilepsy control depends upon the completeness of the surgical resection, but many patients are free of seizures postoperatively and for many years thereafter without ASMs. After the immediate postoperative period, it is useful to repeat neuropsychological testing to compare with preoperative data. Some patients may require special education at school and home.

RELATION BETWEEN CORTICAL DYSPLASIA TYPE II AND HEMIMEGALENCEPHALY

Hemimegalencephaly is an overgrowth of half the brain with dysplasia of supratentorial structures, especially but not confined to the cerebral cortex. Rarely, the ipsilateral brainstem and cerebellum also are enlarged and dysplastic. The diagnosis may be made prenatally by fetal ultrasound and MRI. Hemimegalencephaly may occur as an isolated malformation or may be associated with some neurocutaneous syndromes, especially epidermal nevus syndromes (both keratinocytic and sebaceous types), proteus syndrome with overgrowth of facial structures, visceral organs and extremities, and TSC. Hemimegalencephaly is a highly epileptogenic lesion. It affects both genders and all ethnic groups.

The histopathology of hemimegalencephaly is identical to that of FCD IIb, including balloon cells. Both FCD II and hemimegalencephaly are postzygotic somatic mutations with the same genetic basis of mTOR pathway overexpression. The closely related AKT and PK3CA pathways are primarily involved in epidermal nevus syndromes. From a neuroembryological perspective, hemimegalencephaly and FCD II have the same microscopic findings because they are the same disorder, and the difference in extent of the lesion depending on how early or late in the normal 33 mitotic cycles of periventricular neuroepithelium needed to generate all cortical neurons (on an exponential basis) is the somatic mutation from mTOR or related pathways expressed. Early expression leads to more extensive lesions of hemimegalencephaly, whereas late expression produced smaller lesions of FCD II. In sum, neuroembryological, neuropathological, and genetic data all are consistent with hemimegalencephaly with FCD II being the same fundamental disorder and the difference being the *timing* of developmental events.

FOCAL CORTICAL DYSPLASIA TYPE III

FCD III is usually type II but also sometimes type I FCD is associated with another principal lesion. Subtypes are identified.

FCD IIIa is associated with hippocampal sclerosis and the FCD is always in the temporal neocortex, usually the parahippocampal gyrus. FCD is a congenital developmental lesion whereas hippocampal sclerosis is always acquired postnatally. Hippocampal sclerosis thus cannot induce the formation of FCD. The issue still debated as to whether chronic seizure discharges from the mesial temporal lobe neocortex can induce hippocampal sclerosis remains incompletely resolved but if true could explain FCD IIIa. Hippocampal sclerosis refers not to gliosis, which may also be present, but rather to neuronal loss in Ammon's horn and sometimes also the dentate gyrus. Subtypes of hippocampal sclerosis are well-defined neuropathologically.

FCD IIIb is associated with a nearby tumor, usually a cortical neuroblastic neoplasm such as ganglioglioma or dysembryoplastic neuroepithelial tumor. Ganglioglioma also shows overexpression of tau protein, similar to FCD I and II and hemimegalencephaly.

FCD IIIc is associated with a primary vascular malformation of the cortex or overlying leptomeninges, either arterial or venous. It is seen in some cases of Sturge–Weber disease.

FCD IIId is associated with a variety of other lesions. Fetal cerebral infarcts including porencephalic cysts may show FCD Ia in preserved tissue adjacent to the cyst. FCD IIId also can be associated with areas of inflammation or vasculitis, prenatal infections, or other primary lesions of brain.

Minimal Focal Cortical Dysplasias (mFCD). This term is still somewhat controversial among neuropathologists and is not currently part of the classification scheme of the ILAE Commission on Neuropathology. It is a neuropathological diagnosis in which neither FCD I nor II is demonstrated in the cortical gray matter, but there are excessive subcortical U-fiber neurons at the site of an electrographic epileptic focus and the patient has a clinical course consistent with FCD. MRI may show no abnormalities but at times blurring of the gray/white junction is seen.

Mild malformation of cortical development with oligodendroglial hyperplasia in frontal lobe epilepsy (**MOGHE**) is a recently neuropathologically described entity in which there is a proliferation of nonneoplastic oligodendrocytes in the white matter. Intractable focal epilepsy occurs and the diagnosis is established by neuropathological examination of the brain resection, including immunoreactivities specific to glial cells. Preoperative MRI examination may show nonspecific white matter gliosis but is not diagnostic.

TUBEROUS SCLEROSIS COMPLEX (TSC)

TSC is a genetically complex disease because it is both a germline mutation with the autosomal dominant transmission in 2/3 of cases and occurs sporadically in 1/3. It is also an mTOR pathway disorder as a postzygotic somatic mutation with multiorgan involvement – indeed the most frequent mTORopathy of all. The two chromosomal mutations are nonhomologous tumor-suppressor genes: *TSC1* at locus 9q34 encoding a 130kDA protein, hamartin, and *TSC2* at 16p13.3 encoding a 200kDa protein, tuberin. The most frequent systemic lesions are congenital cardiac rhabdomyomata, renal dysgenesis, and postnatal development of various types of cutaneous lesions. The brain shows *cortical tubers* that appear progressively in late prenatal life and over years postnatally. Neuropathologically, these hamartomatous tubers are almost indistinguishable from FCD IIb but often include microcalcifications not found in FCD II. Other subtle details also distinguish them histopathologically.

Some tubers are highly epileptogenic and others less so, enabling surgical resection of the most epileptogenic lesions even though it does not cure the disease or ensure total freedom from seizures postnatally. The subventricular neuroectodermal tumors (subependymal giant cell astrocytoma or SEGA) are characteristic brain lesions in TSC that contain no neurons, only dysplastic and neoplastic glial cells; hence, they do not contribute to epilepsy. Infants with TSC have a high risk of developing infantile (epileptic) spasms with a hypsarrhythmic EEG, usually at 3–4 months of age, which often is responsive to the administration of vigabatrin. Patients with TSC have cognitive impairment to variable degrees. TSC is discussed in greater depth in Chapter 27.

CLINICAL PEARLS

- FCDs are developmental lesions from fetal life and vary in size, from involving one gyrus to hemimegalencephaly involving an entire cerebral hemisphere.
- All FCDs are epileptogenic and usually refractory to ASMs. They present clinically in the neonatal period, infancy, or childhood as focal onset epilepsy.
- FCD type I is a disorder of lamination with microcolumnar cortical architecture similar to that seen normally in the first half of gestation; neurons are normal in size and morphology. The genetic basis is not yet known.
- FCD type II involves focal dyslamination and disorganization of the cortex, but many neurons and glial cells are abnormally enlarged (megalocytic) and have abnormal shapes of the soma and processes (dysplastic). The genetic basis is an upregulation of the mTOR signaling pathway and related upstream pathways such as AKT and PIK1C/PI3K. Disorders of mTOR are postzygotic somatic mutations.

- The difference between subtypes IIa and IIb is that IIb includes balloon cells of mixed lineage, which express both glial and neuronal proteins and also primitive proteins of progenitor cells.
- FCD IIb and hemimegalencephaly are the same disorder, the difference being in timing of onset of in which of the mitotic cycles of progenitor neuroepithelial cells, the earlier the onset the more extensive the cerebral lesion. Not all clones of neuroepithelial cells are involved.
- FCD III is FCD I or II adjacent to another principal brain lesion, such as hippocampal sclerosis (IIIa), cerebral tumor (IIIb), vascular malformation (IIIc), or another lesion (IIId).
- Neuroimaging, particularly MRI, is better for identifying lesions of FCD II than I; definitive diagnosis is by neuropathological examination of surgical resections.
- Minimal FCD (mFCD) behaves clinically as an FCD but neuropathologically does not fulfill the criteria of either FCD I or II, though it shows other features in common: excessive heterotopic neurons in the subcortical U-fiber layer form synaptic plexi that can contribute to cortical epileptic networks. One recently recognized variant of mFCD is MOGHE, a proliferation of nonneoplastic oligodendrocytes in the subcortical white matter.
- EEG and intraoperative ECoG or depth recordings help localize the epileptic focus but do not distinguish the type of FCD.
- Treatment of FCD after the failure of multiple ASMs is surgical resection.
- If residual seizures occur postoperatively, the ketogenic diet may be effective in controlling them.
- Neuropathological examination of the resected tissue using modern techniques is essential for definitive diagnosis and contributes to prognosis.
- TSC shares many neuropathological and genetic features of an mTOR pathway disorder with FCD II and hemimegalencephaly.
- mTOR inhibitors may have a future supplementary role in FCD II, hemimegalencephaly, and TSC.
- Prognosis for seizure control of all FCDs postoperatively depends in large part on whether the brain resection was total or subtotal. Some patients require a second surgery.
- In addition to standard ASMs and surgical resection, a promising supplementary approach in the treatment of FCD II, hemimegalencephaly, and TSC is the administration of mTOR inhibitors.

Funding: Alberta Children's Hospital Research Institute, Grant #60–28450, Project 10027949.

REFERENCES

Besson P., Andermann F., Dubeau F., Bernasconi A. Small focal cortical dysplasia lesions are located at the bottom of a deep sulcus. *Brain* 2008;131: 3246–55.

Blümcke I., Coras R., Busch R.M., Morita-Sherman M., Lal D., Prayson R., Cendes F., Lopes-Cendes I., Rogerio F., Almeida V.S., Rocha C.S., Sim N.S., Lee J.H., Kim S.H., Baulac S., Baldassari S., Adle-Biassette H., Walsh C.A., Bizzotto S., Doan R.N., Morillo K.S., Aronica E., Mühlebner A., Becker A., Cienfuegos J., Garbelli R., Giannini C., Honavar M., Jacques T.S., Thom M., Mahadevan A., Miyata H., Niehusmann P., Sarnat H.B., Söylemezoglu F., Najm I. Toward a better definition of focal cortical dysplasia: An iterative histopathological and genetic agreement trial. *Epilepsia* 2021;62(6): 1416–28.

Blumcke I., Spreafico R., Haaker G., Coras R., Kobow K., Bien C.G., Pfäfflin M., Elger C., Widman G., Schramm J., Becker A., Braun K.P., Leijten F., Baayen J.C., Aronica E., Chassoux F., Hamer H., Stefan H., Rössler K., Thom M., Walker M.C., Sisodiya S.M., Duncan J.S., McEvoy A.W., Pieper T., Holthausen H., Kudernatsch M., Meencke H.J., Kahane P., Schulze-Bonhage A., Zentner J., Heiland D.H., Urbach H., Steinhoff B.J., Bast T., Tassi L., Lo Russo G., Özkara C., Oz B., Krsek P., Vogelgesang S., Runge U., Lerche H., Weber Y., Honavar M., Pimentel J., Arzimanoglou A., Ulate-Campos A., Noachtar S., Hartl E., Schijns O., Guerrini R., Barba C., Jacques T.S., Cross J.H., Feucht M., Mühlebner A., Grunwald T., Trinka E., Winkler P.A., Gil-Nagel A., Toledano Delgado R., Mayer T., Lutz M., Zountsas B., Garganis K., Rosenow F., Hermsen A., von Oertzen T.J., Diepgen T.L., Avanzini G.; EEBB Consortium. Histopathological findings in brain tissue obtained during epilepsy surgery. *N Engl J Med* 2017;377: 164856.

Blümcke I., Thom M., Aronica E., Armstrong D.D., Vinters H.V., Palmini A., Jacques T.S., Avanzini G., Barkovich A.J., Battaglia G., Becker A., Cepeda C., Cendes F., Colombo N., Crino P., Cross J.H., Delalande O., Dubeau F., Duncan J., Guerrini R., Kahane P., Mathern G., Najm I., Ozkara C., Raybaud C., Represa A., Roper S.N., Salamon N., Schulze-Bonhage A., Tassi L., Vezzani A., Spreafico R. The clinical-pathological spectrum of focal cortical dysplasias: A consensus classification proposed by an ad hoc Task Force of the ILAE Diagnostic Methods Commission. *Epilepsia* 2011;52: 158–74.

Coras R., Holthausen H., Sarnat H.B. Focal cortical dysplasia type I (in mini-symposium, Epilepsy-Associated Neuropathology, Blümcke I, editor). *Brain Pathology* 2021;31: e2964.

Curatolo P., Moavero R. mTOR inhibitors as a new therapeutic option for epilepsy. *Expert Rev Neurother* 2013;13: 627–38.

D'Gama A.M., Woodworth M.B., Hossain A.A., Bizzotto S., Hatem N.E., LaCoursiere C.M., Najm I., Ying Z., Yang E., Barkovich A.J., Kwiatkowski D.J., Vinters H.V., Madsen J.R., Mathern G.W., Blümcke I., Poduri A., Walsh C.A. Somatic mutations activating the mTOR pathway in dorsal telencephalic progenitors cause a continuum of cortical dysplasias. *Cell Rep* 2017;21(13): 3754–66.

D'Gama A.M., Geng Y., Couto J.A., Martin B., Boyle E.A., LaCoursiere C.M., Hossain A., Hatem N.E., Barry B.J., Kwiatkowski D.J., Vinters H.V., Barkovich A.J., Shendure J., Mathern G.W., Walsh C.A., Poduri A. mTOR pathway mutations cause hemimegalencephaly and focal cortical dysplasia. *Ann Neurol* 2015;77: 720–5.

Flores-Sarnat L. Epilepsy in neurological phenotypes of epidermal nevus syndrome. *J Pediatr Epilepsy* 2016;5: 97–110.

Flores-Sarnat L., Sarnat H.B., Dávila-Gutiérrez G., Álvarez A. Hemimegalencephaly: Part 2. Neuropathology suggests a disorder of cellular lineage. *J Child Neurol* 2003;18: 776–85.

Galanopoulou A.S., Gorter J.A., Cepeda C. Finding a better drug for epilepsy: The mTOR pathway as an antiepileptogenic target. *Epilepsia* 2012;53: 1119–30.

Jansen L.A., Mirzaa G.M., Ishak G.E., O'Roak B.J., Hiatt J.B., Roden W.H., Gunter S.A., Christian S.L., Collins S., Adams C., Rivière J.B., St-Onge J., Ojemann J.G., Shendure J., Hevner R.F., Dobyns W.B. P13K/AKT pathway mutations cause a spectrum of brain malformations from megalencephaly to focal cortical dysplasia. *Brain* 2015;138: 1613–28.

Krsek P., Maton B., Korman B., Pacheco-Jacome E., Jayakar P., Dunoyer C., Rey G., Morrison G., Ragheb J., Vinters H.V., Resnick T., Duchowny M. Different features of histopathological subtypes of pediatric focal cortical dysplasia. *Ann Neurol* 2008;63: 758–69.

Lee J.H., Huynh M., Silhavy J.L., Kim S., Dixon-Salazar T., Heiberg A., Scott E., Bafna V., Hill K.J., Collazo A., Funari V., Russ C., Gabriel S.B., Mathern G.W., Gleeson J.G. De novo somatic mutations in components of thePI3K-AKT3-mTOR pathway cause hemimegalencephaly. *Nat Genet* 2012;44: 941–45.

Lim J.S., Kim W.I., Kang H.C., Kim S.H., Park A.H., Park E.K., Cho Y.W., Kim S., Kim H.M., Kim J.A., Kim J., Rhee H., Kang S.G., Kim H.D., Kim D., Kim D.S., Lee J.H. Brain somatic mutations in mTOR cause focal cortical dysplasia type II leading to intractable epilepsy. *Nat Med* 2015;21: 395–400.

Lindhurst M.J., Sapp J.C., Teer J.K., Johnston J.J., Finn E.M., Peters K., Turner J., Cannons J.L., Bick D., Blakemore L., Blumhorst C., Brockmann K., Calder P., Cherman N., Deardorff M.A., Everman D.B., Golas G., Greenstein R.M., Kato B.M., Keppler-Noreuil K.M., Kuznetsov S.A., Miyamoto R.T., Newman K., Ng D., O'Brien K., Rothenberg S., Schwartzentruber D.J., Singhal V., Tirabosco R., Upton J., Wientroub S., Zackai E.H., Hoag K., Whitewood-Neal T., Robey P.G., Schwartzberg P.L., Darling T.N., Tosi L.L., Mullikin J.C., Biesecker L.G. A mosaic activating mutation in AKT1 associated with the Proteus syndrome. *N Engl J Med* 2011;365: 611–9.

Mühlebner A., Bongaarts A., Sarnat H.B., Scholl T., Aronica E. New insights into a spectrum of developmental malformations related to mTOR dyregulations: Challenges and perspectives. *J Anat* 2019;235: 521–42.

Najm I.M., Tassi L., Sarnat H.B., Holthausen H., LoRusso G. Epilepsies associated with focal cortical dysplasias (FCDs*). Acta Neuropathol* 2014;128: 5–19.

Najm I., Lal D., Alonso Vanegas M., Cendes F., Lopes-Cendes I., Palmini A., Paglioli E., Sarnat H.B., Walsh C.A., Wiebe S., Aronica E., Baulac S., Coras R., Kobow K., Cross J.H., Garbelli R., Holthausen H., Rössler K., Thom M., El-Osta A., Lee J.H., Miyata H., Guerrini R., Piao Y.S., Zhou D., Blümcke I. The ILAE consensus classification of focal cortical dysplasia (FCD): An update proposed by an *ad hoc* task force of the ILAE Diagnostic Methods Commission. *Epilepsia* 2022;63(8): 1899–1919.

Najm I., Sarnat H.B., Blümcke I. The international consensus classification of focal cortical dysplasia – A critical update 2018. *Neuropathol Appl Neurobiol* 2018;44: 18–31.

Watanabe K., Ohba C., Tsurusaki Y., Miyake N., Zheng Y., Sato T., Takebayashi H., Ogata K., Kameyama S., Kakita A., Matsumoto N. Somatic mutations in the mTOR gene cause focal cortical dysplasia type IIb. *Ann Neurol* 2015;78: 375–86.

Nishikawa S., Goto S., Hamasaki T., Yamada K., Ushio Y. 2002. Involvement of *Reelin* and Cajal-Retzius cells in the developmental formation of vertical columnar structures in the cerebral cortex: Evidence from the study of mouse presubicular cortex. *Cereb Cortex* 2002;12: 1024–30.

Palmini A., Holthausen H. Focal malformations of cortical development: A most relevant etiology of epilepsy in children. *Handb Clin Neurol* 2013;111: 549–65.

Palmini A., Najm I., Avanzini G., Babb T., Guerrini R., Foldvary-Schaefer N., Jackson G., Luders H.O., Prayson R., Spreafico R., Vinters H.V. Terminology and classification of the cortical dysplasias. *Neurology* 2004;62: S2–8.

Poduri A., Evrony G.D., Cai X., Elhosary P.C., Beroukhim R., Lehtinen M.K., Hills L.B., Heinzen E.L., Hill A., Hill R.S., Barry B.J., Bourgeois B.F., Riviello J.J., Barkovich A.J., Black P.M., Ligon K.L., Walsh C.A. Somatic activation of AKT3 causes hemispheric developmental brain malformations. *Neuron* 2012;74: 41–8.

Sarnat H.B., Flores-Sarnat L. α-B-crystallin: A tissue marker of epileptic foci in paediatric resections. *Can J Neurol Sci* 2009;36: 566–74.

Sarnat H.B., Flores-Sarnat L., Trevenen C.L. Synaptophysin immunoreactivity in the human fetal hippocampus and neocortex from 6 to 41 weeks of gestation. *J Neuropathol Exp Neurol* 2010;69: 234–45.

Sarnat H.B., Flores-Sarnat L., Crino P., Hader W., Bello-Espinosa L. Hemimegalencephaly: Foetal tauopathy with mTOR hyperactivation and neuronal lipidosis. *Folia Neuropathol* 2012;50: 330–45.

Sarnat H.B., Flores-Sarnat L. Radial micro-columnar cortical architecture: Maturational arrest or focal cortical dysplasia? *Pediatr Neurol* 2013;48: 259–270.

Sarnat H.B. Clinical Neuropathology Practice Guide 5–2013: Markers of neuronal maturation. *Clin Neuropathol* 2013;32: 340–69.

Sarnat H.B., Flores-Sarnat L. Morphogenesis timing of genetically-programmed brain malformations in relation to epilepsy. *Progr Brain Res* 2014;213: 181–98.

Sarnat H.B., Philippart M., Flores-Sarnat L., Wei X.-C. Timing in neural development: Arrest, delay, precociousness and temporal determination of malformations. *Pediatr Neurol* 2015;52: 473–86.

Sarnat H.B., Flores-Sarnat L. Infantile tauopathies: Hemimegalencephaly; tuberous sclerosis complex; Focal cortical dysplasia 2; ganglioglioma. *Brain Dev* 2015;37: 553–62.

Sarnat H.B. Immunocytochemical markers of neuronal maturation in human diagnostic neuropathology. *Cell Tiss Res* 2015;359: 279–94.

Sarnat H.B., Hader W., Flores-Sarnat L., Bello-Espinosa L. Synaptic plexi of the U-fibre layer beneath focal cortical dysplasias: Role in epileptic networks. *Clin Neuropathol* 2018;37: 262–76.

Sarnat H.B. New neuropathological concepts in focal cortical dysplasias (Chapter 20). In: *Wyllie's Treatment of Epilepsy*, 7th edition. Wyllie E., editor. Philadelphia, PA: Lippincott Williams & Wilkins 2021:263–71.

Sarnat H.B., Flores-Sarnat L. Excitatory/inhibitory synaptic ratios in polymicrogyria and Down syndrome help explain epileptogenesis in malformations. *Pediatr Neurol* 2021;116: 41–54.

Schurr J., Coras R., Rössler K., Pieper T., Kudernatsch M., Holthausen H., Winkler P., Woermann F., Bien C.G., Polster T., Schulz R., Kalbhenn T., Urbach H., Becker A., Grunwald T., Huppertz H.J., Gil-Nagel A., Toledano R., Feucht M., Mühlebner A., Czech T., Blümcke I. Mild malformation of cortical development with oligodendroglial hyperplasia in frontal lobe epilelpsy: A new clinico-pathological entitly. *Brain Pathol* 2017;27: 26–35.

Taylor D.C., Falconer M.A., Bruton C.J., Corsellis J.A. Focal dysplasia of the cerebral cortex in epilepsy. *J Neurol Neurosurg Psychiatry* 1971;34: 369–87.

Tsai V., Parker W.E., Orlova K.A., Baybis M., Chi A.W., Berg B.D., Birnbaum J.F., Estevez J., Okochi K., Sarnat H.B., Flores-Sarnat L., Aronica E., Crino P.B. Fetal brain mTOR pathway activation in tuberous sclerosis complex. *Cerebr Cortex* 2014;24: 315–27.

Xu Q., Uliel-Sibony S., Dunham C., Sarnat H., Flores-Sarnat L., Brunga L., Davidson S., Lo W., Shlien A., Connolly M., Boelman C., Datta A. mTOR inhibitors as a new therapeutic strategy in treatment resistant epilepsy in hemimegalencephaly: A case report. *J Child Neurol* 2019;34: 132–8.

Yasin S.A., Latak K., Becherini F., Ganapathi A., Miller K., Campos O., Picker S.R., Bier N., Smith M., Thom M., Anderson G., Helen Cross J., Harkness W., Harding B., Jacques T.S. Balloon cells in human cortical dysplasia and tuberous sclerosis: Isolation of a pathological progenitor-like cell. *Acta Neuropathol* 2010;120: 85–96.

Zillhardt J.L., Poirier K., Broix L., Lebrun N., Elmorjani A., Martinovic J., Saillour Y., Muraca G., Nectoux J., Bessieres B., Fallet-Bianco C., Lyonnet S., Dulac O., Odent S., Rejeb I., Ben Jemaa L., Rivier F., Pinson L., Geneviève D., Musizzano Y., Bigi N., Leboucq N., Giuliano F., Philip N., Vilain C., Van Bogaert P., Maurey H., Beldjord C., Artiguenave F., Boland A., Olaso R., Masson C., Nitschké P., Deleuze J.F., Bahi-Buisson N., Chelly J. Mosaic parental germline mutations causing recurrent forms of malformations of cortical development. *Eur J Hum Genet* 2016;24: 611–4.

10 Malformations of Cortical Development

Marilisa M. Guerreiro
University of Campinas

Maria Augusta Montenegro
UC San Diego School of Medicine

CONTENTS

Malformations of cortical development (MCDs) comprise a large, heterogeneous group of disorders of disrupted cerebral cortex formation caused by various genetic, infectious, vascular, or metabolic etiologies. MCDs are characterized by abnormal cortical structure or presence of heterotopic gray matter, sometimes associated with abnormal brain size. Although MCDs usually manifest in childhood with epilepsy, developmental delay, and focal neurological signs, some patients may have normal or near-normal cognitive function and no seizures, depending on the extent of the cortical malformation.

The different types of MCDs are the result of abnormalities that occurred at different stages of cortical development, and their classification is based on the three main stages of cortical development (Table 10.1):

- Cell proliferation and apoptosis.
- Neuronal migration.
- Postmigrational development.

However, because cortical development is a dynamic process where there is an overlap of one or more stages during several weeks, it is likely that all three stages of cortical development are involved in the pathogenesis of some MCDs.

DOI: 10.1201/9781003296478-11

TABLE 10.1

Classification of the Malformations of Cortical Development

Malformations due to Abnormal Neuronal and Glial Proliferation or Apoptosis

A. Decreased proliferation/increased apoptosis or increased proliferation/decreased apoptosis – abnormalities of brain size
   - Microcephaly with normal to thin cortex
   - Microlissencephaly (extreme microcephaly with thick cortex)
   - Microcephaly with extensive polymicrogyria
   - Megalencephalies

B. Abnormal proliferation (abnormal cell types)
   - Nonneoplastic
     a. Cortical hamartomas of tuberous sclerosis
     b. Cortical dysplasia with balloon cells (focal cortical dysplasia type II)
     c. Hemimegalencephaly
   - Neoplastic (associated with disordered cortex)
     d. Dysembryoplastic neuroepithelial tumor
     e. Ganglioglioma
     f. Gangliocytoma

Malformations due to Abnormal Neuronal Migration

A. Lissencephaly/subcortical band heterotopia spectrum
B. Coblestone complex/congenital muscular dystrophy syndromes
C. Heterotopia
   - Subependymal (periventricular)
   - Subcortical (other than band heterotopia)
   - Marginal glioneural

Malformations due to Abnormal Postmigrational Development

A. Polymicrogyria and schizencephaly
   - Bilateral polymicrogyria syndromes
   - Schizencephaly (polymicrogyria with clefts)
   - Polymicrogyria or schizencephaly as part of multiple congenital anomaly/mental retardation syndromes
B. Cortical dysplasia without balloon cell and without dysmorphic neurons
C. Cortical dysgenesis secondary to inborn errors of metabolism

Source: Modified from Barkovich (2012).

The diagnosis of MCD is based on detailed visual analysis of high-resolution MRI, and sometimes subtle lesions are identified only by image postprocessing with techniques such as multiplanar reconstruction. The complete list of more than 200 entities included in the classification of MCD is presented in the paper by Barkovich et al. (2012); however, since then, other types of MCD have been described. In this chapter, we approach only some of those conditions due to their frequency and importance. Nevertheless, before addressing some MCDs, we briefly explain the process of normal cortical development.

NORMAL CORTICAL DEVELOPMENT

1. **Cell proliferation** starts around the 5th and 6th weeks of gestation in the periventricular germinal area after the formation of the neural tube during the first 4 weeks. During cell proliferation, differentiation between neuronal and glial cells occurs. If this process of differentiation does not proceed normally, primitive, indifferentiate, and aberrant cells will be formed. Those are the so-called balloon cells. They appear abundantly in focal cortical dysplasia (FCD) type II, hemimegalencephaly, and tuberous sclerosis complex.

2. **Neuronal migration** starts around the 5th and 6th weeks of gestation as well, when a neuron starts moving out of the germinal zone. For this purpose, the neuron will be adherent to one glial cell that plays an important role in directing the neuron to its final cortical destination. Therefore, the glial cell acts as a bridge to facilitate the migrational process. Migration is highly dependent on several genetically determined steps. It occurs mainly until the 22nd week of gestation, although some studies have shown that migration may occur even during the first months of postnatal life. An abnormality during this stage may lead to several heterotopias (focal/nodular or diffuse heterotopia, depending on the extent of the abnormality), culminating with lissencephaly and its variants. The thick cortex caused by the arrested migration of neurons prevents the normal cortical morphology because the amount of neurons that reach the cortex is an important stimulus for sulcal and gyral formation.

3. **Postmigrational development.** When the migrational process brings the neurons to the cortical surface, the cells are organized into six anatomically distinct layers. The external layer is the first one to be formed (layer I). It contains Cajal–Retzius cells, which will die, soon leaving a molecular layer that limits the migrational process. The other five layers will receive neurons following an inside-out process, that is, after layer I is formed the next migrational wave will be allocated in the inner layer (layer VI) and the next migrational wave will be allocated in the following layer V and so on. This highly complex process occurs mostly during the 16th and 24th weeks of gestation and is very vulnerable to genetically determined vascular insults. The two main malformations are polymicrogyria and schizencephaly (Figure 10.1).

MALFORMATIONS DUE TO CELL PROLIFERATION AND APOPTOSIS

As mentioned above, FCD type II is the hallmark malformation of this stage. The abnormal and undifferentiated balloon cells depict the early injury that took place. FCD is usually related to epilepsy and is considered, in some surgical series, to be the most common etiology of refractory focal epilepsy in children. The occurrence of rhythmic epileptiform discharges on intraoperative electrocorticography and scalp electroencephalogram (EEG) correlates with the intrinsic epileptogenicity of FCD. Positron emission tomography became a powerful tool in detecting unsuspected

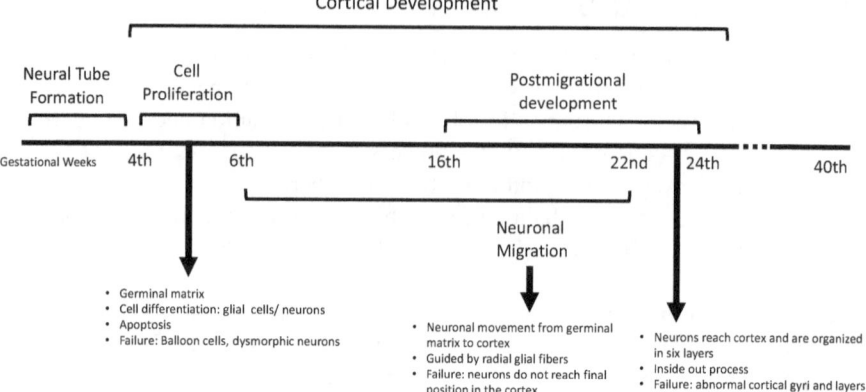

FIGURE 10.1 Timeline describing the most important hallmarks of normal cortical development.

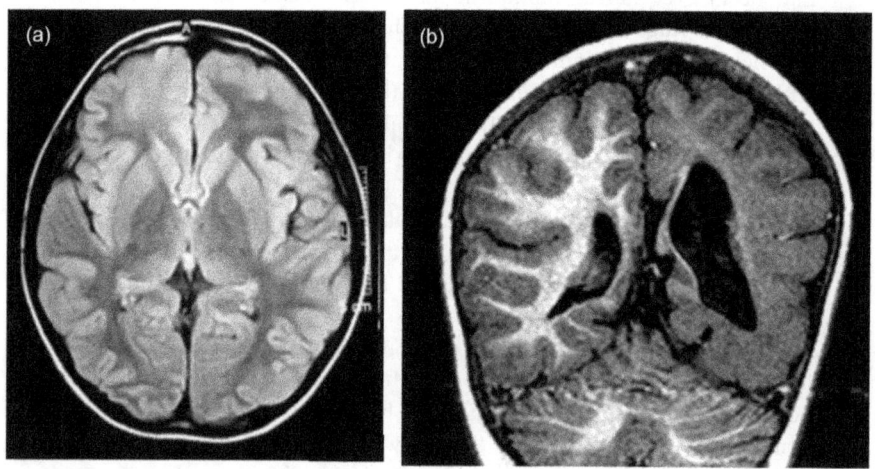

FIGURE 10.2 (a) FCD in the right frontal lobe, characterized by cortical thickening and blurring between gray and white matter. (b) Hemimegalencephaly in the left hemisphere characterized by diffuse hemispheric enlargement, cortical thickening and simplified gyral pattern, and abnormal white matter signal.

brain malformations (particularly cortical dysplasia) in infants with spasms. The reader can find more on FCD in Chapter 9 of this book.

Hemimegalencephaly should be suspected early in life if the infant presents with drug-resistant epilepsy and focal motor signs such as hemiparesis, in keeping with a hemispheric disorder. Surgical treatment is the best therapeutic option to enable optimal development for those children. Tuberous sclerosis complex is classically related to cognitive, behavioral, and epilepsy manifestations, but no motor signs are usually detected (Figure 10.2).

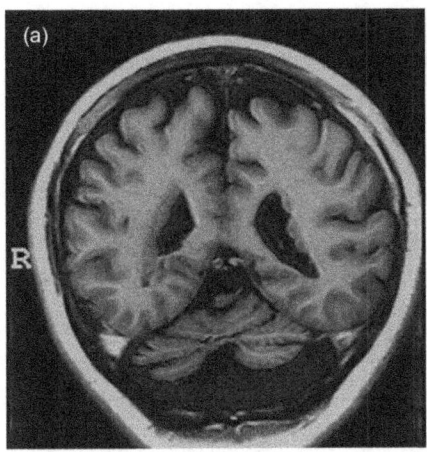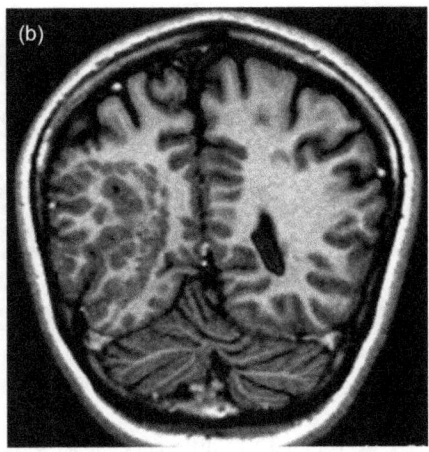

FIGURE 10.3   (a) Periventricular nodular heterotopia, characterized by gray matter nodules lining the ventricular wall. (b) Subcortical heterotopia, characterized by a bulky mass of gray matter in a swirling pattern in the right temporooccipital region.

MALFORMATIONS DUE TO ABNORMAL NEURONAL MIGRATION

Neuroimaging and clinical features are highly dependent on the extent of the abnormal neuronal migration. If just a small number of neurons stop their migration, the patient will have a heterotopia (gray matter in abnormal locations) that may be silent or cause minor symptoms such as treatable epilepsy. However, if the number of neurons is more pronounced, patients may present with drug-resistant epilepsy, variable degrees of cognitive deficits, and focal neurological motor signs (Figure 10.3). If a whole migrational wave does not reach the cortex, a patient may have a laminar/band heterotopia (also called double cortex), which is also dependent on the number of neurons that did not properly migrate.

The most severe neuroimaging and clinical pictures are seen in lissencephaly when most or all migrational waves do not succeed in reaching their final destination in the cortex, hence not forming the six cortical layers. Brain MRI typically shows a very thick abnormal cortex, with simplified gyri or complete absence of sulcation. We can find lissencephaly and pachygyria occurring in different brain areas of the same patient. The preferred term, in this case, is agyria (no gyria)/pachygyria (few broad gyria) complex.

Lissencephaly, pachygyria, and subcortical band heterotopia represent different ends of the spectrum of the same disorder, and heterogeneity of these malformations may occur in different patients within the same family (Figure 10.4). Patients frequently have drug-resistant epilepsy and cognitive impairment.

MALFORMATIONS DUE TO POSTMIGRATIONAL DEVELOPMENT

The term polymicrogyria is applied when multiple small gyri are grouped together which sometimes resemble a large gyrus. Polymicrogyria may occur in

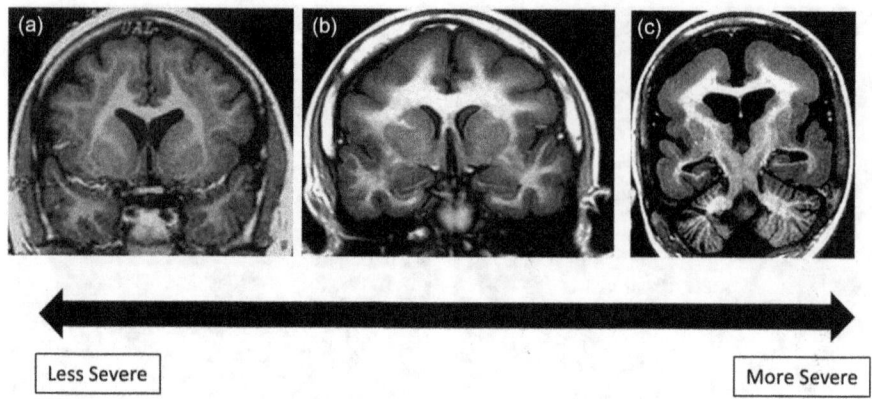

FIGURE 10.4   Three different patients with MCDs showing different ends of the spectrum of subcortical laminar heterotopia, agyria–pachygyria, and lissencephaly. (a) Subcortical laminar heterotopia (double cortex). (b) Diffuse cortical thickening and pachygyria. (c) Lissencephaly.

any part of the cortex but it is more commonly found around the Sylvian fissure. Polymicrogyria with a clear vascular etiology has been reported in some cases and when occurring in both perisylvian regions, often presents with the clinical picture of acquired faciopharyngoglossomasticatory diplegia or congenital bilateral perisylvian syndrome.

Epilepsy is considered a frequent symptom in patients with polymicrogyria. Nevertheless, several studies have shown that the frequency of epilepsy is lower than previously reported, and the occurrence of epilepsy in patients with polymicrogyria depends on the extent of the cortical involvement and the interrelationships between genetics and prenatal injury. Yet, when present, epilepsy is more easily controlled in patients with polymicrogyria than in other types of MCDs.

Most patients with polymicrogyria present with bilateral and symmetric cortical abnormalities. Although less frequent, unilateral and asymmetrical lesions may also be found. A variable extent of polymicrogyric cortex, cortical unfolding, and disruption of the gyral architecture is observed, representing a broad radiological spectrum usually with a corresponding spectrum of clinical features. It is interesting to note that polymicrogyria can be associated with electrographic *status epilepticus*. If there is an improvement in EEG discharges after introduction of an antiseizure medication (ASM), there will be an improvement in the pseudobulbar symptoms.

Due to severe dysarthria or anarthria, patients with perisylvian polymicrogyria are often labeled as presenting with severe cognitive impairment, when in fact most patients actually have normal cognition. Developmental language disorder can be associated with polymicrogyria and the clinical manifestation varies according to the extent of the cortical abnormality. A subtle form of posterior parietal polymicrogyria presenting as developmental language disorder is a mild form of perisylvian syndrome.

Polymicrogyria and schizencephaly seem to share the same etiology, suggesting a common or similar vascular and/or genetic insult. The presence of polymicrogyria

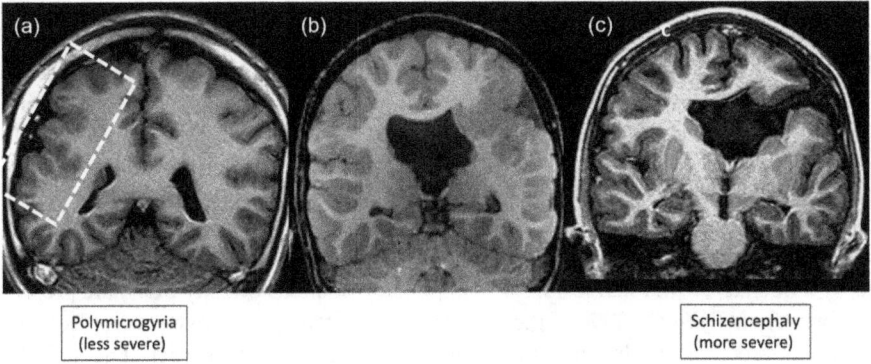

FIGURE 10.5   Three different patients with MCD showing different ends of the spectrum of polymicrogyria and schizencephaly. (a) Left perisylvian polymicrogyria (box). (b) Polymicrogyria with cortical folding. (c) Schizencephaly.

in the schizencephalic borders reinforces this concept of a common pathophysiology. Another association can be demonstrated in patients with polymicrogyria in one hemisphere and schizencepahly in the other. Yet, another similarity is the main location in the cerebral cortex – that is, around the Sylvian fissure for both entities (Figure 10.5).

Patients with schizencephaly often have epilepsy, variable degrees of cognitive impairment, and focal neurological motor deficits, making schizencephaly a frequent cause of hemiplegic cerebral palsy.

TYPE OF EPILEPSY SYNDROME IN PATIENTS WITH MCD

The type of epilepsy syndrome associated with MCD can be variable, and the patient's age is one of the most important aspects for its determination. Epilepsy in the first 3 months of life tends to be of the focal-onset type. West syndrome is characterized by epileptic spasms, hypsarrthymia, and developmental delay, and its onset occurs mainly from the fourth to the seventh months of life. The age range of expression of hypsarrhythmia correlates with the differentiation of the intracortical synchronizing mechanism provided by intrinsically bursting neurons. Burst-suppression patterns shown on the EEG reflect the dysfunction of thalamocortical connections. In the second year of life, there is a sufficient degree of maturation to support sustained rhythmic spike-and-wave discharges. Lennox–Gastaut syndrome is the best recognized clinical example of this EEG ontogeny.

The EEG evaluation of patients with MCD clearly reflects these three main stages of cerebral maturation: (1) focal discharges in the first 3 months of life and onset of hypsarrhythmia between 4 and 7 months of age, (2) generalized epileptiform discharges characterized by slow spike-and-wave complexes after 2 years of life and during the first decade of life, and (3) multifocal and generalized discharges are seen throughout life. These changes are associated with the degree of cerebral maturation (myelination and synaptogenesis).

Treatment Approach

MCDs are usually associated with drug-resistant epilepsy. Treatment should be aimed at optimizing seizure control, and the type of ASM depends on the seizure subtype, which may vary according to the patient's age. Patients with schizencephaly and polymicrogyria have their seizures more easily controlled by ASM than patients with other types of MCDs.

When treatment with ASM fails, epilepsy surgery should be considered. For several decades, epilepsy surgery has been the treatment of choice for drug-resistant epilepsy associated with focal lesions. Cortical malformations (mostly FCD) are present in approximately 20%–30% of the specimens reported by epilepsy surgery centers. It is believed that, in children, these numbers might be even higher. The surgical outcome of patients with drug-resistant epilepsy due to a single dysplastic lesion is usually dependent upon the completeness of lesion resection. Notwithstanding the development of new ASM and improvements in surgical techniques and approaches, seizure control remains a challenge in patients with MCD.

SUGGESTED REFERENCES

Barkovich J.A., Guerrini R., Kuzniecky R.I., Jackson G.D., Dobyns W.B. A developmental and genetic classification for malformations of cortical development: Update 2012. *Brain* 2012;135: 1348–69.

Guerreiro M.M., Andermann E., Guerrini R., Dobyns W.B., Kuzniecky R., Silver K., Van Bogaert P., Gillain C., David P., Ambrosetto G., Rosati A., Bartolomei F., Parmeggiani A., Paetau R., Salonen O., Ignatius J., Borgatti R., Zucca C., Bastos A.C., Palmini A., Fernandes W., Montenegro M.A., Cendes F., Andermann F. Familial perisylvian polymicrogyria: A new familial syndrome of cortical maldevelopment. *Ann Neurol* 2000;48: 39–48.

Guerreiro M.M., Hage S.R., Guimaraes C.A., Abramides D.V., Fernandes W., Pacheco P.S., Piovesana A.M., Montenegro M.A., Cendes F. Developmental language disorder associated with polymicrogyria. *Neurology* 2002;59: 245–50.

Montenegro M.A., Guerreiro M.M., Lopes-Cendes I., Guerreiro C.A., Cendes F. Interrelationship of genetics and prenatal injury in the genesis of malformations of cortical development. *Arch Neurol* 2002;59: 1147–53.

Severino M., Geraldo A.F., Utz N., Tortora D., Pogledic I., Klonowski W., Triulzi F., Arrigoni F., Mankad K., Leventer R.J., Mancini G.M., Barkovich J.A., Lequin M.H., and Rossi A., on behalf of the European Network on Brain Malformations (Neuro-MIG). Definitions and classification of malformations of cortical development: Practical guidelines. *Brain* 2020;143: 2874–94.

Section II

The Neonate

11 Self-Limited Neonatal Epilepsy Syndromes

Maria Augusta Montenegro and Jong M. Rho
University of California

CONTENTS

CASE PRESENTATION

A 4-day-old baby girl was brought to the emergency department due to an episode of rhythmic clonic movements of the left arm witnessed by her mother during breastfeeding. The episode lasted 1 minute. She was a full-term baby, the product of a normal pregnancy and delivery, with Apgar scores of 9 and 10, and had no perinatal medical issues. Her mother had experienced seizures during the first month of her life, but they were easily controlled with phenobarbital. A work-up including serum glucose, electrolytes, brain magnetic resonance imaging (MRI) scan, cerebrospinal fluid (CSF) studies, and electroencephalogram (EEG) were all normal. She was admitted for observation and phenobarbital was started. Despite treatment with this antiseizure medication (ASM), she still had several brief focal seizures for 2 days, but since then she became seizure free. She was diagnosed with self-limited (familial) neonatal epilepsy. During follow-up, she did not present with other types of clinical seizures and a repeat EEG at 1 month of age was normal. She was weaned off of phenobarbital, and at last follow-up, when she was 2 years old, she had normal development and remained seizure free.

DIFFERENTIAL DIAGNOSIS

Neonatal seizures are frequently caused by metabolic disturbances or brain injury (ischemic stroke, hemorrhage, brain malformations, infection, etc.), and the most common cause of neonatal seizures is hypoxic-ischemic encephalopathy (HIE). Prenatal and perinatal history can be a valuable tool to access possible risk factors such as congenital malformations, infection, and HIE. Laboratory testing will help to identify possible electrolyte disturbances and hypoglycemia, and CSF analysis should be performed if CNS infection is suspected. Brain MRI can identify structural lesions such as stroke, hemorrhage, brain malformation, or central venous thrombosis.

If the etiology of the seizure activity is not identified by the tests described above (especially in the setting of a normal brain MRI), a genetic epilepsy syndrome should be considered. The most common genetic conditions associated with neonatal onset seizures are as follows:

- Pyridoxine-dependent epilepsy.
- Pyridox(am)ine-phosphate deficiency.
- Maple syrup urine disease.
- Non-ketotic hyperglycinemia.
- CDKL5-associated developmental and epileptic encephalopathy.
- Glucose transporter 1 (GLUT1) deficiency syndrome.
- KCNQ2 developmental and epileptic encephalopathy.
- Self-limited neonatal epilepsies.

Next-generation sequencing (NGS) epilepsy gene panels or whole exome sequencing (WES) has the highest yield to establish the diagnosis of neonatal seizures; however, these tests are not always readily available. Some clinical findings are useful to help establish the diagnosis in some patients, especially in disorders that require specific treatment (Table 11.1).

DIAGNOSTIC APPROACH

The most recent position statement from the International League Against Epilepsy (ILAE) established two self-limited epilepsy syndromes:

- Self-limited (familial) neonatal epilepsy (previously called benign familial neonatal seizures).
- Self-limited familial neonatal-infantile epilepsy.

The clinical characteristic of both epilepsy syndromes can overlap, and the diagnosis of self-limited familial neonatal-infantile epilepsy is established based on the history

---

TABLE 11.1
Clinical Findings That Are Helpful in the Diagnosis of Neonatal Seizures

Disease	Useful Clinical Finding
Pyridoxine-dependent epilepsy	Positive response to pyridoxine/folinic acid (or pyridoxal phosphate) trial
Pyridox(am)ine-phosphate deficiency	Positive response to pyridoxal phosphate trial
Maple syrup urine disease	Characteristic urine odor
Nonketotic hyperglycinemia	Glycine peak on magnetic resonance spectroscopy
Glucose transporter 1 deficiency syndrome	CSF/blood glucose ratio

TABLE 11.2

Clinical Features of Self-Limited Neonatal Epilepsies

Characteristic	Self-Limited (Familial) Neonatal Epilepsy	Self-Limited Familial Neonatal-Infantile Epilepsy
Onset	2 and 7 days (but can start later in the first month of life)	Neonatal or infancy (1 day to 23 months)
Type of Seizures	Focal tonic or clonic	Focal tonic or clonic
Interictal EEG	Normal, might have interictal spikes	Normal, might have interictal spikes
Family history of seizures	Negative (in patients with self-limited neonatal epilepsy) Positive for self-limited neonatal seizures (in patients with self-limited familial neonatal epilepsy)	Positive for self-limited epilepsy in the neonatal period and other family members with self-limited epilepsy in the infantile period
Genetics	Possibly autosomal dominant with incomplete penetrance (*KCNQ2*, 80%; *KCNQ3* and *SCN2*A less frequent) *De novo* mutations in nonfamilial cases	Autosomal dominant with incomplete penetrance (*SCN2A*, *KCNQ2*) *De novo* mutations in nonfamilial cases

of other family members with neonatal and infantile epilepsies. Table 11.2 shows the most important characteristics of both epilepsy syndromes:

Self-limited (familial) neonatal epilepsy is divided into familial and nonfamilial subtypes, but they share the same genetic etiology. The nonfamilial cases are probably caused by *de novo* mutations. Figure 11.1 shows the diagnostic pathway for self-limited neonatal epilepsies.

TREATMENT STRATEGY

Self-limited neonatal epilepsy and self-limited familial neonatal-infantile epilepsy are, as the names denote, transient conditions and the use of ASMs is believed to not affect remission or long-term outcome of the epilepsy. However, the favorable prognosis is not obvious at the time of initial presentation, and seizures can be very frequent, or at times severe (e.g., *status epilepticus*). Therefore, most patients are treated with intravenous ASMs such as phenobarbital and benzodiazepines.

More recent studies have indicated that sodium channel blockers such as carbamazepine or phenytoin are effective in patients with neonatal seizures associated with loss-of-function *KCNQ2* mutations. They are associated with fewer cardiorespiratory side effects and are a valuable treatment option for these patients.

LONG-TERM OUTCOME

The prognosis is usually very favorable, with complete seizure remission by 6 months of life in most patients; however, seizure clusters, very frequent seizures, and even *status epilepticus* can occur in the neonatal period. Up to 30% of the patients with *KCNQ2* mutations can present with seizures later in life, mostly febrile seizures,

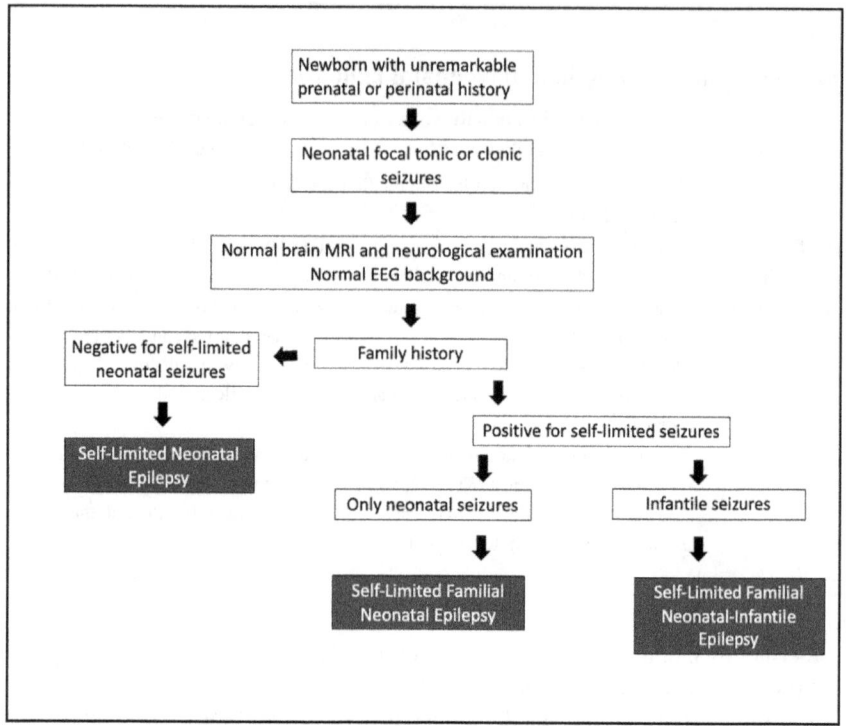

FIGURE 11.1   Diagnostic pathway for self-limited neonatal epilepsies.

CLINICAL PEARLS

- Self-limited neonatal syndromes are divided into two syndromes with overlapping phenotypes: (1) self-limited (familial) neonatal epilepsy and (2) self-limited familial neonatal-infantile epilepsy.
- The mutations more frequently associated with self-limited neonatal syndromes are *KCNQ2* and *SCN2A*, possibly inherited as an autosomal dominant trait with incomplete penetrance. The nonfamilial cases probably have *de novo* mutations.
- Prognosis is usually favorable, with complete seizure remission by 6 months.
- Although phenobarbital is still considered the first-line therapy for neonatal seizures, sodium channel blockers can be highly effective in patients with neonatal seizures due to loss-of-function *KCNQ2* mutations.

generalized tonic-clonic seizures, or self-limited epilepsy with centrotemporal spikes. Drug-resistant epilepsy is rare.

PATHOPHYSIOLOGY/NEUROBIOLOGY OF DISEASE

Most self-limited neonatal epilepsies are due to mutations in the *KCNQ2* and *SCN2A*, possibly inherited as an autosomal dominant trait with incomplete penetrance. The nonfamilial cases probably have *de novo* mutations. For loss-of-function *KCNQ2* mutations, it is generally believed that failure of potassium channel repolarization of the cell membrane (e.g., preventing the down stroke of the action potential) contributes to hyperexcitability. *SCN2A* is localized to excitatory neurons, and hence gain-of-function mutations would be expected to result in increased activity of these cells and contribute to seizure genesis.

SUGGESTED REFERENCES

Grinton B.E., Heron S.E., Pelekanos J.T., Zuberi S.M., Kivity S., Afawi Z., Williams T.C., Casalaz D.M., Yendle S., Linder I., Lev D., Lerman-Sagie T., Malone S., Bassan H., Goldberg-Stern H., Stanley T., Hayman M., Calvert S., Korczyn A.D., Shevell M., Scheffer I.E., Mulley J.C., Berkovic S.F. Familial neonatal seizures in 36 families: Clinical and genetic features correlate with outcome. *Epilepsia* 2015;56: 1071–80.

Ronen G.M., Rosales T.O., Connolly M., Anderson V.E., Leppert M. Seizure characteristics in chromosome 20 benign familial neonatal convulsions. *Neurology* 1993;43: 1355–60.

Sands T.T., Balestri M., Bellini G., Mulkey S.B., Danhaive O., Bakken E.H., Taglialatela M., Oldham M.S., Vigevano F., Holmes G.L., Cilio M.R. Rapid and safe response to low-dose carbamazepine in neonatal epilepsy. *Epilepsia* 2016;57: 2019–30.

Sharpe C., Reiner G.E., Davis S.L., Nespeca M., Gold J.J., Rasmussen M., Kuperman R., Harbert M.J., Michelson D., Joe P., Wang S., Rismanchi N., Le N.M., Mower A., Kim J., Battin M.R., Lane B., Honold J., Knodel E., Arnell K., Bridge R., Lee L., Ernstrom K., Raman R., Haas R.H.; NEOLEV2 Investigators. Levetiracetam versus phenobarbital for neonatal seizures: A randomized controlled trial. *Pediatrics* 2020;145: e20193182.

Zuberi S.M., Wirrell E., Yozawitz E., Wilmshurst J.M., Specchio N., Riney K., Pressler R., Auvin S., Samia P., Hirsch E., Galicchio S., Triki C., Snead O.C., Wiebe S., Cross J.H., Tinuper P., Scheffer I.E., Perucca E., Moshé S.L., Nabbout R. ILAE classification and definition of epilepsy syndromes with onset in neonates and infants: Position statement by the ILAE task force on nosology and definitions. *Epilepsia* 2022;63: 1349–1397.

12 Self-Limited (Familial) Infantile Epilepsy

Heather Pekeles and Kenneth A. Myers
McGill University Health Center

CONTENTS

CASE PRESENTATION

A 6-month-old girl was brought to the emergency room by her parents after multiple paroxysmal events. On history, she was an infant of an unremarkable term pregnancy with no complications in the perinatal period. She did not have other medical problems. The episodes consisted of staring and rhythmic arm shaking, which could involve either her left or right sides. The events started 24 hours earlier and were occurring up to five times per day. Her parents were unable to suppress these movements with pressure to the limb. There was never a clear loss of consciousness or impaired awareness. Family history was significant for a mother and maternal aunt who had similar events in infancy; in both cases, the events resolved at approximately 2 years of age. On assessment in the emergency room, the girl was afebrile with normal vital signs and appeared well with a normal neurological examination. Given the frequency of the episodes, she was admitted for further workup. Brain magnetic resonance imaging (MRI) was normal. A lumbar puncture was done given the frequency and focality of her seizures, and results showed no signs of an infectious process. An interictal electroencephalogram (EEG) was normal in wakefulness and sleep; however, during one of the events, rhythmic focal epileptiform discharges were observed. The girl was started on carbamazepine which controlled the seizures, and she was discharged home in the next few days. A trio epilepsy gene panel was ordered, which identified a maternally inherited pathogenic variant in PRRT2. The girl's seizures were well controlled on medication and she continued to develop normally. At 18 months of age, her medication was weaned and seizures did not recur.

DOI: 10.1201/9781003296478-14

DIAGNOSTIC APPROACH AND DIFFERENTIAL DIAGNOSIS

The diagnosis of self-limited (familial) infantile epilepsy (SeLIE) is clinical, based almost entirely on history, examination, and EEG. Pregnancy and perinatal history are usually unremarkable and the infant has usually been previously well. Development is typically normal. Family history is positive for other individuals with seizures as infants, most often following a pattern of autosomal dominant inheritance. The onset of seizures is typically between 3 and 20 months of age, with a peak at 6 months. Seizures are typically frequent at onset; however, they are usually easily controlled with an antiseizure medication (ASM). Seizures usually remit within 1 year of onset.

Baseline neurological exam is normal. Focal seizures occur with behavioral arrest, impaired awareness, automatisms, head/eye version, and clonic movements, often progressing to a hemiclonic or focal to bilateral tonic-clonic seizure. The seizures are brief, usually less than 3 minutes, but frequent, usually 5–10 per day over a period of 1–3 days at onset.

A key feature of SeLIE is the self-limited course, but this is obviously not clear at the time of initial presentation. For this reason, even if there is a reassuring family history, it is usually necessary to undertake at least some additional investigations in order to rule out other causes. When an infant initially presents with focal seizures, the differential diagnosis is broad, including meningitis, intracranial abscess, stroke, inborn error of metabolism, brain malformation, neoplastic processes, and other, more severe genetic epilepsy syndromes. With respect to the latter, epilepsy syndromes that might initially present in a similar manner to SeLIE include Dravet syndrome and epilepsy of infancy with migrating focal seizures (EIMFS).

Dravet syndrome often initially presents with focal motor seizures; however, at least some of the events occur in association with fever and status epilepticus is common. Over time, Dravet syndrome and SeLIE are easily differentiable, as Dravet patients usually have drug-resistant epilepsy with multiple seizure types, and eventually experience developmental plateau or regression. The interictal EEG in Dravet syndrome may be normal at the time of initial presentation, but eventually develops multifocal and/or generalized epileptiform discharges, as well as diffuse background slowing.

Similarly, clinical evolution allows differentiation of SeLIE from EIMFS, a syndrome in which there is usually some associated developmental plateau or regression, and seizures are more commonly drug resistant. The interictal EEG can be variable in EIMFS, but signs of severe encephalopathy such as burst suppression may be seen.

In SeLIE, the background EEG is normal, including normal sleep activity. If there is diffuse slowing of the EEG background, it is important to consider other epilepsy syndromes or etiologies. Alternatively, if persistent focal slowing is seen in one area, a structural brain abnormality must be ruled out. With respect to ictal EEG patterns, seizures in SeLIE are accompanied by focal rhythmic discharges that may start in either hemisphere, and sometimes show interhemispheric migration. Brain MRI is typically normal. Finally, known genetic causes can be investigated with genetic testing including targeted gene testing, gene panels or whole genome or exome sequencing depending on local center practices and resources. Specific genetic etiologies are discussed below.

TREATMENT STRATEGY

Since SeLIE is a self-limited syndrome, one could theoretically consider not treating patients' seizures; however, the seizure frequency is usually so high at initial presentation that all patients are prescribed an ASM. The choice of agent does not seem to be especially important, with most medications having apparent equal efficacy. The ASMs most commonly reported in the literature include carbamazepine, valproic acid, phenobarbital, and zonisamide; however, other ASMs would likely work just as well. A more important consideration is ensuring that the patient does not experience any unnecessary side effects of the medication. Given that a primary mitochondrial disorder could mimic the initial presentation of SeLIE, one should avoid valproic acid unless the diagnosis is completely certain.

Given the gene mutations associated with the disease (see below), some believe that certain ASMs are more effective because of their sodium channel blocking mechanism of action. A single ASM is typically sufficient to control seizures and polytherapy is rarely necessary. Given that seizures remit in infancy or early childhood, lifelong treatment is not required.

LONG-TERM OUTCOME

The outcome for infants with SeLIE is favorable. In most cases, seizures remit within 1 year of onset and development is normal. The diagnosis of SeLIE is important, especially for counseling to relieve parental anxiety and to avoid aggressive ASM treatment if not warranted. A small proportion of infants will have epilepsy later in life. In addition, a minority of infants with the *PRRT2* mutation are noted to develop paroxysmal movement disorders including paroxysmal dyskinesia later in life.

PATHOPHYSIOLOGY

Familial SeLIE has autosomal dominant inheritance and may be associated with pathogenic variants in several different genes. *PRRT2* pathogenic variants are identified in approximately 80% of cases; however, *SCN2A*, *SCN8A*, *KCNQ2*, and *KCNQ3* have also been associated. Importantly, other epilepsies, including other self-limited epilepsies, as well as epileptic encephalopathies, have overlapping genes that have been implicated. In contrast to certain epileptic encephalopathies, it is not yet clearly established why this disease typically remits early and has favorable prognosis.

Most cases of self-limited familial infantile epilepsy are associated with pathogenic variants in *PRRT2*, a gene that provides instructions for making the proline-rich transmembrane protein 2. This protein interacts with the presynaptic protein synaptosomal-associated protein 25 (SNAP-25), which is involved in neurotransmitter release from synaptic vesicles.

The *SCN2A* and *SCN8A* encode for subunits of voltage-gated sodium channels, which are transmembrane glycoprotein complexes composed of a large alpha subunit with four repeat domains, each of which is composed of six membrane-spanning segments, and one or more regulatory beta subunits. Voltage-gated sodium channels function in the generation and propagation of action potentials in neurons and

CLINICAL PEARLS

- Familial SeLIE is characterized by infantile onset of seizures, in the context of a family history of epilepsy.
- Seizures typically remit within 1 year of onset, and development is normal.
- Seizures are usually easily controlled with a single ASM.
- Pathogenic variants in *PRRT2* are the most common cause, but *SCN2A*, *SCN8A*, *KCNQ2*, and *KCNQ3* have also been associated.

muscle. Of note, pathogenic variants in both *SCN2A* and *SCN8A* can also be associated with severe early-onset developmental and epileptic encephalopathies.

The *KCNQ2* and *KCNQ3* genes encode subunits of a voltage-gated potassium channel. These channels open in response to membrane depolarization and allow potassium ions to leave the cell resulting in hyperpolarization. In SeLIE, *KCNQ2* and *KCNQ3* pathogenic variants reduce potassium channel function. Pathogenic variants in *KCNQ2* and *KCNQ3* may also both be associated with self-limited familial neonatal epilepsy. Additionally, *KCNQ2* pathogenic variants may cause a severe early-onset developmental and epileptic encephalopathy while *KCNQ3* pathogenic variants have also been associated with intellectual disability with or without seizures and/or cortical visual impairment.

SUGGESTED REFERENCES

Bayat A., Bayat M., Rubboli G., Moller R. Epilepsy syndromes in the first year of life and usefulness of genetic testing for precision therapy. *Genes* 2021;12: 1051.

Ebrahimi-Fakhari D., Saffari A., Westenberger A., Klein C. The evolving spectrum of PRRT2-associated paroxysmal diseases. *Brain* 2015;138: 3476–95. doi: 10.1093/brain/awv317.

Heron S.E., Grinton B.E., Kivity S., Afawi Z., Zuberi S.M., Hughes J.N., Pridmore C., Hodgson B.L., Iona X., Sadleir L.G., Pelekanos J., Herlenius E., Goldberg-Stern H., Bassan H., Haan E., Korczyn A.D., Gardner A.E., Corbett M.A., Gécz J., Thomas P.Q., Mulley J.C., Berkovic S.F., Scheffer I.E., Dibbens L.M. PRRT2 mutations cause benign familial infantile epilepsy and infantile convulsions with choreoathetosis syndrome. *Am J Hum Genet* 2012;90: 152–60.

Specchio N., Vigevano F. The spectrum of benign infantile seizures. *Epilepsy Res* 2006;70(Suppl 1): S156–67.

Van Roest A., Van de Vel A., Lederer D., Ceulemans B. The clinical and genetic spectrum in infants with (an) unprovoked cluster(s) of focal seizures. *Eur J Paediatr Neurol* 2020;24: 148–53.

Vigevano F. Benign familial infantile seizures. *Brain Dev* 2005;27: 172–7.

Zhao Q., Liu Z., Hu Y., Fang S., Zheng F., Li X., Li F., Lin Z. Different experiences of two PRRT2-associated self-limited familial infantile epilepsy. *Acta Neurol Belg* 2020;20: 1025–8.

Zuberi S.M., Wirrell E., Yozawitz E., Wilmshurst J.M., Specchio N., Riney K., Pressler R., Auvin S., Samia P., Hirsch E., Galicchio S., Triki C., Snead O.C., Wiebe S., Cross J.H., Tinuper P., Scheffer I.E., Perucca E., Moshé S.L., Nabbout R. ILAE classification & definition of epilepsy syndromes in the neonate and infant: Position statement by the ILAE task force on nosology and definitions. *Epilepsia* 2022;63: 1349–97.

13 Early Myoclonic Encephalopathy (Ohtahara Syndrome)

Reega Purohit
Northwestern University Feinberg School of Medicine

Linda Laux
Northwestern University, Feinberg School of Medicine

CONTENTS

CASE PRESENTATION

*The male patient was born to a healthy 33-year-old mother at 39-week gesta-
tion via C-section, with Apgar scores of 9 and 9. His postdelivery course was
uncomplicated, and patient was discharged home on day of life 2 from the newborn nursery. At 1 week of life, the patient began displaying abnormal movements that were concerning for seizures. Each episode lasted approximately
1–2 minutes and occurred 2–3 times per hour. The events were described as
tonic extension of the extremities with eye deviation. The second seizure semiology involved right arm and leg flexion, with eye fluttering. This would occur
at least hourly and would last for 10 seconds. A loading dose of phenobarbital
was administered but the events continued, and the patient was admitted to
the intensive care unit for escalation of care. On EEG, he was noted to have
a burst suppression pattern (Figure 13.1), with greater suppression seen over
the left hemisphere compared to the right and bursts with more epileptiform
discharges embedded over the left as well. He also had very frequent tonic
seizures arising from the left frontal temporal head region (Figure 13.2) and
subclinical seizures arising from left temporal occipital region. Patient was*

DOI: 10.1201/9781003296478-15

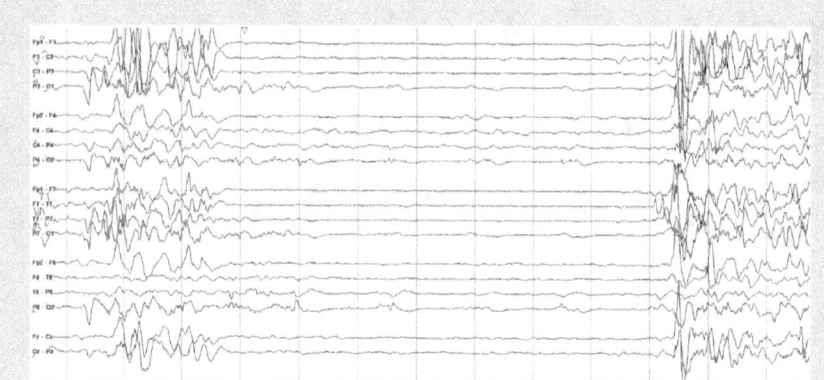

FIGURE 13.1 Burst suppression background. There is greater suppression seen over the left compared to the right hemisphere. Additionally, the bursts had more epileptiform discharges embedded over the left hemisphere (sensitivity 10 μV/mm, time base 30 mm/seconds).

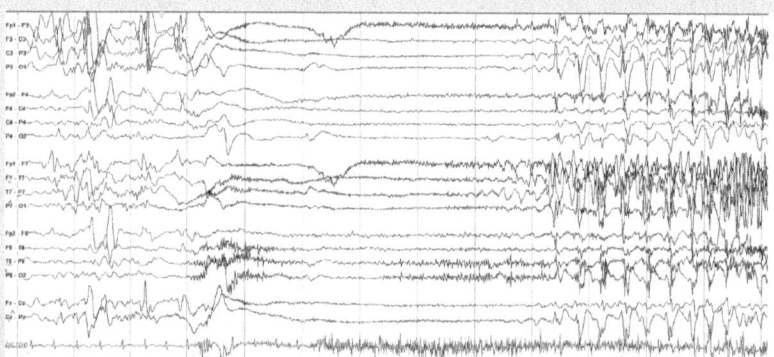

FIGURE 13.2 Tonic seizure arising from left frontal temporal region. Tonic stiffening noted on the deltoid channel (sensitivity 10 μV/mm, time base 30 mm/seconds).

quickly given fosphenytoin and levetiracetam loads as well. In response, the seizure burden improved with a seizure lasting approximately 10 seconds presenting every hour in frequency, but the background was still highly abnormal. A pyridoxine challenge was also trialed without improvement in the EEG. In addition to full septic evaluation, patient had an expedited brain MRI. This revealed a large left hemimegalencephaly with an abnormal gyral pattern throughout most of the left cerebral hemisphere and ventriculomegaly (Figure 13.3). This was the cause of his severe course and explains the laterality seen on EEG. After spending a week in the hospital, the patient was discharged home on high doses of levetiracetam, lacosamide, phenobarbital, and topiramate. He continued to have intractable tonic seizures and soon

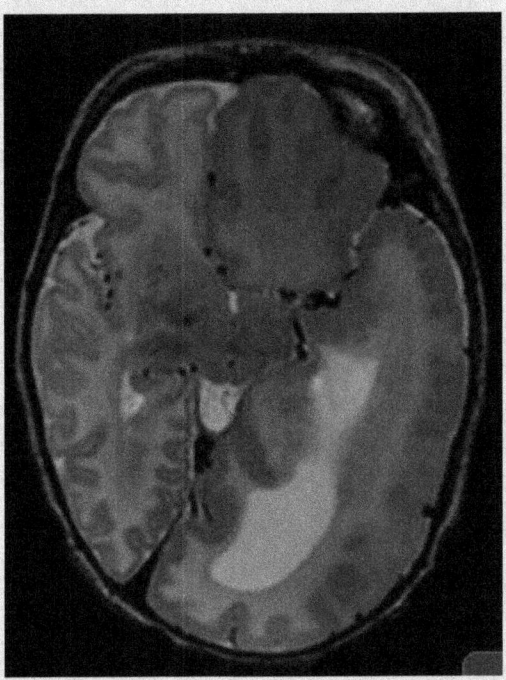

FIGURE 13.3   MRI brain (axial T2) demonstrating left hemimegalencephaly and ventriculomegaly.

thereafter also developed spasms. During hospitalization, the patient was deemed to be an epilepsy surgery candidate with concordant MRI brain, PET, and EEG findings. A hemispherotomy was successfully performed at 3 months of age, without intraoperative or perioperative major complications. Since surgery, the patient has been doing remarkably well with no clinical seizures. He is also gaining more developmental milestones. Previously, the patient had a left gaze preference, but subsequently was tracking more in all directions. He is also using his right-sided extremities more than prior to surgery.

DIFFERENTIAL DIAGNOSIS

Ohtahara syndrome, also referred to as early-infantile epileptic encephalopathy (EIEE), is one of the earliest presenting and most severe age-dependent epileptic encephalopathies. Shunsuke Ohtahara et al. described the clinical and electroencephalographic features in 1976. The incidence is extremely rare. Classically, neonates and infants will acutely present with tonic spasms and a suppression burst pattern on EEG, progressing to intractable epilepsy and significant psychomotor debilitation.

Patients with Ohtahara syndrome present within the early infantile period, often within the first 1–2 weeks of life, but may occur anytime within the first 3 months. On exam, one typically finds an encephalopathic infant with central hypotonia and/or hypertonic extremities. They may develop tonic spasms acutely, with a forward tonic flexion of the body lasting up to 10 seconds, occurring a few to hundreds of times a day.

The differential diagnosis includes other age-dependent epileptic encephalopathies, including infantile spasms and early myoclonic encephalopathy (EME). There are ongoing debates regarding Ohtahara syndrome as a separate entity from EME or whether the two syndromes exist on a spectrum, due to overlapping clinical and EEG features. While the age of presentation is similar, as the name suggests, the distinguishing predominant seizure type in EME is myoclonic seizures.

The infantile spasms seen in West syndrome are extensor or flexor posturing and occur during sleep. This contrasts with the extensor tonic spasms seen in Ohtahara syndrome which can be seen both during awake and sleep periods.

Metabolic derangements are less commonly seen in this syndrome. The disorders presenting as Ohtahara syndrome include nonketotic hyperglycinemia, mitochondrial respiratory chain disorders, pyridoxine dependency, and carnitine palmitoyltransferase deficiency. There is a reported case of Leigh encephalopathy presenting as Ohtahara syndrome.

DIAGNOSTIC APPROACH

A thorough history and physical examination will provide key information attributed to the disorder. Furthermore, the EEG is essential in capturing and characterizing seizures and further narrowing the differential. In benign neonatal conditions causing seizures, the background is often normal and age appropriate. In epileptic encephalopathies, the background is highly abnormal with limited awake and sleep architecture.

Electroencephalographically, Ohtahara syndrome has a suppression burst pattern, with bursts of high amplitude (150–300 μV) sharps/spikes and waves alternating with periods of low-voltage activity. The bursts can last 6 seconds, with suppression intervals of 3–5 seconds. The suppression burst pattern is present during state changes, and normal grapho-elements are not seen. The bursts of activity can correlate with tonic spasms. The EEG will change as the patient clinically evolves as well, with the emergence of other seizure types. In infantile spasms, the patient will have hypsarrhythmia.

All neonates and infants with an abnormal neurological exam and seizures necessitate further work-up with a brain MRI to evaluate potential structural anomalies or insults. Metabolic studies such as serum amino acids, urine organic acids, ammonia, lactate, pyruvate, acylcarnitine profile, and cerebrospinal fluid (CSF) neurotransmitters are often sent. Genetic studies continue to improve and provide a higher diagnostic yield. Initial studies include microarrays and epilepsy gene panels. If these are unrevealing, it is important to consider sending whole exome sequencing.

TREATMENT STRATEGIES

In one-third of patients, the spasms will progress, and patients will develop refractory epilepsy with focal seizures and convulsions. Initially, when etiology is unknown and vitamin dependent epilepsies are on the differential, it is important to consider a trial with pyridoxine, folinic acid or P5P. With respect to other treatment options, no single anti-seizure medication (ASM) has been shown to be more effective than another in treating Ohtahara syndrome.

Given the rarity of the disorder, there are only anecdotal histories regarding medications and their efficacy. Medications trialed include phenobarbital, valproate, zonisamide and benzodiazepines. Adrenocorticotropic hormone may be used, especially in cases progressing to West syndrome. Patients can also be placed on the ketogenic diet as an alternative to control seizures.

Unfortunately, there is limited effectiveness with current therapies. Even in cases where seizures are controlled, there is progression of disease without improvement in development. However, precision medicine in epilepsy and understanding the genetic diagnosis may allow for tailored treatment and improved clinical outcomes. In cases with structural changes, such as with focal cortical dysplasia or hemimegalencephaly, neurosurgical options may help decrease seizure burden.

LONG-TERM OUTCOME

The overall prognosis is grim. Mortality is high during infancy and the surviving patients are neurologically debilitated with profound cognitive and motor deficits. There can be progression to West syndrome by 3–6 months, as well as evolution into Lennox–Gastaut syndrome after 1 year with corresponding EEG findings of hypsarrhythmia and generalized slow spike-and-wave patterns, respectively.

PATHOPHYSIOLOGY/NEUROBIOLOGY OF DISEASE

The pathophysiology is not well understood. When studying the different gene mutations leading to Ohtahara syndrome and their function in the brain, phenotypic pathophysiology is thought to be related to brain dysgenesis or neuronal dysfunction. Prior research has also postulated the syndrome is due to brainstem dysfunction given patients with Ohtahara syndrome have brainstem abnormalities on pathology and tonic seizures are presumed to arise from brainstem dysfunction. Understanding the pathophysiology will ultimately help guide future treatment.

Ohtahara syndrome can present due to a variety of etiologies, most commonly structural brain abnormalities. These include hemimegalencephaly, porencephaly, cerebral migration disorders, and agenesis of the corpus callosum. This is not a comprehensive list of associated structural anomalies. Subtle cerebral migration disorders can be missed on routine imaging.

Recently, with advancements in genetic testing, more cases of Ohtahara syndrome have been linked to specific genetic anomalies. In the study by Olson et al., pathogenic variants in known genes explained 61% of the patients with epileptic encephalopathy, early burst suppression pattern on EEG and without a structural brain malformation. Of note, this study encompasses both Ohtahara syndrome and EME. This is higher than previous reports of a 20%–30% yield from whole exome sequencing. *KCNQ2* was identified in 35.7% of these patients (17/28) as the largest genetic subgroup. Gene mutations in syntaxin binding protein 1 (*STXBP1*), aristaless-related

CLINICAL PEARLS

- Ohtahara syndrome is an extremely rare epileptic encephalopathy presenting in neonates and infants.
- There remains controversy about whether Ohtahara syndrome is a separate entity from early myoclonic encephalopathy, or whether they exist on a clinical continuum together.
- Patients are often encephalopathic with abnormal tone on exam.
- Predominant presentation is tonic spasms with suppression burst patterns on EEG.
- Structural brain malformation is the most common etiologic category.
- More genetic etiologies are being found with advances in genetic testing.
- *KCNQ2* gene mutation may be the largest subgroup of genetic etiologies in patients without structural malformation.
- Prognosis is poor with high morbidity and mortality.

homeobox (*ARX*), sodium voltage-gated channel alpha subunit 2 (*SCN2A*), solute carrier family 25 (*SLC25A22*), and *PNPO* pathogenic variant have all been found in patients with Ohtahara syndrome. Likely pathogenic variants in *PIGA* and *SEPSECS* have also recently been identified in patients with early-onset epileptic encephalopathy. There is not a clear phenotypic correlation to the genetic subgroups. These may also have concurrent structural brain abnormalities.

SUGGESTED REFERENCES

Beal J.C., Cherian K., Moshe S.L. Early-onset epileptic encephalopathies: Ohtahara syndrome and early myoclonic encephalopathy. *Pediatr Neurol* 2012;47: 317–23.

Olson H.E., Kelly M., LaCoursiere C.M., Pinsky R., Tambunan D., Shain C., Ramgopal S., Takeoka M., Libenson M.H., Julich K., Loddenkemper T., Marsh E.D., Segal D., Koh S., Salman M.S., Paciorkowski A.R., Yang E., Bergin A.M., Sheidley B.R., Poduri A. Genetics and genotype-phenotype correlations in early onset epileptic encephalopathy with burst suppression. *Ann Neurol* 2017;81: 419–29.

Pavone P., Spalice A., Polizzi A., Parisi P., Ruggieri M. Ohtahara syndrome with emphasis on recent genetic discovery. *Brain Dev* 2012;34: 459–68.

Yamatogi T., Ohtahara S. Early-infantile epileptic encephalopathy with suppression-bursts, Ohtahara syndrome; its overview referring to our 16 cases. *Brain Dev* 2002;24: 13–23.

14 Early Myoclonic Encephalopathy

Juan Ignacio Appendino
Hospital Italiano de Buenos Aires

Juan Pablo Appendino
University of Calgary

CONTENTS

CASE PRESENTATION

A 6-day-old term infant, product of a first uncomplicated pregnancy and normal vaginal delivery presented to the emergency department with decreased feeding effort, lethargy, and erratic myoclonus – including unilateral facial, limbs, wrists, and single fingers along with clonic movements of either limb. Family history was negative. On exam, axial hypotonia without dysmorphic features or focal deficits was observed. Most of the primitive reflexes were preserved, although moro and root reflexes were weak. Reactivity to touch and sound stimulations were decreased suggesting a moderate degree of encephalopathy. An EEG was done showing a burst-suppression pattern mainly in sleep with occasional spikes or polyspikes, at times associated with myoclonus, although not consistently (Figure 14.1). A brain MRI/MRS showed a small corpus callosum and an abnormal peak at 3.55 ppm (TE = 144 ms; Figure 14.2). Laboratory investigations revealed glycine peaks in CSF and serum. Finally, a pathogenic variant in the GLDC gene confirmed the diagnosis of early myoclonic epilepsy associated with nonketotic hyperglycinemia.

DOI: 10.1201/9781003296478-16

123

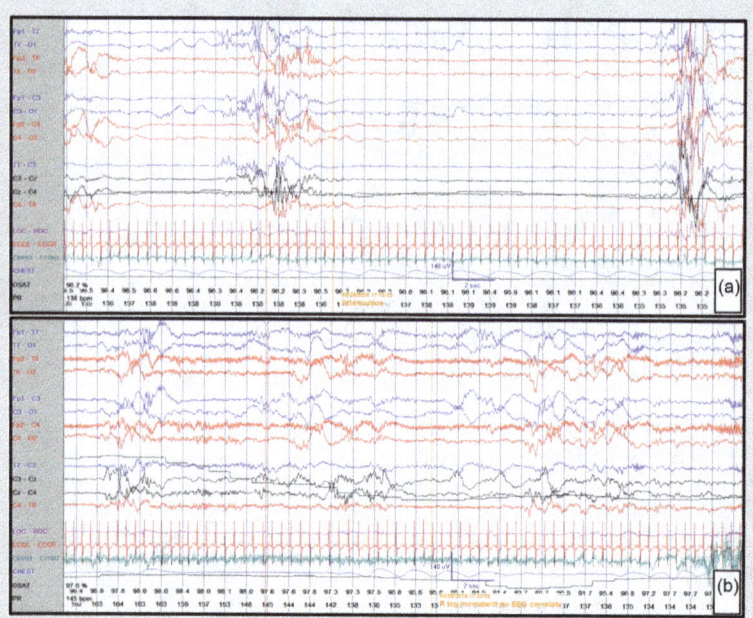

FIGURE 14.1 EEG showing a burst-suppression pattern during sleep (a) and continuous background activity while awake (b). Settings: 1 Hz LFF, 70 Hz HFF, notch 60 Hz on, sensitivity 7 μV/mm, paper speed 15 mm/s.

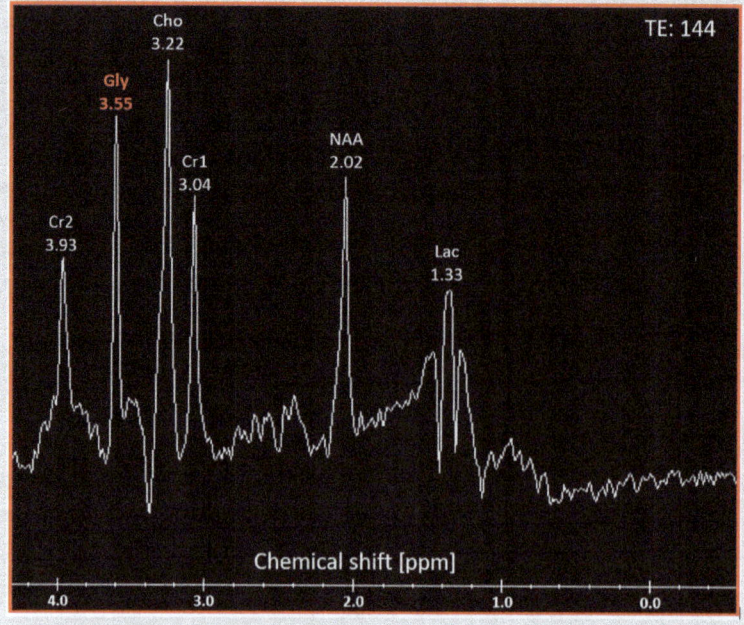

FIGURE 14.2 MRS at TE 144 showing a clear glycine peak (red at 3.55 ppm) and a suspicious lactate peak at 1.33 ppm.

DIFFERENTIAL DIAGNOSIS

- Ohtahara syndrome (EEG and MRI are very helpful in distinguishing from EME).
- Self-limited familial and nonfamilial neonatal seizures (the presence of myoclonic seizures excludes this diagnosis).
- KCNQ2 encephalopathy (this etiology could show a range of phenotypes including Ohtahara syndrome and EME, but at times it is difficult to differentiate).
- DEND syndrome (developmental delay, epilepsy, and neonatal diabetes, last characteristic helps in the diagnostic consideration).

DIAGNOSTIC APPROACH

Early myoclonic epilepsy (EME) was first described in 1978 (2 years after the description of Ohtahara syndrome). It has received different names over time: myoclonic epilepsy with neonatal onset, neonatal epileptic encephalopathy with periodic electroencephalographic paroxysms, and early myoclonic epileptic encephalopathy. In 2001, the Task Force on Classification and Terminology of the International League Against Epilepsy (ILAE) included EME in the category of epileptic encephalopathies with the name early myoclonic encephalopathy.

In 2022, the ILAE launched the "Methodology for classification and definition of epilepsy syndromes with list of syndromes: Report of the ILAE Task Force on Nosology and Definitions" where EME was included in early infantile developmental and epileptic encephalopathy (EIDEE). The concept of "epileptic encephalopathy" implies that the epileptic activity by itself contributes to generating cognitive and behavioral alterations.

EME is characterized by frequent and intractable seizures, severe early-onset epileptic encephalopathy (usually in the neonatal period), and a markedly decreased life expectancy (with patients often dying in the first 2 years of life). EME has an incidence of 1/1000 live births. The characteristic and fundamental seizure type needed to make the diagnosis is the myoclonic seizure. They are erratic, asynchronous and asymmetrical (they change from one body segment to another without following a defined pattern) and are very frequent (at times almost continuous). The face and limbs are usually affected but other more specific sites such as eyelids, fingers, or lips can also be affected. In addition to the myoclonic seizures, these patients may subsequently present with both clonic and tonic focal seizures and in some cases epileptic spasms.

No predominance of gender is observed with EME (1:1 ratio). Most patients have no significant history during pregnancy or childbirth. The head circumference at birth is usually normal and, in some cases, acquired microcephaly is observed (i.e., with nonketotic hyperglycinemia). The physical examination usually draws attention to the presence of an axial hypotonia (usually severe). Marked developmental and behavioral delay is observed, at times seen before the onset of clinical seizures.

The interictal EEG shows a pattern of "burst suppression" which is usually captured only during sleep (unlike Ohtahara syndrome, which is usually documented during both sleep and wakefulness). It is characterized by 1–5 second bursts of spike-and-sharp-waves intermingled with high amplitude (150–300 μV) slow waves

---

TABLE 14.1
Metabolic Disorders Associated With EME

- Nonketotic hyperglycinemia (most common cause)
- Urea cycle disorders
- D-glyceric aciduria
- Methylmalonic acidemia
- Carbamoyl phosphate synthetase hyperammonemia
- Pyridoxine and pyridoxal-5-phosphate deficiency
- Propionic acidemia
- Molybdenum cofactor deficiency
- Sulfite oxidase deficiency
- Xanthine oxidase deficiency
- Menkes disease
- Zellweger syndrome

---

combined with epochs of suppression lasting 3–10 seconds each. During the awake state, the background becomes continuous and symmetric but disorganized, with a mixture of delta and theta activity.

The ictal EEG shows spikes and polyspikes at times associated with clinical myoclonic seizures; however, the myoclonus is not always associated with EEG changes (subcortical myoclonus). Focal seizures show focal rhythmic discharges superimposed on the background activity, including burst suppression if seizures occur during sleep.

Family history in EME is usually unremarkable. Most patients present with a metabolic disorder, and less common genetic or brain malformation etiologies (Tables 14.1 and 14.2). Investigations should include but are not limited to urine organic acids, serum and urine uric acid, plasma amino acids, serum lactate, very-long-chain fatty acids, a lumbar puncture to evaluate the glycine CSF/blood ratio, neurotransmitters, and CSF lactate levels. Genetic panels for epileptic encephalopathies or whole-exome sequencing (WES) are also considered. In addition, a brain MRI with spectroscopy and continuous video-EEG are helpful to guide therapy.

TREATMENT STRATEGY

There is no specific treatment for EME. As it is generally associated with metabolic/genetic disorders, an exhaustive search focused on finding a potentially treatable metabolic etiology must be carried out.

LONG TERM PROGNOSIS

Unfortunately, EME presents an ominous prognosis. Approximately 50% of patients die during their first 2 years of life.

TABLE 14.2
Genetic Disorders Associated with EME

- *CDKL5* (Encodes the cyclin-dependent kinase-like 5. It is a member of Ser/Thr protein kinase family and encodes a phosphorylated protein with protein kinase activity. AD)
- *ERBB4* (Encodes the Erb-B2 receptor tyrosine kinase 4. Encodes the tyrosine kinase receptor HER4, a critical regulator of normal cell function, and neurodevelopmental processes in the brain. AD)
- *KCNQ2* (Encodes the Potassium voltage-gated channel subfamily Q member 2. This protein forms part of the M channels which deactivate and decrease excitability in neurons. AD)
- *SCN2A* (Encodes the sodium voltage-gated channel alpha subunit 2. Voltage-gated sodium channels function in the generation and propagation of action potentials in neurons and muscle. AD)
- *SETBP1* (Encodes the SET binding protein 1. It has been shown to bind the SET nuclear oncogene, which is involved in DNA replication. AD)
- *SIK1* (Encodes the salt-inducible kinase 1. Serine/threonine-protein kinase involved in various processes such as cell cycle regulation, gluconeogenesis and lipogenesis regulation, muscle growth and differentiation, and tumor suppression. AD)
- *SLC25A22* (Encodes the solute carrier family 25, member 22. Involved in transport of glutamate across the inner mitochondrial membrane. AR)
- *SPTAN1* (Encodes the spectrin alpha, nonerythrocytic 1. It has been implicated in other cellular functions including DNA repair and cell cycle regulation. AD)
- *STXBP1* (Encodes the syntaxin binding protein 1. It appears to play a role in the release of neurotransmitters via regulation of syntaxin, a transmembrane attachment protein receptor. AD)
- *PIGA* (Encodes the phosphatidylinositol glycan anchor biosynthesis class A protein. Involved in the catalytic subunit of the glycosylphosphatidylinositol-N-acetylglucosaminyltransferase complex. XLR)

AD, Autosomal Dominant; AR, Autosomal Recessive; XLR, X-linked Recessive.

CLINICAL PEARLS

- A "burst-suppression" pattern is most commonly seen during sleep, but it could be intermittently present during the awake state. A third of patients have it only during sleep. In Ohtahara syndrome, more often seen in both, wakefulness and sleep and tonic seizures are more frequent than myoclonic seizures.
- "Burst-suppression" pattern may transiently evolve into "atypical hypsarrhythmia" in approximately 50% of patients at 3–5 months of age, returning afterward to a definitive "burst-suppression" pattern. Patients usually do not progress to West syndrome, although this could happen.
- EME is generally not associated with structural brain malformations, in contrast to Ohtahara syndrome.

SUGGESTED REFERENCES

Hwang S.K. Genetic basis of early-onset developmental and epileptic encephalopathies. *J Int Gen* 2021;3: 13–20.

Lee S., Kim S.H., Kim B., Lee S.T., Choi J.R., Kim H.D., Lee J.S., Kang H.C. Genetic diagnosis and clinical characteristics by etiological classification in early-onset epileptic encephalopathy with burst suppression pattern. *Epilepsy Res* 2020;163: 106323.

Morrison-Levy N., Borlot F., Jain P., Whitney R. Early-onset developmental and epileptic encephalopathies of infancy: An overview of the genetic basis and clinical features. *Pediatr Neurol* 2021;116: 85–94.

Pressler R.M., Cilio M.R., Mizrahi E.M., Moshé S.L., Nunes M.L., Plouin P., Vanhatalo S., Yozawitz E., de Vries L.S., Puthenveettil Vinayan K., Triki C.C., Wilmshurst J.M., Yamamoto H., Zuberi S.M. The ILAE classification of seizures and the epilepsies: Modification for seizures in the neonate. Position paper by the ILAE Task Force on Neonatal Seizures. *Epilepsia* 2021;62: 615–28.

van Karnebeek C.D.M., Sayson B., Lee J.J.Y., Tseng L.A., Blau N., Horvath G.A., Ferreira C.R. Metabolic evaluation of epilepsy: A diagnostic algorithm with focus on treatable conditions. *Front Neurol* 2018;9: 1016.

Yang H., Gong P., Jiao X., Zhou Q., Zhang Y., Jiang Y., Yang Z. The relationship between the characteristics of burst suppression pattern and different etiologies in epilepsy. *Sci Rep* 2021;11: 15903.

Zuberi S.M., Wirrell E., Yozawitz E., Wilmshurst J.M., Specchio N., Riney K., Pressler R., Auvin S., Samia P., Hirsch E., Galicchio S., Triki C., Snead O.C., Wiebe S., Cross J.H., Tinuper P., Scheffer I.E., Perucca E., Moshé S.L., Nabbout R. ILAE classification and definition of epilepsy syndromes with onset in neonates and infants: Position statement by the ILAE Task force on nosology and definitions. *Epilepsia* 2022;63: 1349–97.

15 Hypoxic-Ischemic Encephalopathy (Neonatal Seizures)

Jeffrey J. Gold
UC San Diego School of Medicine

CONTENTS

CASE PRESENTATION

A 23-year-old primigravida woman presented in active labor at 39-week gestation based on the last menstrual period. The mother was on prenatal vitamins prior to conception and throughout pregnancy, which was uncomplicated with full prenatal care. Initial fetal monitoring was reassuring, but after 14 hours of labor, fetal distress was evidenced by bradycardia and loss of variability on the tracings. Delivery was vacuum assisted, and the infant was handed to the pediatrics team, limp and cyanotic with no respiratory effort and a heart rate of 60. Chest compressions were started, and the child was successfully intubated on the second attempt at 2 minutes of life. Heart rate began to improve around 10 minutes of life and the child was extubated to nasal cannula oxygen around 20 minutes of life. Birthweight was recorded as 3,400 g and Apgar scores were 1, 3, 4, and 7 at 1, 5, 10, and 20 minutes, respectively. The child was transferred to the Neonatal Intensive Care Unit (NICU) and started on therapeutic hypothermia, with EEG monitoring began around 2 hours of life after umbilical lines were secured. Brief, independent left and right hemisphere seizures were seen lasting 30–60 seconds immediately after the EEG was started and the neonate received a 20 mg/kg bolus of phenobarbital over 1 hour, after which seizures were no longer seen. A phenobarbital standing dose was started at 2.5 mg/kg twice daily. The EEG was discontinuous and suppressed for the duration of therapeutic hypothermia but

DOI: 10.1201/9781003296478-17

improved when rewarming was undertaken around 72 hours of life. Brain MRI performed at 96 hours of life indicated mild ischemic changes in the bilateral basal ganglia and subcortical white matter, and DWI changes were seen in the splenium of the corpus callosum. The child began feeding shortly after the MRI and was discharged on the 10th day of life on 2.5 mg/kg phenobarbital twice daily with a discharge blood level of 25. Subsequent examination at 6 months of life revealed a developmentally and neurologically normal infant. Routine EEG was normal and phenobarbital was discontinued at that time.

DIFFERENTIAL DIAGNOSIS

Neonatal seizures are more typically a symptom than a cause of brain injury in the newborn period. Any injury or malformation of the brain can cause neonatal seizures. When a cause is discovered, the most common is hypoxic-ischemic encephalopathy (HIE, about 40%), perinatal stroke (about 20%), or intracranial hemorrhage (about 10%). The remainder of neonatal seizures is due to infection, congenital malformation, metabolic disorders, and genetic mutations such as ion channelopathies, and congenital tumors. About half of all neonatal seizures are subclinical (i.e., without any correlated movement, behavioral change, or vital sign disturbance) which likely results in an underestimate of their frequency. Therefore, screening for neonatal seizures with continuous video-EEG monitoring should be undertaken whenever neonatal seizures are suspected, or when neonates are identified with a condition that places them at high risk for neonatal seizures. Back arching from acid reflux, exaggerated startle, Moro reflex, and benign sleep myoclonus of infancy are common mimics of neonatal seizures.

DIAGNOSTIC APPROACH

Neonatal seizures are a medical emergency, and the first priority is treatment (see below). Laboratory testing should be undertaken immediately to rule out electrolyte disturbances and hypoglycemia as causes of seizures that would not require anti-seizure medications (ASMs). If galactosemia is suspected, the child should be denied further feeding until the urine can be tested with a glucose strip and for reducing substances (negative glucose strip in the presence of positive reducing substances suggests this diagnosis).

Lumbar puncture should be performed if central nervous system (CNS) infection is on the differential (with Group B *Streptococcus*, *Escherichia Coli*, and herpes simplex virus making up the bulk of CNS infections in the newborn). Newborn screening should be sent to look for rare metabolic conditions that can cause seizures. Bedside head ultrasound is typically performed to look for large malformations, symptomatic hydrocephalus, and cerebral hemorrhage. Once the neonate is stable enough, a brain MRI scan is typically obtained to look for ischemic injury or subtle malformations. More extensive genetic and metabolic testing can be undertaken on a case-by-case basis once the more common causes of neonatal seizures are ruled out.

HIE is the most common cause of neonatal seizures. It should be suspected when there is concern that the fetus has suffered from a lack of oxygenation, blood flow, or metabolic substrate as might occur when:

- There is a "sentinel event" during labor such as placental abruption, cord prolapse, or tight nuchal cord.
- Fetal monitoring reveals loss of heart tones, late or variable decelerations, or labor is markedly prolonged.
- Cord blood or neonatal blood gas testing reveals acidemia.

To qualify for a diagnosis of HIE, neonates must also demonstrate encephalopathy as defined by the Sarnat scale of neonatal encephalopathy which assigns points when (among other symptoms) neonates are hypotonic, hypo or hyperreflexic, or have abnormal dilation of the pupils. Seizures are considered a sign of (at least) moderate neonatal encephalopathy.

TREATMENT STRATEGIES

If it can be determined that neonatal seizures are due to a transient, reversible cause such as hyponatremia or hypoglycemia, the underlying condition should be treated, and an ASM may not be needed. If seizures are provoked by a treatable underlying condition, specific treatment for that condition should be given (e.g., antibiotics for CNS infection and dietary therapy for specific metabolic conditions), whether or not ASMs are given for treatment of symptomatic seizures.

There is no definite consensus about the use of ASMs for the treatment of neonatal seizures, in part because there is a relative lack of evidence of high-quality clinical trials demonstrating the efficacy and utility of seizure medications in the neonatal age group. A seminal study established that phenobarbital and phenytoin are equally effective at stopping neonatal seizures (about 45% individually and 60% together). Subsequently, the NEOLEV2 trial showed that phenobarbital was more effective than levetiracetam (80% vs 24% at 24 hours). The loop diuretic bumetanide has been trialed several times with possible but not definitive efficacy established. Most practitioners start neonates having seizures on phenobarbital with the goal of discontinuing treatment as soon as possible (interpreted alternately as before NICU discharge or after a few months of seizure freedom depending on the institution and patient factors.)

Neonates with HIE should be considered for therapeutic hypothermia. The exact criteria vary between institutions and clinical trials, but typically neonates must be more than 35 weeks gestation, have HIE identified in the first 6 hours of life, demonstrate at least one sign of hypoxia/ischemia (such as an Apgar score of <6 at 10 minutes, cord blood pH <7.0 or base deficit ≥12) and have moderate-or-worse Sarnat encephalopathy scoring to qualify for cooling. Neonates are typically cooled to 33–34°C for 72 hours and then rewarmed over 6–8 hours. It is thought that therapeutic hypothermia affords a measure of protection against seizures.

LONG-TERM OUTCOME

Long-term outcomes after neonatal seizures are highly dependent on the cause of seizures. Seizures associated with transient electrolyte disturbances rarely result in neurodevelopmental disability, while seizures associated with genetic disorders, brain malformations, and high-grade cerebral hemorrhages are universally correlated with poor outcomes. While it has been established that a high seizure burden predisposes neonates to poor neurodevelopmental outcome, it has been difficult to show the negative impact of brief, rare, or subclinical seizures in neonates with HIE. Overall, it is felt that the cause of the seizures has a greater impact on outcomes than characteristics of the seizures themselves, although most practitioners agree status epileptics is often correlated with worse outcomes.

HIE accounts for 5%–10% of neonatal deaths (all gestational ages) and up to 25% of term neonatal deaths. Prior to the widespread use of therapeutic hypothermia, 50%–60% of neonates with HIE had evidence of brain injury on MRI, with rates of cerebral palsy and epilepsy estimated at about 40% and 20%, respectively. Cooling is thought to reduce the rates of brain injury on MRI, cerebral palsy, and epilepsy by about half. There is some evidence to suggest that hypothermia is more efficacious in neonates with mild to moderate HIE than severe HIE.

PATHOPHYSIOLOGY/NEUROBIOLOGY OF DISEASE

The causes of HIE can be divided into maternal, placental, and fetal factors. Maternal factors include maternal hypoglycemia and maternal diabetes (when the infant receives a high degree of insulin from the mother but loses access to glucose after birth, resulting in profound neonatal hypoglycemia). Placental factors include abruption or occlusion of the cord (due to clots, knots, or compression). Fetal factors are rare but include inborn errors of metabolism and bleeding (such as subgaleal hemorrhage and bleeding dyscrasias).

Whether deprived of oxygen or glucose, neurons lose the ability to create ATP via the electron transport chain and cellular processes stall. In particular, the Na^+/K^+

CLINICAL PEARLS

- Neonatal seizures are a symptom more than a cause of brain injury. Outcomes after neonatal seizures depend more on the etiology of seizures than the characteristics of the seizures themselves.
- Neonatal seizures are difficult to discover. All neonates at risk for seizures should be screened with continuous video-EEG monitor to facilitate rapid identification and treatment.
- Phenobarbital has the most evidence of efficacy in the treatment of neonatal seizures, but the duration of therapy should be as short as possible.
- Neonates with HIE should be treated with therapeutic hypothermia and should be monitored for seizures during therapy.

pumps that maintain the neuronal membrane potential gradient fail, causing an increase in the resting membrane potential toward the Nerst potential of sodium. These hyper-excitable neurons are thus prone to seizures. Seizures result in the excessive accumulation of glutamate which produces further influx of calcium and sodium into the cell, thereby raising the membrane potential and predisposing neurons to hyperexcitability and more seizure activity. Other energy-dependent cellular activities not specific to neurons (peroxisomal and ribosomal activity, for example) also fail. Neurons become edematous as they attempt to dilute toxic solutes, eventually resulting in failure of the cell membrane and finally necrosis or apoptosis.

SUGGESTED REFERENCES

Glass H.C., Shellhaas R.A., Wusthoff C.J., Chang T., Abend N.S., Chu C.J., Cilio M.R., Glidden D.V., Bonifacio S.L., Massey S., Tsuchida T.N., Silverstein F.S., Soul J.S.; Neonatal Seizure Registry Study Group. Contemporary profile of seizures in neonates: A prospective cohort study. *J Pediatr* 2016;174: 98–103.

Jacobs S.E., Berg M., Hunt R., Tarnow-Mordi W.O., Inder T.E., Davis P.G. Cooling for newborns with hypoxic ischaemic encephalopathy. *Cochrane Database Syst Rev* 2013;2013(1): CD003311.

Painter M.J., Scher M.S., Stein A.D., Armatti S., Wang Z., Gardiner J.C., Paneth N., Minnigh B., Alvin J. A comparison of the efficacy of phenobarbital and phenytoin in the treatment of neonatal seizures. *N Engl J Med* 1999;341: 485–9.

Sarnat H.B., Sarnat M.S. Neonatal encephalopathy following fetal distress. A clinical and electroencephalographic study. *Arch Neurol* 1976;33: 696–705.

Sharpe C., Reiner G.E., Davis S.L., Nespeca M., Gold J.J., Rasmussen M., Kuperman R., Harbert M.J., Michelson D., Joe P., Wang S., Rismanchi N., Le N.M., Mower A., Kim J., Battin M.R., Lane B., Honold J., Knodel E., Arnell K., Bridge R., Lee L., Ernstrom K., Raman R., Haas R.H.; NEOLEV2 INVESTIGATORS. Levetiracetam versus phenobarbital for neonatal seizures: A randomized controlled trial. *Pediatrics* 2020;145: e20193182.

16 Epilepsy of Infancy with Migrating Focal Seizures

Danielle deCampo
Children's Hospital of Philadelphia

Eric Marsh
University of Pennsylvania

CONTENTS

CASE PRESENTATION

A family brings their 4-month infant to the emergency room (ER) after witnessing the baby having jerking on one side of the body. Labs and exam in the ER were unremarkable so the child was referred to a pediatric neurologist. In the few weeks prior to the visit, the parents noticed a few more of these events, with jerking only on the right side of the body (with a few episodes captured on mobile phone video). The baby was born at term, with no complications and had a normal development course. Neurological exam was unremarkable. The neurologist obtained a routine EEG which showed a diffusely slow background with multifocal spike-wave discharges. The child was started on levetiracetam, but the events continued to increase in frequency. A subsequent video-EEG study captured a few seizures of focal body jerking with an ictal pattern of rhythmic theta activity that progressively involved adjacent areas as the frequency of the discharges decreased. The child was discharged on a higher dose of levetiracetam. One week later, the infant developed seizures associated with apnea, drooling, and flushing. Shortly thereafter, focal motor seizures were observed on the other side of the body which became more frequent. A repeat EEG showed a diffusely slow background with prevalence of slow waves shifting from one hemisphere to another. Ictal EEG showed seizures with the same rhythmic theta activity at onset noted previously but

DOI: 10.1201/9781003296478-18

arising from each hemisphere independently and in some cases, sequentially. The location varied not only from side to side but from also within a hemisphere. Seizures were typically short (1–4 minutes), but at times clustered, lasting more than an hour at a time. Some events evolved to bilateral tonic-clonic seizures. A brain MRI after discharge demonstrated mildly increased CSF spaces and mild ventricular prominence of undetermined significance. One month after onset, seizures were occurring up to 25 times daily and were intractable to the antiseizure medications (ASMs) levetiracetam, oxcarbazepine, and topiramate. The infant demonstrated significant psychomotor decline losing eye contact, inability to grasp objects, and had increased hypotonia. Head growth stagnated with progressive crossing of head circumference percentiles over the ensuing months. A genetic workup which included an epilepsy panel and whole exome sequencing was unremarkable. Repeat EEGs showed a slow background with multifocal sharps. At the 1-year follow-up, the child had a severe static encephalopathy with persistent seizures. He was able to inconsistently track objects, made some sounds, and was able to grasp objects but was unable to sit independently. Head circumference was in the 18th percentile. During the following year, seizures decreased in frequency, and the child started to slowly acquire new milestones including ability to babble; however, illnesses would easily trigger seizures with some resulting in status epilepticus.

DIFFERENTIAL DIAGNOSIS

Focal motor seizures occurring in infants should be considered an emergency until acute causes are ruled out. Acute causes of focal seizures in infancy consist of infection (meningitis/encephalitis), stroke, bleeding, metabolic derangement, electrolyte imbalance, or mass lesion. In this case, with a child that appeared otherwise well with no signs of illness or focal findings on neurological exam, these can generally be ruled out.

The differential of focal epilepsy in an infant consists of seizures due to a malformation of cortical development, vascular anomaly, or genetic epilepsy, with many potential genes. In this case, where the focal motor seizures began to alternate hemispheres along with autonomic seizures, the differential was between self-limited (familial) neonatal epilepsy (SeLNE) (formerly known as benign familial neonatal epilepsy) or a more malignant syndrome. In SeLNE, seizures typically start shortly after birth (2–7 days of life) and infants have a normal developmental course or only mild developmental delay. Seizures remit by 6 weeks to 6 months of age.

Frequent drug-resistant seizures along with moderate-to-profound psychomotor impairment during infancy point toward a developmental and epileptic encephalopathy (DEE) such as early-infantile developmental and epileptic encephalopathy (EIDEE; this syndrome includes patients with Ohtahara syndrome and early myoclonic encephalopathy), or Dravet syndrome (formerly known as severe myoclonic of infancy). EIDEE commences before 3 months of age, and infants have multiple seizure types including tonic, myoclonic, focal clonic, and epileptic spasms. Abnormal development is typically seen *before* the presentation of seizures. Infants often have co-existing movement disorders including myoclonus, chorea, dystonia, and tremor. EEG has a burst suppression pattern that also helps to distinguish it from other DEE syndromes.

Infants with Dravet syndrome generally have seizures beginning at 3–9 months of age and have normal development/mild delay up until seizure onset. Patients have focal hemi-clonic, generalized clonic, and generalized tonic-clonic seizures; however, seizures do not have a migratory pattern on EEG, with multiple seizure foci on the same EEG. Patients with Dravet syndrome also have other seizure types including myoclonic seizures. Seizures can be triggered by elevated body temperature and physical activity.

Mitochondrial cytopathies and metabolic syndromes should also be considered, and empirical treatment with pyridoxine should be trialed to rule out pyridoxine-dependent epilepsy. Both these etiologies typically do not have alternating seizure patterns but can have multiple seizure types with multifocal onsets.

DIAGNOSTIC APPROACH

Epilepsy of infancy with migrating focal seizures (EIMFS; formerly known as malignant migrating partial seizures of infancy) was first described in 1995 by Coppola in a series of 14 infants over an 11-year period. It is classified as a DEE under the ILAE task force. It is a rare syndrome with prevalence of 0.11/10,000 children. The age of presentation, EEG pattern, and clinical course are valuable in making the diagnosis. The key features of this syndrome are as follows:

- Onset of focal motor seizures within the first 6 months.
- Focal motor seizures that arise from both hemispheres and migrate from one cortical region to another that can be prolonged with episodes of *status epilepticus.*
- Initially normal or mildly abnormal development followed by stagnation/delay.

Coppola's original description divided the natural history in three phases:

- Phase 1 (0–7 months of age, mean age 3 months in previously normal developing infants): sporadic focal motor seizures that can evolve to bilateral tonic-clonic seizures and sometimes occur in clusters with seizure-free periods (days–weeks). Autonomic manifestations (apnea, flushing, cyanosis) during seizures can also occur.
- Phase 2 ("stormy phase"; 3 weeks–10 months of age): increased seizure frequency occurring in clusters (5–30 clusters/day) that may be near continuous leading to focal *status epilepticus.* During this stage, there may be some response to drug therapy, but eventually seizures return.
- Phase 3 (age of onset varies from 1 year to >5 years): seizure-free period, although seizures can be precipitated by illness. Developmental delay/stagnation is established with hypotonia, peripheral spasticity, as well as postnatal acquired microcephaly.

Initially, EEG background can be normal or excessively slow for age but with development of multifocal epileptogenic foci within 6 months of presentation. Ictal EEG demonstrates rhythmic sharp discharges in the theta-alpha range starting from one cortical region with expansion to contiguous regions or "migrating" independently to different areas of the same or opposite hemisphere, so that on one recording, there were sequential shifting areas of ictal onset between hemispheres or overlapping seizures with different areas of onset. Clinically, patients may have unilateral focal tonic or clonic activity that can evolve to the contralateral side over the course of the seizure, lateral eye gaze/head deviation, or maybe autonomic (drooling, flushing, and apnea). *Status epilepticus* is common. Myoclonic seizures are typically exclusionary. Although originally described as rare, several recent reports suggest that hysparrhythmia and burst suppression EEG patterns can occur in cases of EIMFS but are not common.

Imaging can be normal, but over time there may be diffuse cerebral atrophy with increased extra-axial fluid. Pathology shows hippocampal gliosis and neuronal loss, and delayed myelination with white matter hyperintensity. There are also decreased *N-acetyl aspartate* peaks on MRI spectroscopy.

Originally, no etiology for EIMFS was identified. More recently, multiple genes have been associated with this phenotype. Therefore, sending an epilepsy panel and/or whole exome sequencing is warranted. Ultimately, understanding the genetic basis of EIMFS (see Neurobiology/Pathophysiology for more details) will open the door toward more targeted or precision therapies.

TREATMENT STRATEGY

The great majority of cases of EIMFS have drug-resistant epilepsy. Seizure control or seizure reduction has been reported in select cases with levetiracetam, cannabidiol, adrenocorticotropic hormone (ACTH), rufinamide, ketogenic diet in combination with topiramate and prednisolone, lacosamide, topiramate, oxcarbazepine, phenytoin, and vigabatrin. High doses of potassium bromide are reported to be effective in a handful of patients, either in isolation or in conjunction with ketogenic diet or other ASMs (topiramate, clonazepam, and stiripentol), but its use is limited by skin toxicity (bromoderma) and sedation.

LONG-TERM OUTCOME

The prognosis for EIMFS is poor. Clinically, patients with EIMFS may be normal appearing or with low tone at birth but go on to develop abnormal neurological features during the first year of life including axial hypotonia, spasticity, and intellectual disability. Postnatal acquired microcephaly with a reduction of the circumference up to two standard deviations can occur by the first year of life. Infants can also have gut motility disorders and movement disorders including dystonia leading to scoliosis, choreoathetosis, and acute dyskinesia.

While seizures decrease in frequency with age, patients rarely become seizure free. During seizure-free periods, patients may advance in developmental milestones but may decline during periods of increased seizure frequency. There are reports of select patients who have less severe long-term outcomes of only borderline intellectual disability following a plateau period during the intractable phase or rarely have a largely normal outcome.

Nevertheless, the long-term outcome for most children remains poor with pharmaco-resistant seizures, intellectual disability, and early death with reports of mortality rates ranging 17%–50%. In a recent study of 14 patients, 57% (8/14) of patients died between 2 and 9 years of age with median age of death at 2 years and 7 months from complications of infections and respiratory insufficiency.

PATHOPHYSIOLOGY/NEUROBIOLOGY OF DISEASE

There is no singular underlying cause of EIFMS. Instead, this syndrome may represent a heterogenous encephalopathy with more than one etiology. Likely, the greatest advancement in understanding the neurobiology of this syndrome is the association with several *de novo*/mosaic variant genetic mutations with up to 33 pathogenic gene variants identified as of 2019. In one study of 135 patients, up to 69% had a pathogenic association with the most frequent being *KCNT1* (27%) and *SCN2A* (7%). Other genes associated with this syndrome include *SCN1A*, *SCN2A*, *SLC12A5*, *SLC25A22*, *BRAT1*, *PLCB1*, and *TBC1D24*.

Apart from these known genetic associations, cases of EIFMS have also been attributed to congenital disorders of glycosylation. Obtaining this genetic information can potentially guide treatment. For example, quinidine, a known sodium channel blocker is a candidate treatment for gain-of-function *KCNT1* mutations in

CLINICAL PEARLS

- EIFMS is a DEE characterized by seizure onset within the first 6 months of life with focal seizures that can be associated with autonomic manifestations arising from both hemispheres and migrating from one cortical region to another.
- Infants may have normal to mildly abnormal development at birth but exhibit psychomotor plateau/decline following seizure onset, manifesting as hypotonia, spasticity, intellectual disability, and postnatal acquired microcephaly.
- Characteristic features of the EEG include an ictal pattern with rhythmic sharp discharges starting from one region and migrating independently to different areas of the same or opposite hemisphere, within the same recording.
- Most cases of EIFMS are resistant to drugs. There may be partial response with several ASMs but no single effective treatment.
- Long-term outcome is poor with drug-resistant seizures, intellectual disability, and early death.
- There is no singular underlying cause, but pathogenic variants have been associated with EIFMS, particularly *KCNT1* and *SCN2A*. Targeted treatment may help to improve the outcome for these patients.

EIFMS, but more studies are needed to validate this as a treatment. Ultimately, these types of data provide a framework for a more tailored therapeutic approach.

SUGGESTED REFERENCES

Barba C., Darra F., Cusmai R., Procopio E., Vici C.D., Keldermans L., Vuillaumier-Barrot S., Lefeber D.J., Guerrini R., CDG Group. Congenital disorders of glycosylation presenting as epileptic encephalopathy with migrating partial seizures in infancy. *Dev Med Child Neurol* 2016;58: 1085–1091.

Burgess R., Wang S., McTague A., Boysen K.E., Yang X., Zeng Q., Myers K.A., Rochtus A., Trivisano M., Gill D.; EIMFS Consortium, Sadleir L.G., Specchio N., Guerrini R., Marini C., Zhang Y.H., Mefford H.C., Kurian M.A., Poduri A.H., Scheffer I.E. The genetic landscape of epilepsy of infancy with migrating focal seizures. *Ann Neurol* 2019;86: 821–31.

Caraballo R.H., Fontana E., Darra F., Cassar L., Negrini F., Fiorini E., Arroyo H., Ferraro S., Fejerman N., Dalla Bernardina B. Migrating focal seizures in infancy: Analysis of the electroclinical patterns in 17 patients. *J Child Neurol* 2008;23: 497–506.

Coppola G., Plouin P., Chiron C., Robain O., Dulac O. Migrating partial seizures in infancy: A malignant disorder with developmental arrest. *Epilepsia* 1995;36: 1017–24.

Gross-Tsur V., Ben-Zeev B., Shalev R.S. Malignant migrating partial seizures in infancy. *Pediatr Neurol* 2004;31:287–90.

Hmaimess G., Kadhim H., Nassogne M.C., Bonnier C., van Rijckevorsel K. Levetiracetam in a neonate with malignant migrating partial seizures. *Pediatr Neurol* 2006;34: 55–59.

Marsh E., Melamed S.E., Barron T., Clancy, R.R. Migrating partial seizures in infancy: expanding the phenotype of a rare seizure syndrome. *Epilepsia* 2005;46: 568–72.

McTague A., Appleton R., Avula S., Cross J.H., King M.D., Jacques T.S., Bhate S., Cronin A., Curran A., Desurkar A., Farrell M.A., Hughes E., Jefferson R., Lascelles K., Livingston J., Meyer E., McLellan A., Poduri A., Scheffer I.E., Spinty S., Kurian M.A., Kneen R. Migrating partial seizures of infancy: Expansion of the electroclinical, radiological and pathological disease spectrum. *Brain* 2013;136: 1578–91.

Milligan C.J., Li M., Gazina E.V., Heron S.E., Nair U., Trager C., Reid C.A., Venkat A., Younkin D.P., Dlugos D.J., Petrovski S., Goldstein D.B., Dibbens L.M., Scheffer I.E., Berkovic S.F., Petrou S. KCNT1 gain of function in 2 epilepsy phenotypes is reversed by quinidine. *Ann Neurol* 2014;75: 581–90.

Okuda K., Yasuhara A., Kamei A., Araki A., Kitamura N., Kobayashi Y. Successful control with bromide of two patients with malignant migrating partial seizures in infancy. *Brain Dev* 2000;22: 56–59.

Poisson K., Wong M., Lee C., Cilio M.R. Response to cannabidiol in epilepsy of infancy with migrating focal seizures associated with KCNT1 mutations: An open-label, prospective, interventional study. *Eur J Paediatr Neurol* 2020;25: 77–81.

Vendrame M., Poduri A., Loddenkemper T., Kluger G., Coppola G., Kothare S.V. Treatment of malignant migrating partial epilepsy of infancy with rufinamide: Report of five cases. *Epileptic Disord* 2011;13: 18–21.

Section III

The Infant

17 Febrile Seizures

Morris H. Scantlebury
University of Calgary

CONTENTS

CASE PRESENTATION

The patient presented to the emergency room at 2 years of age with a 24-hour history of diarrhea. Parents noted he had a tactile temperature, and they gave him acetaminophen. Four hours later mother noticed he was tachypneic and when she picked him up, he was warm, unresponsive with his eyes open and he was limp. Emergency medical services (EMS) was called and, in the ambulance, he developed generalized tonic-clonic shaking. The seizure waxed and waned for 30 minutes without a return to baseline in between. The seizures were finally aborted with multiple (x4) doses of midazolam and fosphenytoin. The patient was tired and sleepy for 4–5 hours postictally. On examination, the patient was febrile (39°C), sleepy but rousable and irritable. The patient moved all limbs symmetrically. A Babinski sign was elicited in the left great toe. His deep tendon reflexes were normal and symmetric. Otherwise, the patient was born to a 30-year-old Gravida 7 Para 1 mother who had 4 elective abortions and one spontaneous abortion due to her father's death. There were no complications during the pregnancy, delivery, or postnatally. The patient had a prior history of a single brief generalized febrile seizure. Family history was notable for the father having had febrile seizures starting around 2 years of age. The patient also had a 9-year-old paternal cousin who was recently diagnosed with epilepsy. The parents are nonconsanguineous. Development was normal. In the hospital, the patient was treated with intravenous fluids and empirically started on meningitic doses of ceftriaxone and vancomycin. The EEG showed focal sharp waves and slowing recorded in the right temporal region (Figure 17.1). The head CT and MRI brain were normal. The cerebral spinal fluid (CSF) analysis did not show abnormalities. The antibiotics were subsequently stopped, and the patient was discharged from hospital within 24 hours. Since discharge, the patient was febrile seizure free

DOI: 10.1201/9781003296478-20

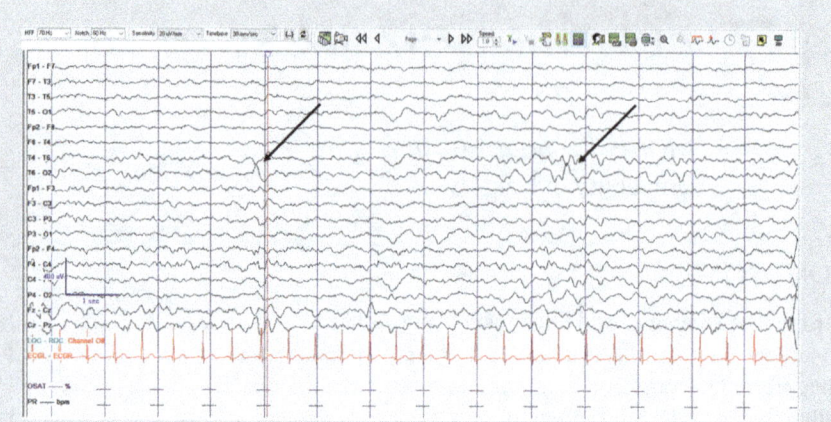

FIGURE 17.1   Bipolar longitudinal montage showing focal sharp waves recorded over the right temporal T6 head region.

until 3 years of age when he represented to the ED following a cluster of three brief febrile seizures in 24 hours. The patient is now 4 years old and has some mild expressive language delays but is otherwise normal. He has not had any further febrile seizures.

DIFFERENTIAL DIAGNOSIS AND DIAGNOSTIC APPROACH

Febrile seizures are the most common seizure disorder to affect children and can either be simple or complex. Simple febrile seizures account for 75% of febrile seizure (FS) and are brief (lasting less than 5 minutes), isolated in 24 hours, and generalized. Complex febrile seizures are either prolonged (>5 minutes), recurrent within 24 hours, or focal or a combination thereof. It is important to make the distinction between simple and complex febrile seizures as simple febrile seizures are most commonly benign whereas complex febrile seizures may have a more guarded outcome regarding the development of brain damage and emergence of epilepsy.

Febrile seizures occur in 2%–5% of the pediatric population in North America, but there is significant geographic variability in its prevalence. The peak age of onset is around 18 months of age. This 2-year-old boy was diagnosed with febrile *status epilepticus* which is a form of complex febrile seizure defined as seizures with fever lasting >30 minutes; ~5% of patients with complex febrile seizures will present as febrile *status epilepticus*.

The American Academy of Pediatrics does not recommend blood testing, imaging, or EEGs in patients with their first simple febrile seizure. The updated guideline recommends lumbar puncture as an option ("consider strongly" was the term used previously) and only in patients unimmunized against *Haemophilus influenzae* type b (Hib) or *Streptococcus pneumoniae*, in whom immunization status cannot be determined and in those patients pretreated with antibiotics. Instead, efforts should be directed at determining the cause of the fever in patients with their first febrile seizure. There is no consensus recommendation for what testing should be done in complex febrile seizures, but it is prudent that every effort should be taken to determine the cause of the complex febrile seizure which may include a full septic work-up, EEG, and imaging (CT and/or MRI brain) where clinically indicated.

TREATMENT STRATEGY

Febrile *status epilepticus* is a neurological emergency as brain damage and epilepsy may ensue which can be mitigated with prompt control of the seizures. Operationally, febrile *status epilepticus* should be considered after a seizure lasting 5 minutes as after this time-point it is less likely for the seizure to stop without intervention. Thus, abortive treatments for febrile seizures lasting ~5 minutes that can be given in the prehospital setting should be prescribed. Many options are available (e.g., sublingual lorazepam, intra-nasal, or buccal midazolam, which are preferred over rectal diazepam because of ease of use and cost). This patient was prescribed sublingual lorazepam.

Should prophylactic treatments be started? Consideration could be given to starting this patient on prophylactic treatments for febrile seizures. However, currently, there are no effective strategies identified that would prevent febrile seizures in children who are ill. Interestingly, tepid sponging and antipyretics to control the fever have not been shown to be effective. Benzodiazepines given for the duration of an illness may be effective, but the risks outweigh the benefits. Other antiseizure medications (ASMs) have not been shown to be particularly effective except for perhaps phenobarbital but the side effects prohibit its use. One placebo-controlled study has supported the use of clobazam. However, one major concern of this study is that the recurrence rates in the control group were extremely high (83%), and therefore, this study requires repeating. Levetiracetam may also have benefits and is probably safe.

Febrile *status epilepticus* is a neurological emergency, and every effort should be taken to promptly abort the seizures to prevent brain damage. Recurrence risks are high and therefore patients with febrile *status epilepticus* should be prescribed abortive treatments. Greater efforts are needed to identify prophylactic treatments for febrile seizures for those at highest risk of having a seizure with every fever.

LONG-TERM OUTCOME

Generally, 30% of patients will have a second febrile seizure after the first one and 50% of these patients will have a third. About 7% of patients with febrile seizures will have three or more seizures. The risk factors for recurrence of febrile seizures are as follows:

- Early age at onset (<1 year).
- First-degree consanguinity of parents.
- Epilepsy in a first-degree relative.
- Initial complex (prolonged) febrile seizure.

Our patient has a family history of epilepsy and a second febrile seizure which was complex; therefore, his risk of recurrence is very high. Luckily, our patient did not have abnormal brain imaging which is a risk factor for recurrent episodes of febrile *status epilepticus*. As febrile seizures occur in children between 3 months and 6 years of age this patient is expected to eventually outgrow this condition.

Will the seizures negatively impact the brain? With simple febrile seizures, it is unlikely the seizures will damage the brain. However, long-term cognitive consequences have been reported with simple febrile seizures in babies less than 1 year. Patients with three or more lifetime simple febrile seizures may have a mildly elevated risk of developing epilepsy. However simple febrile seizures are generally benign, and the parents should be reassured.

In contrast, complex febrile seizures including febrile *status epilepticus* are associated with a high risk of developing brain damage. Approximately 10% of the patients with febrile *status epilepticus* will develop hippocampal abnormalities (atrophy or sclerosis). MRI brain T2 or DWI hyperintense signal and swelling identified acutely in the hippocampus following febrile *status epilepticus* may be predicative of developing irreversible hippocampal injury.

Regarding EEG, focal slowing and attenuation have been correlated with increased hippocampal T2 signal abnormalities, while early development of EEG abnormalities has been found to increase the risk for recurrent non-febrile seizures and epilepsy. The risk of developing epilepsy following complex febrile seizures is 10%–20% as opposed to 2%–7.5% following simple febrile seizures.

PATHOPHYSIOLOGY/NEUROBIOLOGY OF DISEASE

The cause of febrile seizures is poorly understood. The role of ionic channel dysfunction, heat-sensitive ionic channels, inflammation, fever-induced respiratory alkalosis, and abnormal thermoregulation is being actively investigated. Genetic factors likely play a role in this patient with a family history of febrile seizures and epilepsy. However, genetic testing is not routinely recommended in patients with solely febrile seizures as no definitive susceptibility gene for febrile seizures has been identified.

CLINICAL PEARLS

- Febrile seizures are the most common seizure disorder to affect children and occur in 2%–5% of the pediatric population in North America.
- Simple febrile seizures account for 75%.
- Blood testing, imaging, or EEGs are not recommended in patients with their first simple febrile seizure.
- Febrile *status epilepticus* is a neurological emergency, and every effort should be taken to promptly abort the seizures to prevent brain damage. Recurrence risks are high and therefore patients with febrile *status epilepticus* should be prescribed abortive treatments.

Interestingly, the risk factors for febrile *status epilepticus* have not been well studied. Subtle developmental brain abnormalities have been identified in patients with temporal lobe epilepsy and a remote history of febrile *status epilepticus*. Preclinical studies have supported the sequence of preexisting brain lesion, an increased risk of febrile *status epilepticus*, and subsequent development of epilepsy.

SUGGESTED REFERENCES

Berg A.T., Shinnar S. Complex febrile seizures. *Epilepsia* 1996;37: 126–33.

Lewis D.V., Shinnar S., Hesdorffer D.C., Bagiella E., Bello J.A., Chan S., Xu Y., MacFall J., Gomes W.A., Moshé S.L., Mathern G.W., Pellock J.M., Nordli Jr. D.R., Frank L.M., Provenzale J., Shinnar R.C., Epstein L.G., Masur D., Litherland C., Sun S.; FEBSTAT Study Team. Hippocampal sclerosis after febrile status epilepticus: The FEBSTAT study. *Ann Neurol* 2014;75: 178–85.

Nordli Jr. D.R., Moshé S.L., Shinnar S., Hesdorffer D.C., Sogawa Y., Pellock J.M., Lewis D.V., Frank L.M., Shinnar R.C., Sun S.; FEBSTAT Study Team. Acute EEG findings in children with febrile *status epilepticus*: Results of the FEBSTAT study. *Neurology* 2012;79: 2180–6.

Offringa M., Bossuyt P.M., Lubsen J., Ellenberg J.H., Nelson K.B., Knudsen F.U., Annegers J.F., el-Radhi A.S., Habbema J.D., Derksen-Lubsen G., Hauser W.A., Kurland L.T., Banajeh S.M.A., Larsen S. Risk factors for seizure recurrence in children with febrile seizures: A pooled analysis of individual patient data from five studies. *J Pediatr* 1994;124: 574–84.

Offringa M., Newton R., Nevitt S.J., Vraka K. Prophylactic drug management for febrile seizures in children. *Cochrane Database Syst Rev* 2021;6: CD003031.

Scantlebury M.H., Gibbs S.A., Foadjo B., Lema P., Psarropoulou C., Carmant L. Febrile seizures in the predisposed brain: A new model of temporal lobe epilepsy. *Ann Neurol* 2005;58: 41–9.

Subcommittee on Febrile Seizures; American Academy of Pediatrics. Neurodiagnostic evaluation of the child with a simple febrile seizure. *Pediatrics* 2011;127: 389–94.

18 Genetic Epilepsy with Febrile Seizures Plus (GEFS+)

Michaela Castello and Aliya Frederick
UC San Diego School of Medicine

CONTENTS

CASE PRESENTATION

The index patient is a 9-year-old girl with a history of approximately 30 generalized tonic-clonic seizures beginning at 5 months of age. The seizures initially began with fever, but later occurred spontaneously in the absence of fever or intercurrent illness. From 3 to 4 years of age, she experienced absence seizures. An initial EEG demonstrated generalized 3 Hz spike-and-slow-wave discharges. She was given the diagnosis of childhood absence seizures and treated with lamotrigine. Despite adequate doses, she continued to have occasional seizures. A repeat EEG was interpreted as normal. Lamotrigine was discontinued in lieu of valproic acid which made her seizure free. All along, her neurological examination was normal. Interestingly, her family history was positive for seizures in her older brother, who experienced a total of 50 generalized tonic-clonic seizures with and without fever beginning at age 7 months. He also had generalized myoclonic seizures from age 7 months to 3 years. His EEG at age 4 years was notable for mild background slowing, but similar to his younger sister, a repeat study was normal, as was his neurological exam. Notably, other family members experienced seizures with and without fever, including another brother (from 1 to 25 years of age), an aunt, and

DOI: 10.1201/9781003296478-21

two first cousins. One of the aunt's sons was diagnosed with Severe Myoclonic Epilepsy of Infancy (SMEI or Dravet syndrome), while the other had a history of both myoclonic and atonic seizures and was described as having some mild intellectual disability or cognitive delay.

DIFFERENTIAL DIAGNOSIS

The combination of a normal neurological examination, strong positive family history of seizures, and normal or abnormal EEGs with focal or generalized interictal abnormalities suggests a disorder within the spectrum of the genetic epilepsy syndromes. The presence of myoclonic seizures in the patient's brother and the early presentation at age 7 months, however, is not consistent with childhood absence epilepsy, juvenile absence epilepsy, or juvenile myoclonic epilepsy. Furthermore, the diagnosis of SMEI in the cousin suggests a cause other than a simple idiopathic generalized epilepsy syndrome and would be more consistent with the self-limited neonatal-infantile epilepsies.

Genetic Epilepsy with Febrile Seizures Plus (GEFS+) was first described in 1997 by Scheffer and Berkovic, with further revisions to the definition in 2017. GEFS+ has a heterogenous presentation of seizure types with a familial component, most commonly generalized convulsive febrile seizures. In contrast to simple febrile seizures, affected individuals may experience seizures both with and without fever, and seizures persist beyond the age at which simple febrile seizures are expected to remit. They may also exhibit other seizure types including focal, absence, myoclonic, and atonic seizures, and multiple seizure types can be seen within affected families.

In more recent years, GEFS+ has come to be understood as an epilepsy spectrum that includes myoclonic-atonic epilepsy (MAE), severe myoclonic epilepsy of infancy (SMEI or Dravet Syndrome), myoclonic epilepsy of infancy (MEI), and other idiopathic and genetic generalized or focal epilepsies with variable phenotypes. MAE presents between 7 months and 6 years, manifests as myoclonic seizures with an associated atonic component, and has a relatively benign natural history. With MAE, most seizures remit within a few years of onset and upward of 60% of patients are cognitively normal. This is in contrast with SMEI, which presents with prolonged febrile seizures, followed by the development of myoclonic, atypical absence, and sometimes focal-onset seizures associated with variable cognitive decline in the majority of patients.

The EEG background is typically normal in GEFS+. However, focal or generalized interictal epileptiform discharges can occasionally be seen. Brain imaging with magnetic resonance imaging is typically normal. Most patients have a normal neurological examination, except those few with syndromes such as MAE or SMEI, which can be associated with at least some mild degree of encephalopathy. Most patients respond to treatment with antiseizure medications (ASMs) appropriate for generalized epilepsies, including valproic acid, topiramate, lamotrigine, and levetiracetam, although not all patients require treatment. Seizures often remit by puberty.

GEFS+ was initially thought to be inherited in an autosomal dominant manner with variable penetrance. However, we now know that the GEFS+ spectrum of disorders displays a complex inheritance pattern with numerous potential contributory genes. The most commonly known mutations occur in genes encoding subunits of the voltage-gated sodium channel or the ligand-gated GABA$_A$ chloride channel. Sodium channel subunits alpha-1, alpha-2, alpha-9, and beta-1 are often affected (*SCN1A*, *SCN2A*, *SCN9A*, and *SCN1B*, respectively), as are the gamma 2 and delta subunits of the GABA$_A$ channel (*GABRG2* and *GABRD*, respectively). More recently, mutations in syntaxin 1B (*STX1B*), a protein involved in cellular exocytosis, have also been implicated in GEFS+. Pathogenic variants in known GEFS+ genes are identified in one-third of families tested, with 10% of those families harboring variants in *SCN1A*.

DIAGNOSTIC APPROACH

As with all epilepsy syndromes, the history provides important clues for a definitive diagnosis. Seizure types and their age of onset are the most important features, with the presence or absence of family history being especially relevant in GEFS+. Questioning grandparents and more distant relatives can often provide more information about the occurrence of seizures within the family.

Details of cognitive and motor development will help determine whether encephalopathy is present. In GEFS+, the neurological examination is typically normal. An EEG is an essential test, but this may be normal, nonepileptiform (i.e., nonspecific, such as diffuse slowing), or show focal or generalized interictal epileptiform discharges. In patients with simple febrile seizures, a normal EEG is most commonly seen. For those patients with a more severe epilepsy syndrome, such as SMEI, slowing of the background and frequent spike-and-slow-wave discharges are more likely. Neuroimaging usually plays a minor role in the diagnosis of generalized epilepsy and has more utility in focal epilepsies. In the case of patients with GEFS+, brain imaging is usually normal.

Gene tests for the most common mutations associated with GEFS+ are commercially available but given the evolving nature of epilepsy genetics in general, it should be kept in mind that a negative gene test does not rule out the disorder.

TREATMENT STRATEGY

GEFS+ patients with the simple febrile seizure phenotype may not need pharmacotherapy. However, treatment should be considered when afebrile seizures occur, or if febrile seizures are frequent or prolonged and there is a positive family history. The range of treatment options includes chronic daily ASM therapy or abortive medications such as diazepam when seizures occur acutely. Seizures usually respond to ASMs appropriate for generalized epilepsy syndromes. Vagus nerve stimulation or the ketogenic diet may be helpful in selected medically refractory cases. Resective epilepsy surgery is generally not indicated in these patients, although rare individuals with hippocampal sclerosis have been reported in GEFS+ families.

LONG-TERM OUTCOME

The long-term outcome depends upon seizure types, initial presentation, and whether the neurologic examination is normal. Importantly, the specific genetic abnormality may be a critical determinant of the clinical outcome, but no clear genotype/phenotype correlations have been established to date.

Prognosis appears to be related to the actual epilepsy syndrome that the patient exhibits. In the original 1997 report describing a large extended GEFS+ family, most members had benign and self-limited forms of the syndrome, such as febrile seizures persisting beyond the usual age, or febrile seizures with absences. However, one individual had generalized seizures that persisted into middle age and another had severe drug-resistant MAE. As noted previously, SMEI is not a benign disorder, and the majority of such patients have significant cognitive impairment and persistent epilepsy.

PATHOPHYSIOLOGY/NEUROBIOLOGY OF DISEASE

Genetic mutations causing a loss or gain of function are presumed in all cases of GEFS+. Some studies suggest that a mutation in the gamma-2 subunit of the $GABA_A$ receptor leads to a decrease in the inhibitory GABA-induced currents, thus leading to neuronal hyperexcitability. Research involving mutations in genes encoding various subunits of the voltage-gated sodium channel indicates that changes in sodium channel function can range from net increases in inward sodium current (via slowing of inactivation or reduction in the sodium current run-down, seen with *SCN1A* mutations) to a shortening of the refractory period following an action potential (with *SCN1B* mutations).

Gene Name	General Function
SCN1A	Voltage-gated sodium channel
SCN2A	Voltage-gated sodium channel
SCN9A	Voltage-gated sodium channel
SCN1B	Voltage-gated sodium channel
GABRD	$GABA_A$ chloride channel
GABRG2	$GABA_A$ chloride channel
STX1B	Cellular exocytosis

CLINICAL PEARLS

- GEFS+ is a heterogeneous genetic syndrome most often associated with febrile seizures that persist beyond the typical age of remission.
- The diagnosis is suggested on the basis of a strong family history of febrile and afebrile seizures and/or generalized epilepsy, although focal seizures can occur.
- Given the broad spectrum of disease, treatment for GEFS+ should be based on features of the specific epilepsy syndrome affecting the individual.
- Genetic mutations in voltage-gated sodium channels, subunits of $GABA_A$ receptors, and the syntaxin protein have been associated with GEFS+, but the specific type of mutation cannot accurately predict prognosis or response to treatment.

While there remains an absence of clear genotype/phenotype correlations, many of the more benign GEFS+ patients were found to have missense mutations, while the SMEI phenotype was more often associated with truncation defects. Unidentified susceptibility genes probably account for some of the variability and incomplete penetrance is seen in this disorder. This is an evolving area of research, and at present, genotype is not predictive enough of phenotype to be clinically useful. Nevertheless, genetic counseling should be performed in all patients and their families with proven mutations.

SUGGESTED REFERENCES

Audenaert D., Van Broeckhoven C., De Jonghe P. Genes and loci involved in febrile seizures and related epilepsy syndromes. *Hum Mutat* 2006;27: 391–401.

Baulac M., Gourfinkel-An I., Baulac S., Leguern E. Myoclonic seizures in the context of generalized epilepsy with febrile seizures plus (GEFS+). *Adv Neurol* 2005;95: 103–125.

Nakayama J., Arinami T. Molecular genetics of febrile seizures. *Epilepsy Res* 2006;70 (Suppl 1): S190–8.

Scheffer I.D., Berkovic S.F. Generalized epilepsy with febrile seizures plus: A genetic disorder with heterogeneous clinical phenotypes. *Brain* 1997;120: 479–90.

Zhang Y.H., Burgess R., Malone J.P., Glubb G.C., Helbig K.L., Vadlamudi L., Kivity S., Afawi Z., Bleasel A., Grattan-Smith P., Grinton B.E., Bellows S.T., Vears D.F., Damiano J.A., Goldberg-Stern H., Korczyn A.D., Dibbens L.M., Ruzzo E.K., Hildebrand M.S., Berkovic S.F., Scheffer I.E. Genetic epilepsy with febrile seizures plus: Refining the spectrum. *Neurology* 2017;89: 1210–9.

Zuberi S.M., Wirrell E., Yozawitz E., Wilmshurst J.M., Specchio N., Riney K., Pressler R., Auvin S., Samia P., Hirsch E., Galicchio S., Triki C., Snead O.C., Wiebe S., Cross J.H., Tinuper P., Scheffer I.E., Perucca E., Moshé S.L., Nabbout R. ILAE classification and definition of epilepsy syndromes with onset in neonates and infants: Position statement by the ILAE task force on nosology and definitions. *Epilepsia* 2022;63: 1349–97.

19 Myoclonic Epilepsy of Infancy

Douglas R. Nordli, III
Mayo Clinic

Douglas R. Nordli, Jr.
University of Chicago Medicine

CONTENTS

CASE PRESENTATION

A 14-month-old boy presented to the neurology office with the chief complaint of "exaggerated startles" that had been occurring up to 20 times per day. The events began 1 month prior to presentation at the office. A cell phone video was reviewed, which captured the typical events that parents were seeing at home. The video revealed several brief jerks of both arms with upward eye deviation, lasting approximately 2 seconds. The boy was not disturbed by the event and continued to play in his crib. Gestation and birth history were unremarkable, and development has been typical. There was no family history of epilepsy. General physical and neurologic examinations were normal. A routine EEG was performed which captured multiple typical events. The EEG background was normal for age. There were four push button events, which were associated with a burst of diffuse spike-and-wave discharges (Figure 19.1). The discharges lasted approximately 2 seconds and were time locked with bilateral arm jerking and upward eye deviation. The patient rapidly returned to baseline following each event. The video-EEG findings were reviewed with the patient's family who agreed with valproate treatment. An epilepsy next-generation sequencing gene panel was obtained and was unremarkable. After titration to a dose of 30 mg/kg/day, the patient was free of seizures and remained so for the next 2 years. After clinical remission, a repeat

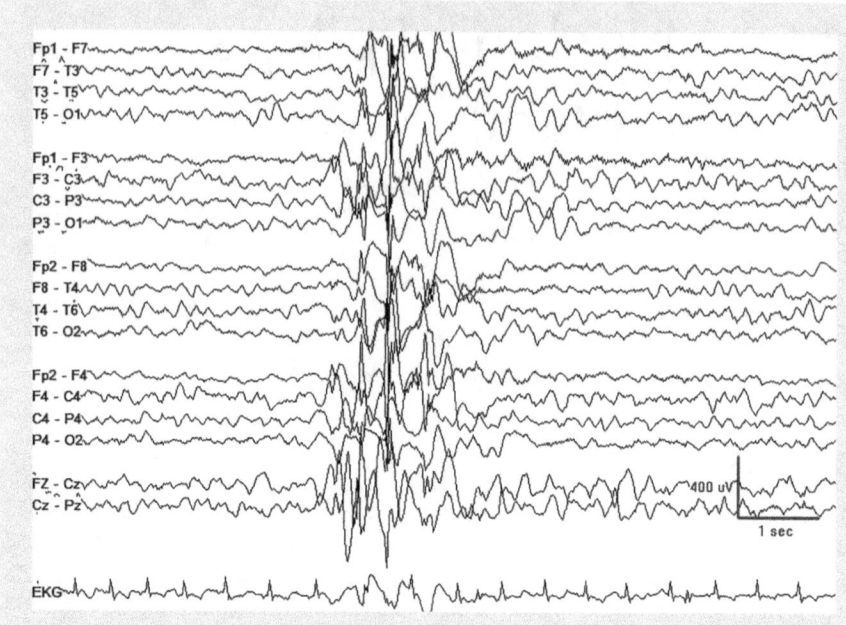

FIGURE 19.1   EEG showing generalized spike-and-wave discharges lasting 1–2 seconds in duration that are time locked with clinical myoclonia on video EEG.

EEG was normal and medication was weaned. On follow-up at 3.5 years of age, he continued to have normal development and had no further seizures off medication.

DIFFERENTIAL DIAGNOSIS

The first consideration when approaching this case should be determining whether the jerks are epileptic in nature. Non-epileptic conditions that mimic myoclonic attacks can often be distinguished from myoclonic epilepsy of infancy (MEI) by a careful history that focuses on time course and a careful description of the events. Hypnic myoclonus must be isolated to sleep and can be excluded if attacks are witnessed during wakefulness. Shuddering attacks may be seen in children as young as 4–6 months of age but are usually characterized by stiffening of the body, adduction of the knees, flexion or extension of the neck, and high-frequency/low-amplitude trembling lasting several seconds. Children with shuddering spells may have a positive family history of essential tremors. Nonepileptic myoclonus can also be seen in association with opsoclonus. However, cases of myoclonus in association with opsoclonus are often progressive and typically begin following the onset of the "dancing" eye movements. Other types of nonepileptic myoclonus, such as those seen in a variety of metabolic and genetic diseases, can be excluded by a normal neurologic examination and developmental assessment.

Once nonepileptic myoclonus has been excluded, an EEG should be obtained. Careful attention should be given to the background of the EEG in addition to any events that are captured. Capturing an event is critical as infants with MEI and other entities within the differential diagnosis may have normal interictal EEGs, at least initially. If there is no EEG correlation, benign infantile myoclonus is the most likely diagnosis, as it is nonepileptic in origin. Infantile spasms may be confused with myoclonic events but can usually be distinguished by several important clinical and electrographic features. Spasms usually consist of a more prolonged tonic contracture rather than the lightening jerk of myoclonus, are more often seen upon awakening, and are usually accompanied by hypsarrhythmia and ictal electrodecrements on EEG. Clinically, patients experiencing spasms may sometimes cry in between events and appear to be in discomfort throughout the cluster.

Severe myoclonic epilepsy of infancy (Dravet syndrome) should also be considered in patients with prolonged febrile convulsions followed by afebrile seizures. Although the interictal EEG may be initially normal, epileptiform discharges and background slowing develop over time. Lennox–Gastaut syndrome usually does not present in this age group and is incompatible with preexisting normal development and unremarkable interictal EEG. Progressive myoclonic epilepsies may also be on the differential diagnosis. Careful attention should be given to exaggerated photic responses or epileptiform discharges provoked by low frequency (1–2 Hz) photic stimulation, which are characteristics of neuronal ceroid lipofuscinosis type 2.

DIAGNOSTIC APPROACH

As discussed above, a careful history and neurologic examination is essential for the diagnosis of this syndrome. The most useful supplement to these clinical tools is the video EEG which, will help classify the myoclonus as epileptic and rule out other epilepsy syndromes. The background of the EEG is normal and interictal discharges are uncommon. The myoclonus is associated with generalized spike-and-wave or polyspike-and-wave discharges usually lasting 1–3 seconds. In some patients, the myoclonus is stimulated by intermittent photic stimulation, while reflex myoclonus may be triggered by a loud sound or other stimulus. Neuroimaging is not indicated in typical cases as this is an idiopathic syndrome not associated with structural malformations. Genetic testing may be considered in patients to help narrow the differential diagnosis, especially in atypical cases. The diagnostic yield of genetic testing is typically lower in patients with normal background compared patients with slow EEG

**BOX 19.1   CLINICAL CHARACTERISTICS OF
MYOCLONIC EPILEPSY OF INFANCY**

A. Brief (1–2) seconds of clinical myoclonia
B. Normal development
C. Normal neurologic examination

BOX 19.2   ELECTROENCEPHALOGRAPHIC CHARACTERISTICS OF MYOCLONIC EPILEPSY OF INFANCY

Interictal findings
- None
- Normal EEG background

Ictal findings
- Diffuse or generalized spike and wave discharges lasting 1–2 seconds in duration that are time-locked with clinical myoclonia on video-EEG.

---

backgrounds. No causal mutations of myoclonic epilepsy of infancy have been found with specialty consensus.

TREATMENT STRATEGY

Treatment of myoclonic epilepsy of infancy with antiseizure medications (ASMs) should be offered to families with the knowledge that its ultimate effect on outcome is uncertain. Based on the latest literature, some authors suggest that an earlier onset of seizures and delay of treatment may be associated with poorer outcomes. However, this association has not been borne out in other studies and there is insufficient evidence to conclude that latency to treatment and age of onset are independent predictors of outcome, especially given the broad underlying spectrum of the condition itself.

Although there is no evidence from randomized controlled trials, the first-line agent for treatment is considered to be valproic acid. Seizure freedom rates using valproic acid range from 77% to 95% of patients. Other commonly prescribed treatments include levetiracetam and clobazam. Given this natural history, adequate monotherapy trials with monitoring of blood levels should be documented before additional agents are added. Routine follow-up should be scheduled to monitor the child's development and screen for other seizure types regardless of whether treatment is pursued. Although isolated reflex myoclonic seizures do not represent a distinct syndrome, the cognitive outcome may be more benign. Therefore, these seizures are often not treated with an ASM.

There is no current consensus regarding the length of treatment for MEI. Most of the published literature recommends a treatment course of several years after which medication can be tapered if the patient has remained seizure free. Patients with isolated reflex myoclonic seizures may avoid treatment altogether or be tapered after a shorter seizure-free interval of 1 year.

LONG-TERM OUTCOME

Myoclonic epilepsy of infancy was once termed benign myoclonic epilepsy of infancy. However, some patients do not achieve remission of epilepsy and have associated

CLINICAL PEARLS

- Benign myoclonic epilepsy of infancy should be considered when a normally developing child between the age of 6 months and 3 years presents with myoclonus during wakefulness.
- A family history of seizures is seen in an estimated 30%–50% of patients and children may often have a preceding history of febrile seizures.
- The EEG demonstrates generalized spike-and-wave discharges associated with the myoclonic seizures, but the background is normal.
- Despite its name, this disorder can be associated with cognitive impairment, neuropsychiatric disturbances, and seizures that require ongoing treatment.

neurodevelopmental delays. Hence, the word "benign" was dropped from the diagnosis. The incidence of neuropsychiatric disturbances in these children ranges from 21% to 58%. In addition to cognitive disturbances, other neurologic abnormalities have been reported, including fine motor deficits, hyperkinesias, attentional deficits, and behavioral problems. Ten reported cases of purely reflex myoclonic epilepsy in one review had normal outcomes.

The prognosis for long-term seizure control is more encouraging with remission seen in the vast majority of cases. Recurrence of seizures has been reported with a frequency of approximately 18% of published cases, and most often consists of generalized tonic-clonic seizures. In patients with marked photosensitivity, the recurrence risk seems to be higher and more prolonged treatment may therefore be advisable.

PATHOPHYSIOLOGY/NEUROBIOLOGY OF DISEASE

The underlying basis of this disorder is not known. There is most likely some genetic contribution as approximately 50% of cases report a family history of epilepsy or febrile seizures.

SUGGESTED REFERENCES

Auvin S., Pandit F., De Bellecize J., et al. Benign myoclonic epilepsy in infants: Electroclinical features and long-term follow-up of 34 patients. *Epilepsia* 2006;47: 387–93.

Balasundaram P., Anilkumar A.C. Myoclonic epilepsy of infancy. [Updated 2022 May 15]. In: *StatPearls [Internet]*. Treasure Island (FL): StatPearls Publishing, 2022. Available from: https://www.ncbi.nlm.nih.gov/books/NBK570566/

Dravet C., Bureau M. Benign myoclonic epilepsy in infancy. In: Roger J., Bureau M., Dravet C., Genton P., Tassinari C.A., Wolf P. (Eds), *Epileptic Syndromes in Infancy, Childhood and Adolescence*, 4th edition. Surrey: John Libbey Eurotext: 2005, pp. 77–88.

Lombroso C.T., Fejerman N. Benign myoclonus of early infancy. *Ann Neurol* 1977;1: 138–43.

Mangano S., Fontana A., Cusumano L. Benign myoclonic epilepsy in infancy: Neuropsychological and behavioural outcome. *Brain Dev* 2005;27: 218–23.

Zuberi S.M., Wirrell E., Yozawitz E., Wilmshurst J.M., Specchio N., Riney K., Pressler R., Auvin S., Samia P., Hirsch E., Galicchio S., Triki C., Snead O.C., Wiebe S., Cross J.H., Tinuper P., Scheffer I.E., Perucca E., Moshé S.L., Nabbout R. ILAE classification and definition of epilepsy syndromes with onset in neonates and infants: Position statement by the ILAE Task Force on Nosology and Definitions. *Epilepsia* 2022;63: 1349–97.

20 Dravet Syndrome

Douglas R. Nordli, III
Mayo Clinic

Douglas R. Nordli, Jr.
University of Chicago Medicine

CONTENTS

CASE PRESENTATION

A 10-month-old boy was seen in neurological consultation for epilepsy of 3-month duration. When he was 6-month old, he had a prolonged right hemi-body febrile convulsion following routine immunizations. One month later, he was admitted to the hospital after a 10-minute afebrile seizure characterized by diffuse clonus. This was aborted with rectal diazepam. Development, general physical, and neurologic examinations at 7 months of age were all normal. A prolonged EEG did not record any seizures but posterior inter-ictal epileptiform discharges were present (Figure 20.1). He was prescribed levetiracetam 30 mg/kg/day. Three months later, he began to have prominent myoclonia, which persisted despite escalating doses of levetiracetam, and his parents reported little developmental progress. An epilepsy next generation sequencing (NGS) gene panel was ordered.

DOI: 10.1201/9781003296478-23

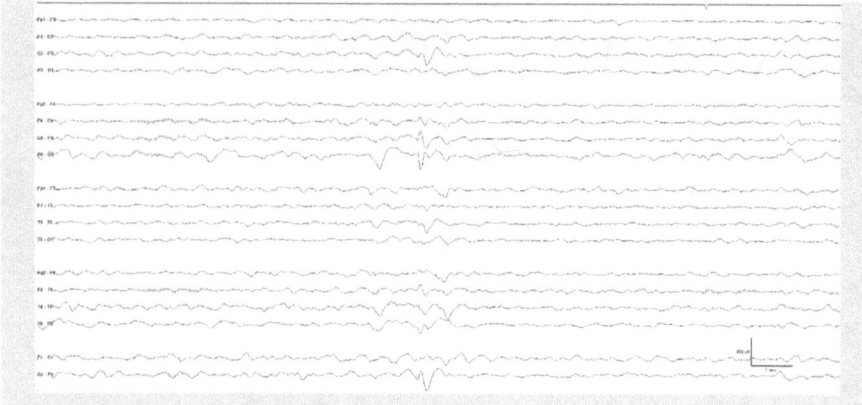

FIGURE 20.1 EEG showing left hemisphere attenuation including reduced amplitude of sleep spindles. There is a right parietal sharp wave seen in the middle of the page. Posterior quadrant epileptiform discharges are present.

DIFFERENTIAL DIAGNOSIS AND DIAGNOSTIC APPROACH

The differential diagnosis for the patient in this case can be approached in several different ways. One typical method is to consider electroclinical syndromes that present in infancy with prominent myoclonic seizures. These include myoclonic epilepsy of infancy, Dravet syndrome, and epilepsy with myoclonic-atonic seizures. The presence of other seizure types, developmental delay, and prominent interictal epileptiform discharges argue against the diagnosis of myoclonic epilepsy of infancy. Typically, no other seizure types other than myoclonia are seen with myoclonic epilepsy of infancy and the diffusely distributed spike-wave discharges are seen only in association with the myoclonia. Epilepsy with myoclonic-atonic seizures usually begins after 1 year of age and there have been no sudden drops following the myoclonia, which is the prototypic seizure for that condition. Severe myoclonic epilepsy of infancy, or Dravet syndrome, is an epilepsy with myoclonus of infancy that contains all the clinical features mentioned in the case.

Another way to approach the patient is to consider possible conditions that could cause a developmental and epileptic encephalopathy (DEE). Classic epileptic encephalopathies as conceptualized by Ohtahara include conditions where the epilepsy itself dramatically contributes to the developmental abnormalities and therefore requires urgent recognition and treatment. A phrase that is borrowed from adult vascular neurologists is "time is brain" in these epilepsies.

Syndromes presenting in infancy in this spectrum include early-infantile developmental and epileptic encephalopathy (EIDEE; this syndrome now includes patients with Ohtahara syndrome and early myoclonic encephalopathy), infantile epileptic spasms syndrome (IESS, which includes West syndrome), and later-onset epileptic encephalopathies. In these disorders, tonic, infantile spasms, and myotonic or spasm-tonic seizures, respectively, are prominent. These are all lacking in the current case.

Also, the EEG background with each of these syndromes shows more prominent multifocal epileptiform discharges, disorganization, and discontinuity, effectively excluding all of these conditions.

Other DEE syndromes could be considered classic epileptogenic encephalopathies where the epilepsy does not clearly contribute to the developmental impairment. One well-recognized syndrome is epilepsy of infancy with migrating focal seizures, but this is excluded by the absence of abundant electrographic ictal events and the lack of earlier encephalographic features. Another well-recognized DEE that presents in infancy is Dravet syndrome, and again prolonged hemi-convulsive seizures with later afebrile seizures and myoclonus are very suggestive.

Within the group of DEEs are other epilepsies that do not necessarily present with named syndromes and are referred to as "nonsyndromic epilepsies". There are many metabolic and genetic disorders within this category and an increasing number has modern treatment implications. Thankfully, most of the metabolic disorders presenting in infancy with seizures that can benefit from immediate treatment can be identified through modern newborn screening. Other conditions can be suspected using simple serum laboratory tests such as glucose, lactate, and ammonia. The largest groups are covered under commercially available NGS epilepsy gene panels. The remaining few conditions can be revealed by selective urinary analyses. If clinically appropriate, treatment with pyridoxine should be initiated pending the results of these diagnostic tests.

Some of these disorders have specific treatments aimed at correcting the enzyme deficiency or changing the consequences of the genetic perturbations. Neuronal ceroid lipofuscinosis (NCL) is one such condition; however, in the current case, there is no progressive microcephaly or optic involvement. Glucose transporter type 1 (GLUT-1) deficiency syndrome, or De Vivo disease can be treated with the ketogenic diet and therefore should always be considered when an infantile DEE is suspected. NGS epilepsy gene panels will reveal a pathogenic variant in *SLC2A1* gene in the vast majority of affected patients, but it is important to recall that about 10% will be missed and therefore a lumbar puncture should be performed if the clinical and EEG features are suggestive.

Finally, a very straightforward and efficient way to approach this case is to consider the interictal EEG features. Tracings that show background slowing with multifocal pleomorphic epileptiform activity are consistent with epilepsies associated with encephalopathy, or DEE. A very simple rule of thumb is to consider diagnostic NGS epilepsy panel testing when patients present early in life, have background EEG slowing and lack any historic or imaging features to suggest an alternative etiology.

TREATMENT STRATEGY

The treatment strategy for Dravet syndrome is rapidly evolving. Historically, treatment has been focused predominantly on diminishing seizure burden and length, typically using more than one medication. In years passed, medications such as valproic acid, clobazam, and stiripentol were widely recommended. Newly approved agents such as fenfluramine and cannabidiol have shown efficacy in both human and animal studies.

Treatment of convulsive seizures may help to lower the risk of sudden unexplained death in epilepsy (SUDEP). Given the high predisposition for status epilepticus, an emergency rescue plan should be provided for all patients. In addition, drugs that inhibit voltage-gated sodium channel function should be used with caution in Dravet syndrome. These drugs are classically contraindicated unless there is a proven gain of function mutation in a sodium channel causing Dravet syndrome. Given that the major of mutations represent loss of function, further inhibiting the few functioning sodium channels is theoretically problematic. The contraindication in use of sodium channel drugs does not apply to patients in status epilepticus unless there is historical information to suggest otherwise. Currently, an antisense oligonucleotide is being studied that increases the number of functioning sodium channels in the brain, which may in the future dramatically change the treatment and outcome of Dravet syndrome.

LONG-TERM OUTCOME

Most children with Dravet syndrome will face intellectual challenges in their lives after seizure onset and are unlikely to live independently. There is a significant risk of SUDEP with approximately 10%–20% of patients passing away before adulthood. Seizure burden does improve over time as patients transition into adulthood.

PATHOPHYSIOLOGY/NEUROBIOLOGY OF DISEASE

Dravet syndrome is predominantly the result of loss-of-function sodium channel mutations in the brain, specifically involving *SCN1A*. Involved sodium channels impact small fast-spiking, parvalbumin-positive interneurons and lead to reduced inhibition onto pyramidal cells.

CLINICAL PEARLS

- Dravet syndrome should be considered in infants and young children presenting with unprovoked afebrile seizures, history of febrile seizures, and developmental delay. Presence of myoclonus increases the possibility of Dravet syndrome or an epileptic encephalopathy.
- Typical EEG shows spike-and-slow wave discharges and background slowing.
- Mutations that cause Dravet syndrome are the result of SCN1A pathogenic variants.
- The use of sodium channel-blocking drugs should be used with extreme caution in most patients with Dravet syndrome.
- Patients with Dravet syndrome face long-term challenges with seizure control and intellectual functioning. Patients with Dravet syndrome are at higher risk of status epilepticus and SUDEP.

SUGGESTED REFERENCES

Chiron C., Dulac O. The pharmacologic treatment of Dravet syndrome. *Epilepsia* 2011;52: 72–5.

Cooper M.S., Mcintosh A., Crompton D.E., McMahon J.M., Schneider A., Farrell K., Ganesan V., Gill D., Kivity S., Lerman-Sagie T., McLellan A., Pelekanos J., Ramesh V., Sadleir L., Wirrell E., Scheffer I.E. Mortality in Dravet syndrome. *Epilepsy Res* 2016;128: 43–7.

Dravet C. Dravet syndrome history. *Dev Med Child Neurol* 2011;53(Suppl 2): 1–6.

Dravet C. The core Dravet syndrome phenotype. *Epilepsia* 2011;52(Suppl 2): S3–S9.

Marini C., Scheffer I.E., Nabbout R., Suls A., De Jonghe P., Zara F., Guerrini R. The genetics of Dravet syndrome. *Epilepsia* 2011;52(Suppl 2): S24–S9.

Scheffer I.E. Diagnosis and long-term course of Dravet syndrome. *Eur J Paediatr Neurol* 2012;16(Suppl 1): S5–8.

Steel D., Symonds J.D., Zuberi S.M., Brunklaus A. Dravet syndrome and its mimics: Beyond SCN1A. *Epilepsia* 2017;58(11): 1807–16.

Ohtahara S., Yamatogi Y. Epileptic encephalopathies in early infancy with suppression-burst. *J Clin Neurophysiol* 2003;20: 398–407.

21 Glucose Transporter-1 Deficiency Syndrome

Joerg Klepper
Children's Hospital Aschaffenburg

CONTENTS

CASE PRESENTATION

A 6-month-old healthy boy presented with a prolonged generalized, nonfebrile convulsion. In the hospital, electroencephalography (EEG) showed prominent epileptiform activity with generalized high-amplitude sharp waves. Family history was negative for epilepsy, but parents reported paroxysmal eye–head movements at 2 months of age. Recurrent seizures and pathological EEG changes prompted treatment with valproic acid and eventually levetiracetam which proved ineffective. Gradual global developmental delay and a complex movement disorder with ataxia, dystonia, and mild spasticity emerged which led to a diagnostic workup at the age of 1 year. Brain imaging was normal, but lumbar puncture showed low glucose concentrations in the cerebrospinal fluid (CSF) with low CSF lactate. A diagnosis of Glut1 Deficiency Syndrome (Glut1DS) was made and a classical 3:1 ketogenic diet was initiated. Seizures stopped with the onset of ketosis and his antiseizure medication (ASM) was eventually tapered off. The diagnosis was confirmed by genetic analysis showing a heterozygous pathogenic SLC2A1-variant.

DIFFERENTIAL DIAGNOSIS

The biochemical hallmark of Glut1DS is *hypoglycorrhachia* (low CSF glucose) in the setting of low-to-normal CSF lactate and normal blood glucose concentrations. Conditions with hypoglycorrhachia are listed in Table 21.1.

DOI: 10.1201/9781003296478-24

TABLE 21.1

Differential Diagnosis of Hypoglycorrhachia

	Blood	CSF			
Condition	Glucose	Glucose	Lactate	Cell Count	Protein
Glut1DS	N	⇩	(⇩)	N	N
Subarachnoid hemorrhage	N	⇩	(⇩)	RBCs	N
Mitochondrial disorder	N	⇩	⇧	N	N
Hypoglycemia	⇩	⇩	N	N	N
Meningitis (bacterial)	N	⇩	⇧	⇧	⇧
Meningitis (viral)	N	(⇩)	N	⇧	(⇧)

Also consider Glut1DS in

- All causes of neonatal seizures and of acquired microcephaly.
- Cryptogenic epileptic encephalopathies with developmental delays.
- Familial epilepsies with autosomal dominant transmission.
- Episodes of paroxysmal neurologic dysfunction responsive to carbohydrate intake.
- Movement disorders (constant or paroxysmal) including dystonia.

DIAGNOSTIC APPROACH

Glut1DS features three basic diagnostic elements: (1) phenotype (epilepsy, movement disorder, developmental delay), (2) genotype (pathogenic variants in *SLC2A1*), and (3) hypoglycorrhachia:

1. Paroxysmal eye–head movements in infants are often the first clinical feature and are considered specific for Glut1DS. Most patients present with seizures within the first 6 months of infancy, followed by global developmental delay and a complex movement disorder with dystonic, ataxic, and spastic elements. Children develop paroxysmal exertion-induced dystonic episodes (PED), often enhanced during puberty. In adolescents and adults impaired speech and dystonia are the predominant impairments of life quality and difficult to treat with ketogenic diets.
2. *SLC2A1* variants are mostly *de novo*, heterozygous and transmitted in an autosomal dominant manner. Deletions and nonsense mutations apparently cause a more severe phenotype. Glut1DS results not from a specific single variant, but from multiple variants with certain "hot spots". In approximately 5%–10% of patients, no variants can be identified (*SLC2A1*-negative).
3. CSF glucose is mostly referred to as being abnormal below 2.2 or 2.5 mmol/L (40 or 45 mg/dL). For the diagnosis of Glut1DS, it is essential to perform the lumbar puncture following a 4–6 hours fast to obtain results under a glucose steady-state condition, to apply age-specific reference values, and to obtain a simultaneous blood glucose level to calculate a CSF/blood glucose ratio

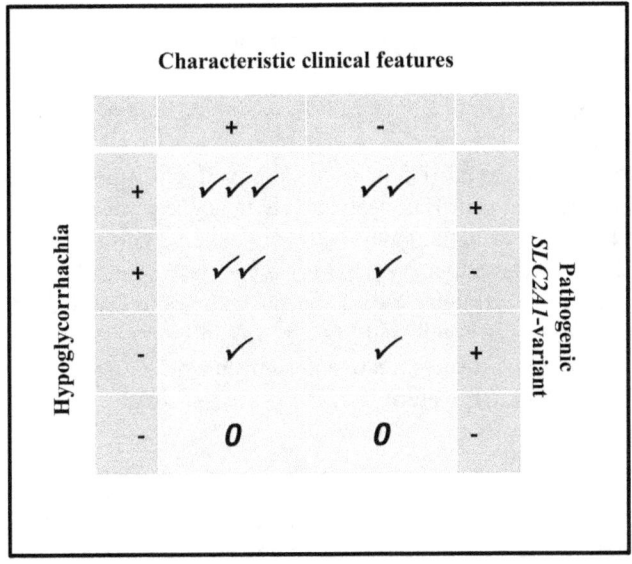

Symbol	diagnosis of Glut1DS	start KDT
✓✓✓	confirmed	yes
✓✓	probable	yes
✓	possible	consider
0	negative	not required

FIGURE 21.1 Consensus recommendation for Glut1DS diagnosis based on three key diagnostic criteria: characteristic clinical features, definite hypoglycorrhachia, and pathogenic *SLC2A1* variants. Reprinted with permission from Klepper et al., *Epilepsia Open* 2020;5: 354–65.

before the lumbar puncture to avoid stress-induced hyperglycemia. The combination of these three elements stratifies Glut1DS as confirmed, probable, or possible (see Figure 21.1).

TREATMENT STRATEGY

A classic ketogenic diet remains the only effective treatment. In contrast to ketogenic diets for childhood epilepsies, ketosis should be maintained as high as possible to provide the maximum fuel for the developing brain. In infants 0–2 years of age, a 3:1 classical ketogenic diet is mandatory. For adolescents and adults, a modified Atkins diet (MAD) offers a good alternative to maintain ketosis. Ketogenic diets are required throughout puberty into adulthood, and presumably for life. Supplements including multivitamins, minerals, calcium and vitamin D, and often carnitine are essential. Symptomatic support (physio-/speech therapy) is warranted. Some patients require additional antiseizure medications (ASMs) despite adequate ketosis, but currently, no

---

CLINICAL PEARLS

- Consider Glut1DS in any child with undefined epilepsy or movement disorder.
- Always consider Glut1DS in isolated low CSF glucose concentrations.
- Remember that Glut 1DS is effectively treatable given the following:
  a. There is a clear pathophysiology: impaired glucose transport into brain causes a brain "energy crisis".
  b. There is a straightforward diagnosis: isolated low CSF glucose (hypoglycorrhachia) and *SLC2A1* variants.
  c. There is an effective treatment: ketogenic diets providing an alternative fuel to the brain.

---

specific recommendations can be given. For potential treatment strategies such as gene/protein replacement or small molecules/biologicals, see Tang et al. (2019).

LONG-TERM OUTCOME

Glut1DS is not a neurodegenerative disease, but long-term data on Glut1DS or ketogenic diet treatments are limited. Symptoms change with age – in infants seizures predominate, in toddlers developmental delay, and a movement disorder. Beyond puberty paroxysmal exertion-induced dystonia (PED) emerges and epilepsy becomes less of an issue. In adults, the phenotypic spectrum and the effects of ketogenic diets is yet undefined.

PATHOPHYSIOLOGY/NEUROBIOLOGY OF DISEASE

Glucose is the essential fuel for the brain. Transport across the blood–brain barrier is exclusively facilitated by the GLUT1 transporter. Consequently, Glut1DS causes neuroglycopenia, e.g., an "energy crisis" in brain resulting in impaired brain angiogenesis, clinical symptoms, and hypoglycorrhachia in the CSF. Ketogenic diets bypass the defect by offering ketones that enter the brain through the MCT transporters and serve as an alternative fuel to the developing brain.

SUGGESTED REFERENCES

Alter A.S., Engelstad K., Hinton V.J., Montes J., Pearson T.S., Akman C.I., De Vivo D.C. Long-term clinical course of Glut1 deficiency syndrome. *J Child Neurol* 2015;30: 160–9.

Klepper J., Akman C., Armeno M., Auvin S., Cervenka M., Cross H.J., De Giorgis V., Della Marina A., Engelstad K., Heussinger N., Kossoff E.H., Leen W.G., Leiendecker B., Monani U.R., Oguni H., Neal E., Pascual J.M., Pearson T.S., Pons R., Scheffer I.E., Veggiotti P., Willemsen M., Zuberi S.M., De Vivo D.C. Glut1 Deficiency Syndrome (Glut1DS): State of the art in 2020 and recommendations of the international Glut1DS study group. *Epilepsia Open* 2020;5: 354–65.

Leen W.G., Wevers R.A., Kamsteeg E.J., Scheffer H., Verbeek M.M., Willemsen M.A. Cerebrospinal fluid analysis in the workup of GLUT1 deficiency syndrome: A systematic review. *JAMA Neurol* 2013;70: 1440–4.

Leen W.G., de Wit C.J., Wevers R.A., van Engelen B.G., Kamsteeg E.J., Klepper J., Verbeek M.M., Willemsen M.A. Child neurology: Differential diagnosis of a low CSF glucose in children and young adults. *Neurology* 2013:81: e178–81.

Tang M., Park S.H., De Vivo D.C., Monani U.R. Therapeutic strategies for glucose transporter 1 deficiency syndrome. *Ann Clin Transl Neurol* 2019:6: 1923–32.

Wang D., Pascual J.M., De Vivo D. Glucose transporter type 1 deficiency syndrome. In: Adam M.P., Ardinger H.H., Pagon R.A., Wallace S.E., Bean L.J.H., Gripp K.W., Amemiya A., editors. *GeneReviews® [Internet]*. Seattle, WA: University of Washington, Seattle 2002 (updated 2018): 1993–2022.

22 Infantile Epileptic Spasms Syndrome

Shaun A. Hussain

UCLA Mattel Children's Hospital and
David Geffen School of Medicine

CONTENTS

CASE PRESENTATION

A 9-month-old girl presented with unusual spells at 7 months of age. Her past history was unremarkable; she was born at term with no pre-, peri-, or postnatal complications. There was no family history of seizures, epilepsy, or neurologic phenomena in youth. Her developmental course was normal at 6 months of age; she was socially engaging, babbling, rolling, scooting, reaching for, and transferring objects between hands. However, since that visit, she seems socially disengaged and her babbling became less robust. There has been no recent illness or infection. Parents described behavioral spells, which began 2 weeks prior to presentation, which occurred daily, several minutes after awakening in the morning. Each event was described as a sudden and brief (approximately 1-second duration) jerk with symmetric extension of both arms, anterior flexion of the neck, and wide opening of the eyes. These jerks tended to repeat in a sequence, recurring every 5–15 seconds, typically over a span of approximately 5 minutes. After each jerk, she would cry for several seconds. Parents reported that she has been generally irritable. On physical examination, vital signs and anthropomorphic measures are normal. General physical examination is unremarkable, excepting the dermatologic exam, which reveals multiple hypopigmented ovoid macules, each 0.5–1.5 cm in diameter, scattered across the trunk and extremities. Comprehensive neurological examination is normal, although she is noted to prefer reaching for objects with her left hand. To

DOI: 10.1201/9781003296478-25

characterize the early-morning events of concern, long-term video-EEG monitoring was performed and demonstrated hypsarrhythmia, manifested by high-voltage (nonepileptiform slow waves with amplitude consistently in the range of 150–250 μV) and abundant multifocal epileptiform discharges, the latter most prominent in the left frontocentral region. Each clinical jerk was accompanied on EEG by a generalized, high-amplitude, and sharply-contoured slow-wave, followed by a generalized relative attenuation of the background lasting 1 second. Each event was thus classified as an epileptic spasm. Brain MRI was performed and revealed numerous cortical tubers throughout the cerebrum, including a rather large (2 cm) tuber along the left frontal convexity, as well as multiple bilateral subependymal nodules along the margins of the lateral ventricles. Genetic testing, via an epilepsy gene panel, identified a heterozygous pathogenic variant in the TSC2 gene. An electroclinical diagnosis of infantile epileptic spasms syndrome (IESS) was substantiated by the history and EEG, and an underlying etiology of tuberous sclerosis complex (TSC) was suggested by dermatologic exam (ash-leaf spots) and confirmed by the radiologic and genetic investigations mentioned above.

DIFFERENTIAL DIAGNOSIS

The typical age of onset of IESS is from 1 to 24 months. The epileptic spasms (seizures) of IESS usually manifest as brief (1–2 seconds), symmetrical contractions of the extremities (arms > legs) and axial musculature (flexion, extension, or both). Asymmetric seizures may occur in the setting of focal structural lesions. The "intensity" of each epileptic spasm ranges from obvious large-amplitude movements to an extremely subtle pause in behavior, sometimes manifesting with only a brief "wide-eyed" stare or subtle head-nod. Within a cluster, there may be a crescendo-decrescendo pattern: at the beginning and end of a cluster, the intensity of each jerk tends to be lower and the interval between events is longer. In contrast, in the middle of a cluster, events tend to be of greater intensity with shorter intervals between events. Although epileptic spasms usually occur in clusters, they may also occur in isolation. Furthermore, whereas epileptic spasms may occur at any time of day, they are by far most frequent upon awakening.

Epileptic spasms are often mistaken for a variety of normal or abnormal infant behaviors, and accordingly, the diagnosis of IESS is often delayed by days, weeks, or even months. The neurological differential diagnosis includes other forms of epilepsy, including benign myoclonic epilepsy of infancy, Ohtahara syndrome (early infantile epileptic encephalopathy), and Dravet syndrome (severe myoclonic epilepsy of infancy). More often, epileptic spasms are confused with (1) episodic, usually postprandial, contortions and crying in the setting of gastroesophageal reflux, (2) benign hypnogogic or hypnopompic jerks (sleep myoclonus), (3) benign myoclonus of infancy, (4) hyperactive Moro response, (5) benign shuddering spells, or (6) infantile colic.

DIAGNOSTIC APPROACH

A diagnosis of IESS is suggested by the clinical history, and in particular, clusters of brief stereotyped movements upon awakening. The definitive diagnosis of IESS requires video-EEG of sufficient duration to both identify epileptic spasms and precisely characterize background epileptiform abnormalities, with hypsarrhythmia being the most common. To identify the underlying etiology of IESS, a general physical examination should include a detailed dermatologic examination to identify various neurocutaneous disorders associated with IESS, especially TSC.

Routine laboratory studies should be conducted to search for infection, although the yield is low. MRI of the brain should be performed promptly to identify structural etiologies of IESS, and if unrevealing or inconclusive, genetic testing should be undertaken to identify the most common genetic etiologies of IESS. The highest yield genetic diagnostic modalities include multiplex epilepsy gene panels and whole exome sequencing, ideally with testing of the child and both parents to maximize the likelihood of identification of rare *de novo* variants.

Chromosomal analysis (i.e., chromosomal microarray) exhibits a lower diagnostic yield, though this may be the most appropriate initial test in a patient with dysmorphic features on physical exam. A variety of metabolic tests may be useful to identify relatively rare causes of IESS. The most common underlying etiologies of IESS include TSC, hypoxic-ischemic encephalopathy, trisomy 21, perinatal stroke/hemorrhage, developmental structural brain malformations (especially focal cortical dysplasia, lissencephaly/pachygyria, polymicrogyria, and absent/dysplastic corpus callosum), Dup15q syndrome, and CDKL5 deficiency disorder.

TREATMENT STRATEGY

Despite substantial historical debate, and highly varied approaches to treatment across centers, there is growing consensus that the most effective therapies include hormonal therapy (high-dose corticosteroids or adrenocorticotropic hormone) or vigabatrin, or both hormonal therapy and vigabatrin administered simultaneously. Perhaps more importantly, given compelling evidence linking treatment delay to adverse long-term developmental outcomes, prompt therapy is essential, at least in the absence of catastrophic developmental status prior to the onset of IESS. Given these data, and the observation that response to most therapies occurs within 1–2 weeks, a systematic treatment protocol is recommended in Figure 22.1.

In case standard therapies fail, there are scant data, and certainly not consensus, to guide the practitioner. Limited data support the use of the ketogenic diet, and an array of anti-seizure medications (ASMs), including benzodiazepines (namely nitrazepam), topiramate, zonisamide, felbamate, rufinamide, and cannabidiol. Among patients with known or suspected focal structural abnormalities (foremost, focal cortical dysplasia), assessment of candidacy for surgical resection is indicated. Similarly, limited data support complete corpus callosotomy for treatment of refractory patients, in some cases as a procedure to aid in the identification of subtle focal cortical dysplasia, and subsequent resection thereof. Lastly, several etiologies should prompt specific therapeutic interventions. These include TSC (for which efficacy of vigabatrin is especially

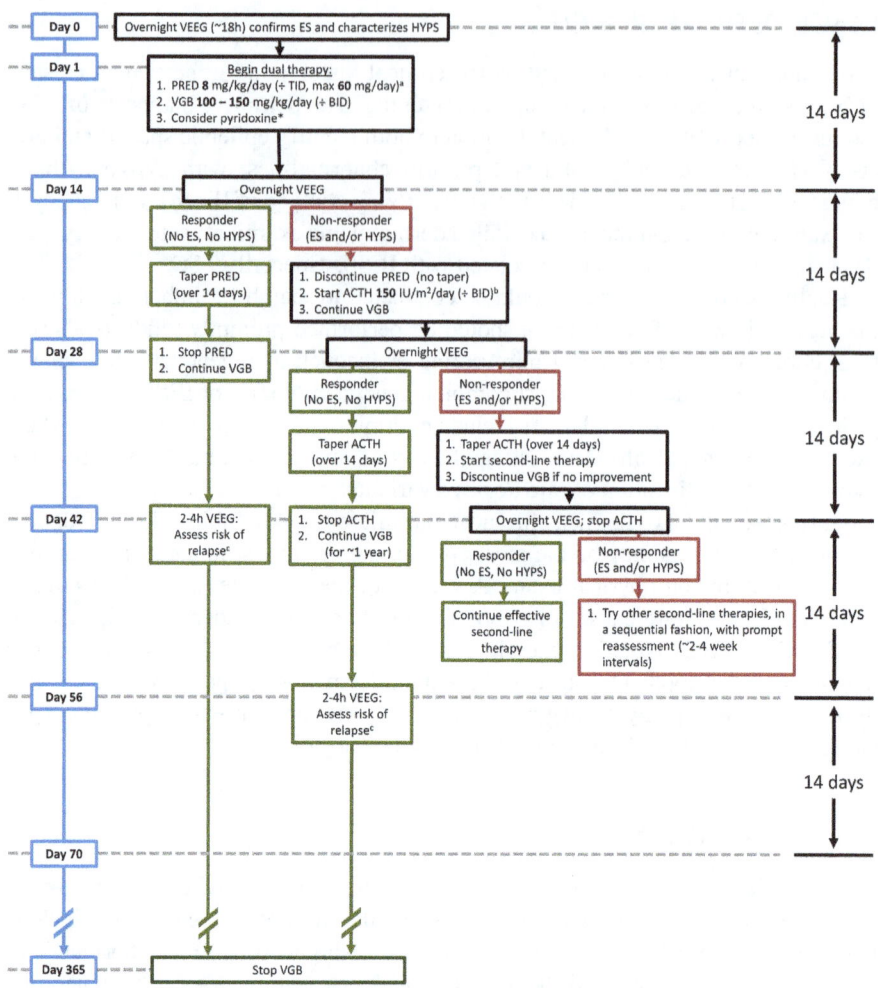

FIGURE 22.1 A proposed treatment protocol for IESS. (a) A weight-independent dosage protocol is a reasonable alternative (i.e., 10 mg four times daily for 1 week, with further titration to 20 mg three times daily among initial nonresponders). (b) If synthetic ACTH is used, the United Kingdom Infantile Spasms Study regimen is suggested (0.5 mg on alternate days for 1 week, with further titration to 0.75 mg on alternate days among initial nonresponders). (c) Relapse risk is associated with multifocal epileptiform discharges on follow-up EEG 1 month after successful treatment. An increasing abundance and multifocality of interictal epileptiform discharges may thus prompt escalation of treatment to reduce relapse risk. Abbreviations: ACTH, adrenocorticotropic hormone; BID, twice-daily administration; ES, epileptic spasms; HYPS, hypsarrhythmia; PRED, prednisolone; TID, thrice-daily administration; VEEG, video-electroencephalogram; VGB, vigabatrin.

TABLE 22.1

Second-Line Therapies for Treatment of IESS

Therapy	Initial Dose	Maximum Maintenance Dose	Minimum Duration of Therapy If No Response	Maximum Duration of Therapy If No Response	Continue Therapy If Response Occurs?
Prednisolone	4–8 mg/kg/day	4–8 mg/kg/day	4 weeks (including 14-day taper)	4 weeks (including 14-day taper)	No
ACTH	150 IU/m² BSA/day	150 IU/m² BSA/day	4 weeks (including 14-day taper)	4 weeks (including 14-day taper)	No
Vigabatrin	50 mg/kg/day	200 mg/kg/day	4 weeks	8 weeks	Yes
Nitrazepam	1 mg/kg/day	10 mg/kg/day	N/A	8 weeks	Yes
Valproic acid	40 mg/kg/day	100 mg/kg/day	N/A	8 Weeks	Yes
Pyridoxine (vitamin B₆)	20 mg/kg/day	50 mg/kg/day	N/A	2 weeks	Yes
Topiramate	10 mg/kg/day	20 mg/kg/day	N/A	8 Weeks	Yes
Zonisamide	10 mg/kg/day	20 mg/kg/day	N/A	8 Weeks	Yes
Rufinamide	10 mg/kg/day	80 mg/kg/day	N/A	8 Weeks	Yes
Felbamate	15 mg/kg/day	80 mg/kg/day	N/A	8 Weeks	Yes
Cannabidiol	5 mg/kg/day	20 mg/kg/day	N/A	8 Weeks	Yes
Intravenous immunoglobulin	400 mg/kg/day × 5 days	400 mg/kg/day × 5 days, every 4–8 weeks	5 days	8 Weeks	Yes
Ketogenic diet	3:1 Ratioᵃ	4:1 Ratioᵃ	3 months	3 months	Yes

ᵃ Ratio refers to the ratio by weight of dietary fat (mg/day) to the sum of dietary carbohydrates and protein (mg/day).

high), pyridoxine (vitamin B6) dependency (treatment with pyridoxine or leucovorin), or pyridoxal-5-phosphate deficiency (treated with pyridoxal-5-phosphate), GLUT1 transporter deficiency syndrome (favorable efficacy of the ketogenic diet), and non-ketotic hyperglycinemia (ameliorated to some extent by sodium benzoate). Table 22.1 summarizes specific therapeutic guidelines for the most common treatments.

The goal of treatment is to quickly eradicate epileptic spasms and the accompanying EEG background abnormalities (hypsarrhythmia and similar) which substantiate the diagnosis. Given this goal, extended (several hours to overnight) video-EEG is the best method to confirm satisfactory response to treatment.

LONG-TERM OUTCOME

With respect to both development and epilepsy, long-term outcomes for IESS are generally poor, with high rates of life-long epilepsy (especially with later-onset

CLINICAL PEARLS

- In an infant 1 month–2 years of age, a clinical history of unusual "jerks," "startles," or "head-nods," especially if occurring in clusters upon awakening, should prompt suspicion of IESS.
- Extended video-EEG monitoring is the procedure of choice to both confirm the diagnosis of IESS and evaluate the impact of treatment.
- The most effective therapies for treatment of IESS are corticosteroids, ACTH, and vigabatrin.
- Prompt and successful treatment is essential to minimize adverse developmental consequences of IESS.
- Among patients with normal or near-normal development at the onset of IESS, and without an underlying etiology that itself adversely impacts development, favorable long-term developmental outcomes are possible with prompt and effective therapy.

Lennox–Gastaut syndrome), intellectual disability, and autism. However, to a great extent, these outcomes reflect etiological factors independent of IESS. Among patients with normal or near-normal development at the time of onset of IESS, who lack an underlying etiology that itself adversely impacts development, favorable long-term outcomes are possible with prompt and successful treatment. Overall, approximately 15%–20% of children with IESS go on to exhibit seizure-freedom and normal (or near-normal) development and behavior.

SUGGESTED REFERENCES

Grinspan Z.M., Mytinger J.R., Baumer F.M., Ciliberto M.A., Cohen B.H., Dlugos D.J., Harini C., Hussain S.A., Joshi S.M., Keator C.G., Knupp K.G., McGoldrick P.E., Nickels K.C., Park J.T., Pasupuleti A., Patel A.D., Shahid A.M., Shellhaas R.A., Shrey D.W., Singh R.K., Wolf S.M., Yozawitz E.G., Yuskaitis C.J., Waugh J.L., Pearl P.L. Management of infantile spasms during the COVID-19 pandemic. *J Child Neurol* 2020;35:828–34.

Hayashi Y., Yoshinaga H., Akiyama T., Endoh F., Ohtsuka Y., Kobayashi K. Predictive factors for relapse of epileptic spasms after adrenocorticotropic hormone therapy in West syndrome. *Brain Dev* 2016;38:32–9.

Hussain S.A. Treatment of infantile spasms. *Epilepsia Open* 2018;3(Suppl 2):S143–54.

Pavone P., Polizzi A., Marino S.D., Corsello G., Falsaperla R., Marino S., Ruggieri M. West syndrome: A comprehensive review. *Neurol Sci* 2020;41:3547–62.

Specchio N., Pietrafusa N., Ferretti A., De Palma L., Santarone M.E., Pepi C., Trivisano M., Vigevano F., Curatolo P. Treatment of infantile spasms: Why do we know so little? *Expert Rev Neurother* 2020;20: 551–66.

23 Gelastic Seizures

Samiya Ahmad
Baylor College of Medicine

Yu-tze Ng
The Children's Hospital of San Antonio
and Baylor College of Medicine

CONTENTS

CASE PRESENTATION

A developmentally normal, 30-month-old boy began having mirthless laughing spells consistent with gelastic seizures at the age of 4 months. His past history was significant only for a Nissen fundoplication which may have been performed for presumptive gastroesophageal reflux disease, or more likely, gelastic seizures have been mistaken for GERD. The seizures were stereotyped and characterized by sucking and laughing. Often, the patient would ask for a drink during the seizure and would drink ferociously if not constrained. At times, the patient would also become violent. The seizures were brief and averaged 30 seconds in duration (range 10–90 seconds) with only occasional, minimal postictal lethargy. He was subsequently diagnosed with a hypothalamic hamartoma (HH) on brain MRI. Seizure frequency had been variable initially but gradually evolved to an average of every 5 minutes, constituting "status gelasticus". The seizures would persist through sleep and awaken the patient throughout the night. The patient had previously failed therapy with phenobarbital, topiramate, and clonazepam. He was treated with levetiracetam, acetazolamide, and nocturnal high-dose lorazepam. None of the antiseizure medications (ASMs) significantly reduced seizure frequency. His neurological examination was otherwise normal. The patient was transferred to a tertiary center for emergent surgical treatment/resection of the HH lesion. Twenty-four-hour scalp video-EEG recording was performed as well as a preoperative brain MRI scan which showed his HH (Figure 23.1a and b). Video-EEG recording confirmed an average of 10 gelastic seizures per hour

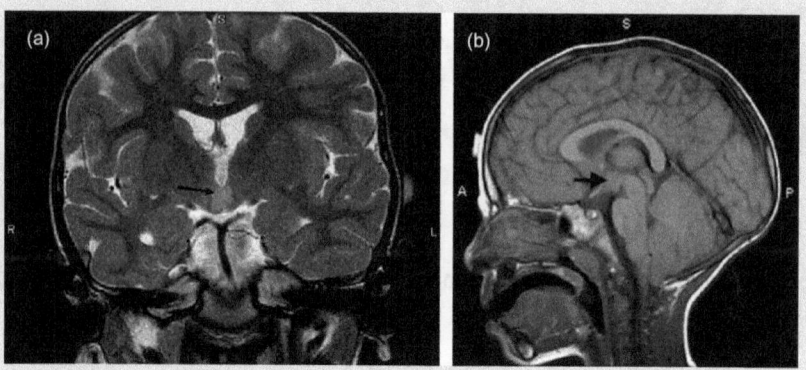

FIGURE 23.1 Preoperative brain MRI T2-weighted coronal (a) and T1-weighted sagittal (b) views of the hypothalamic hamartoma as shown by the arrows.

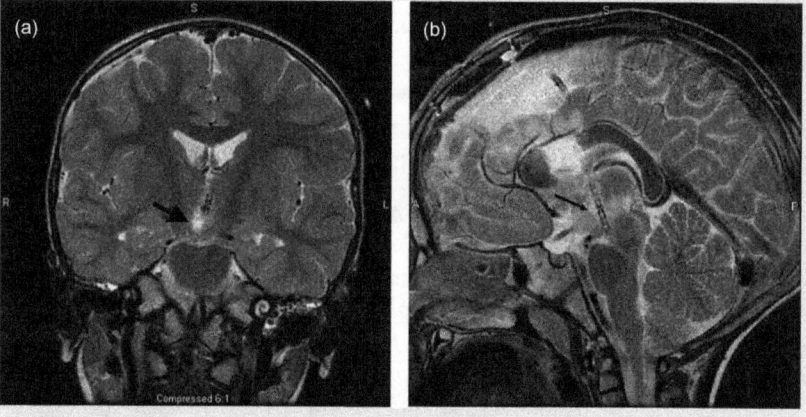

FIGURE 23.2 Postoperative T2-weighted brain MRI coronal (a) and sagittal (b) images of the resected hypothalamic hamartoma shown by the arrows. The postoperative drain tube that was subsequently removed is seen on the sagittal view.

as identified by parents. There were no ictal EEG patterns seen other than muscle and motion artifacts. In addition, the patient's baseline and inter-ictal recordings were normal. The patient then underwent emergent transcallosal interforniceal resection of the HH. The surgery was complicated by a small right-sided thalamic infarct with resultant mild transient left hemiparesis that completely resolved within 2 days. Figures 23.2a and b show the postoperative brain MRI scan. The patient had three brief (less than 30 seconds) stereotypical seizures within the first week after surgery. He became seizure-free for 2 months before the gelastic seizures recurred, but at a much-reduced seizure frequency (i.e., >90% reduction compared to his preoperative base-line). Neuropathological examination of the resected lesion demonstrated subependymal tissue composed of disorganized glial and neuronal elements consistent with a HH. Nineteen months later, endoscopic resection (via the lateral ventricle and through the foramen of Monro) of residual hypothalamic hamartoma tissue was performed for persistent gelastic seizures. The patient has now been seizure-free for more than 12 months and is off all ASMs. He is assessed to be developmentally normal with minor behavioral problems con-sisting of hyperactivity with labile mood.

DIFFERENTIAL DIAGNOSIS

Gelastic (or laughing) seizures were first described by Daly and Mulder in 1957. Gelastic seizures are characterized by bouts of laughter which may be either similar or, more commonly, distinct from the patient's usual laughter, and associated with a slight sensation or appearance of discomfort. A related seizure type may involve crying and/or facial contraction with an exaggerated grimace; these are referred to as dacrystic seizures.

Affected patients may exhibit both forms of seizures, or seizures with mixed fea-tures of both types. Autonomic symptoms such as flushing, tachycardia, and altered respiration are often associated with these seizures. Most (but not all) of these sei-zures are focal onset aware (aka, focal aware or simple partial) in nature with pres-ervation of awareness. The seizures are usually brief (less than 30 seconds) without a postictal phase. *Status gelasticus* is the most severe form, defined as a prolonged cluster of gelastic seizures lasting longer than 20–30 minutes. Patients usually do not report a feeling of mirth. In its mildest form, patients have simply described an urge to laugh that can be self-suppressed.

Scalp EEG monitoring usually does not show any ictal correlate. Typically, the seizure diagnosis is missed or delayed for many years and is often misdiagnosed as a "happy baby", colic or gastroesophageal reflux disease. Patients with gelastic seizures should undergo detailed neuroimaging with particular emphasis on the hypothalamus, including MRI brain scans with fine coronal sections through this region.

Most cases of gelastic seizures represent a symptomatic form of epilepsy. By far the most common etiology for gelastic epilepsy is a HH. HHs are rare developmental malformations of the inferior hypothalamus and tuber cinereum. Other rarer causes include structural lesions impinging upon the floor of the third ventricle, such as tubers of tuberous sclerosis, pituitary tumors, gliomas, meningiomas, and basilar artery aneurysms. Frontal and temporal lobe epilepsy rarely cause gelastic seizures.

In HH patients, gelastic seizures are almost always the first seizure manifestation, which in retrospect often begins shortly after birth. Many of these patients subse-quently develop a refractory mixed epilepsy and epileptic encephalopathy. It is believed that the other evolving seizure types result from a secondary "epileptogenesis" where other parts of the brain "learn" from the HH how to generate seizures.

Intellectual disability and behavioral problems — including rage attacks — are commonly seen. In addition, precocious puberty occurs in approximately half the HH patients. A subset of HH patients has a specific midline syndrome known as Pallister-Hall syndrome. Pallister-Hall syndrome is a rare syndrome that can occur either spontaneously or be inherited in an autosomal dominant fashion through a mutation in the *GLI3* gene. It is associated with polydactly, midline defects, including dysmorphic facial features, hypothalamic hamartoma, and imperforate anus.

DIAGNOSTIC APPROACH

While HH is relatively uncommon with a prevalence of about 1 in 100,000, it is almost certainly underdiagnosed by medical caregivers. The gelastic seizures may initially be atypical and the parents may simply be aware that something is wrong or that they have a baby who "laughs too much." Equally common, the seizures may be more of a dycrastic, or crying seizure, sometimes associated with strained, painful, paroxysmal but stereotypical discomfort spells that may resemble gastroesophageal reflux disease or "colic". Any patient with typical gelastic seizures should be presumed to have an HH – unless shown otherwise – and evaluated with appropriate neuroimaging at an experienced/tertiary medical center.

Central precocious puberty that affects many HH patients is another very distinctive symptom, which should alert one to the diagnosis of an HH. The refractory mixed epilepsy and epileptic encephalopathy that is associated is less specific but certainly part of the clinical picture. Although other seizure types often present later, that is not always the rule and in fact, HHs are an uncommon but important cause of infantile spasms (initial presentation).

TREATMENT STRATEGY AND LONG-TERM OUTCOME

Typically, in HH patients, gelastic seizures (but also other seizure types) are extremely refractory to ASMs and other non-pharmacological therapies. Even as recently as the past decade, experts felt that neurosurgical resection could not be performed safely due to location, and even if it could, may not help the epilepsy. Both these notions have now been dispelled, and a relatively large series of patients have now been cured of their refractory symptomatic gelastic and mixed epilepsy.

For those patients who fail to respond to medications, surgical resection using a transcallosal, interforniceal approach has been shown to be efficacious and generally safe. More recently, many HH surgical resections have been performed using an endoscopic technique with a transventricular approach. Gamma-knife surgery has also been used to treat several HH patients and is often advocated for smaller lesions, particularly in Europe.

The natural history of HHs is generally very poor with a progressive epileptic encephalopathy, severe intellectual disability, and persistent refractory epilepsy. However, variability exists with milder (possibly even asymptomatic) cases never being diagnosed. Indeed, typically with the pedunculated form of HH, some patients may present solely with precocious puberty. More severely affected patients can be significantly improved with surgical therapy resulting in around half the patients becoming seizure-free and nearly 90% with significant seizure reduction.

Newer techniques, including gamma-knife and MR-guided stereotactic laser ablation (SLA), have been found to be beneficial in controlling seizures, and if implemented early, can mitigate behavioral and cognitive decline. Precocious puberty should be evaluated and followed by a pediatric endocrinologist. Leuprolide acetate, a gonadotropin-releasing hormone (GnRH) agonist is effective in treating precocious puberty. Central precocious puberty may resolve following resection of the HH.

NEUROBIOLOGY/PATHOPHYSIOLOGY OF DISEASE

The expression of laughter appears to depend on two different neuronal pathways. One is an involuntary system that involves the deep gray matter structures including the amygdala, thalamic and subthalamic areas, and the dorsal tegmentum. The second and voluntary system originates in the premotor frontal opercular areas and leads through the motor cortex and pyramidal tract to the ventral brainstem. The laughter may result from a laughter-coordination center in the dorsal upper pons.

The pathophysiology of gelastic seizures (and secondary epileptogenesis) arising from HH tissue is poorly understood. However, initial studies have revealed two distinct populations of neurons in surgically resected HH tissue. The first group consists of small γ-aminobutyric acid (GABA)-expressing neurons found principally in nodules that display spontaneous rhythmic firing. The second population is composed of large, quiescent, pyramidal-like neurons with more extensive dendritic and axonal arborization.

It has been proposed that the small, spontaneously firing GABAergic neurons might send inhibitory projections to and drive the synchrony of large output HH neurons.

CLINICAL PEARLS

- Although uncommon, HHs are probably underdiagnosed, and caregivers should be aware of the usual (but not universal) hallmark presentation of gelastic or laughing seizures.
- Other diagnostic clues include central precocious puberty, refractory mixed epilepsy, and an idiopathic psychiatric scenario including autistic features, intellectual disability, and behavioral problems – in particular, rage attacks.
- HHs may present as part of a midline syndrome, in particular Pallister-Hall syndrome with typical clinical features of polydactly, midline defects, including dysmorphic facial features and imperforate anus.
- Medical therapy with ASMs is unlikely to provide seizure freedom and early consideration for surgical treatment should be considered.
- Advances in treatment options include gamma-knife and MR-guided SLA, which can also help improve behavioral and cognitive outcomes, particularly if intervened early in the course of the disease.

Alternatively, the majority of large HH neurons have been found to depolarize in response to $GABA_A$ receptor activation, and such an effect could lead to neuronal excitation.

SUGGESTED REFERENCES

Curry D.J., Raskin J., Ali I., Wilfong A.A. MR-guided laser ablation for the treatment of hypothalamic hamartomas. *Epilepsy Res* 2018;142:131–4.

Daly D., Mulder D. Gelastic epilepsy. *Neurology* 1957;7:189–92.

Fenoglio K.A., Wu J., Kim do Y., Simeone T.A., Coons S.W., Rekate H., Rho J.M., Kerrigan J.F. Hypothalamic hamartoma: Basic mechanisms of intrinsic epileptogenesis. *Semin Pediatr Neurol* 2007;14:51–9.

Freeman J.L., Harvey A.S., Rosenfeld J.V., Wrennall J.A., Bailey C.A., Berkovic S.F. Generalized epilepsy in hypothalamic hamartoma: Evolution and postoperative resolution. *Neurology* 2003;60:762–7.

Kerrigan J.F., Ng Y.T., Chung S., Rekate H.L. The hypothalamic hamartoma: A model of subcortical epileptogenesis and encephalopathy. *Semin Pediatr Neurol* 2005;12:119–31.

Kerrigan J.F., Ng Y.T., Prenger E., Krishnamoorthy K.S., Wang N.C., Rekate H.L. Hypothalamic hamartoma and infantile spasms. *Epilepsia* 2007;48:89–95.

Kim D.Y., Fenoglio K.A., Simeone T.A., Coons S.W., Wu J., Chang Y., Kerrigan J.F., Rho J.M. GABA(A) receptor-mediated activation of L-type calcium channels induces neuronal excitation in surgically resected human hypothalamic hamartomas. *Epilepsia* 2008;49:861–71.

Ng Y.T., Rekate H.L. Coining of a new term, "Status Gelasticus". *Epilepsia* 2006;47:661–2.

Ng Y.T., Rekate H.L., Prenger E.C., Wand N.C., Feiz-Erfan I., Johnsonbaugh R.E., Varland R.V., Chung S.C., Kerrigan J.F. Endoscopic resection of hypothalamic hamartomas for refractory symptomatic epilepsy. *Neurology* 2008;70:1543–8

Sweetman L.L., Ng Y.T., Kerrigan J.F. Gelastic seizures misdiagnosed as gastro-esophageal reflux disease. *Clinic Peds* 2007;46:325–8.

Wild B., Rodden F.A., Grodd W., Ruch W. Neuronal correlates of laughter and humor. *Brain* 2003;126:2121–38.

24 Intractable Epilepsy after Herpes Simplex Encephalitis

Daniel A. Freedman and Dave F. Clarke
The University of Texas at Austin

CONTENTS

CASE PRESENTATION

The patient is a 3-year-old right-handed female with drug-resistant epilepsy who was referred for evaluation and treatment. At 10 months of age, she developed a fever and began having intermittent left hemi-body clonic activity. Initially seen in the emergency department, she was diagnosed with febrile seizures and discharged. Seizures continued the following day and she was admitted for 22 days requiring multiple antiseizure medications (ASMs) to control her seizures. Cerebrospinal fluid polymerase chain reaction (PCR) was positive for herpes simplex virus (HSV). Her initial EEG showed bilateral, independent, periodic discharges (BIPDs; Figure 24.1), and her initial neuroimaging studies revealed bilateral temporal lobe edema.

DOI: 10.1201/9781003296478-27

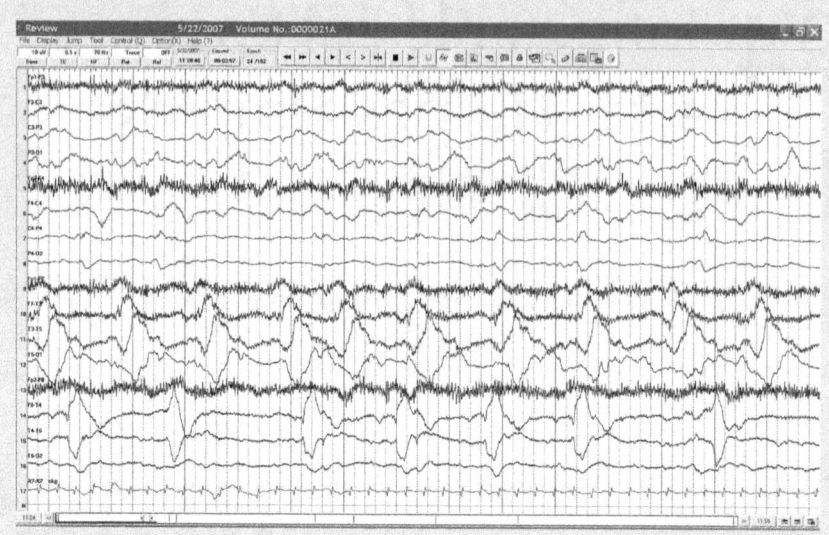

FIGURE 24.1   This is a 2-year-old, 9 days after clinical onset of HSV encephalitis. EEG depicts right temporal periodic sharp waves with contralateral periodic slowing which is maximal in the left temporal head region. These findings are similar to the EEG described above in the case illustration.

Although she was aggressively treated with acyclovir, the encephalitis caused impairment in expressive more than receptive language function, left hemiparesis, and medically intractable epilepsy. Her current seizure semiology consists of predominantly epileptic spasms with flexion of the left arm and tonic events, with a frequency of 10–25 seizures per week. Prior ASMs include vigabatrin, prednisolone, levetiracetam, and zonisamide. She had a prior right parietal resection, but this was also unsuccessful in controlling her seizures. Her present ASM regimen includes clobazam, felbamate, rufinamide, and cannabidiol.

A recent video-EEG study revealed interictal left greater than right frontal epileptiform discharges (Figure 24.2) with rapid bisynchrony. Frequent flexor spasms were captured with left arm flexion suggesting a right hemispheric onset but with rapid bilateral spread, often resulting in falls. A brain MRI study revealed right parietal encephalomalacia, as well as periventricular and subcortical white matter signal hyperintensities in the right more than left temporal and parietal lobes (Figure 24.3). Neuropsychological testing revealed a functional level comparable to a 12–22 month-old child with receptive language as a relative strength. After reviewing the results, a complete corpus callosotomy was recommended.

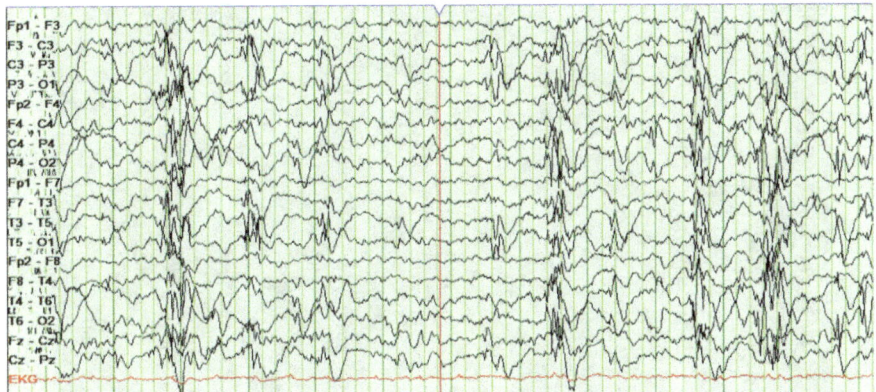

FIGURE 24.2 This EEG shows frequent interictal epileptiform activity with independent right centro-temporo-parietal polyspike bursts and left greater than right centrotemporal discharges.

DIFFERENTIAL DIAGNOSIS

Viral encephalitis is one of the most common causes of symptomatic *status epilepticus*. Herpes simplex virus (HSV), affecting 2–4 cases per 1,000,000 per year, is the most common cause of encephalitis in the United States. HSV acquired congenitally or in the neonatal period (often HSV type 2) is a diffuse process with a different clinical presentation and course than that acquired during infancy or childhood (often HSV type 1).

Though childhood-acquired HSV may have a wide spectrum of clinical presentations, it has a predilection for the limbic system and the temporal lobes. The case discussed above represents a child who acquired herpes simplex encephalitis (HSE) at 3 years of age, which caused intractable structural epilepsy with focal and generalized features and significant neuro-cognitive/neuro-developmental deficits.

Fever and confusion should immediately alert the physician to the possibility of central nervous system (CNS) involvement. Focal seizures, though sometimes seen in other causes of encephalitis, are often a presenting symptom in herpes encephalitis. Meningitis, other viral encephalitides, inflammatory diseases like autoimmune encephalitis, and focal neoplastic lesions are other possible causes of similar presenting symptoms. In a child with known epilepsy, any febrile illness may lower seizure threshold and could mimic some of the symptoms of viral encephalitis. Other suggestive symptoms include headache (irritability in younger children), unusual behavior, lethargy, vomiting, and other neurological symptoms such as cranial nerve findings and localized deficits. Symptoms are more nonspecific in very young children who may present with decreased activity or irritability and inconsolable crying.

DIAGNOSTIC APPROACH

A lumbar puncture is required in anyone in whom a CNS infection is suspected. Lymphocytic pleocytosis, elevated serum protein, and normal blood glucose are often seen in viral encephalitis, but normal values do not rule out the condition and a

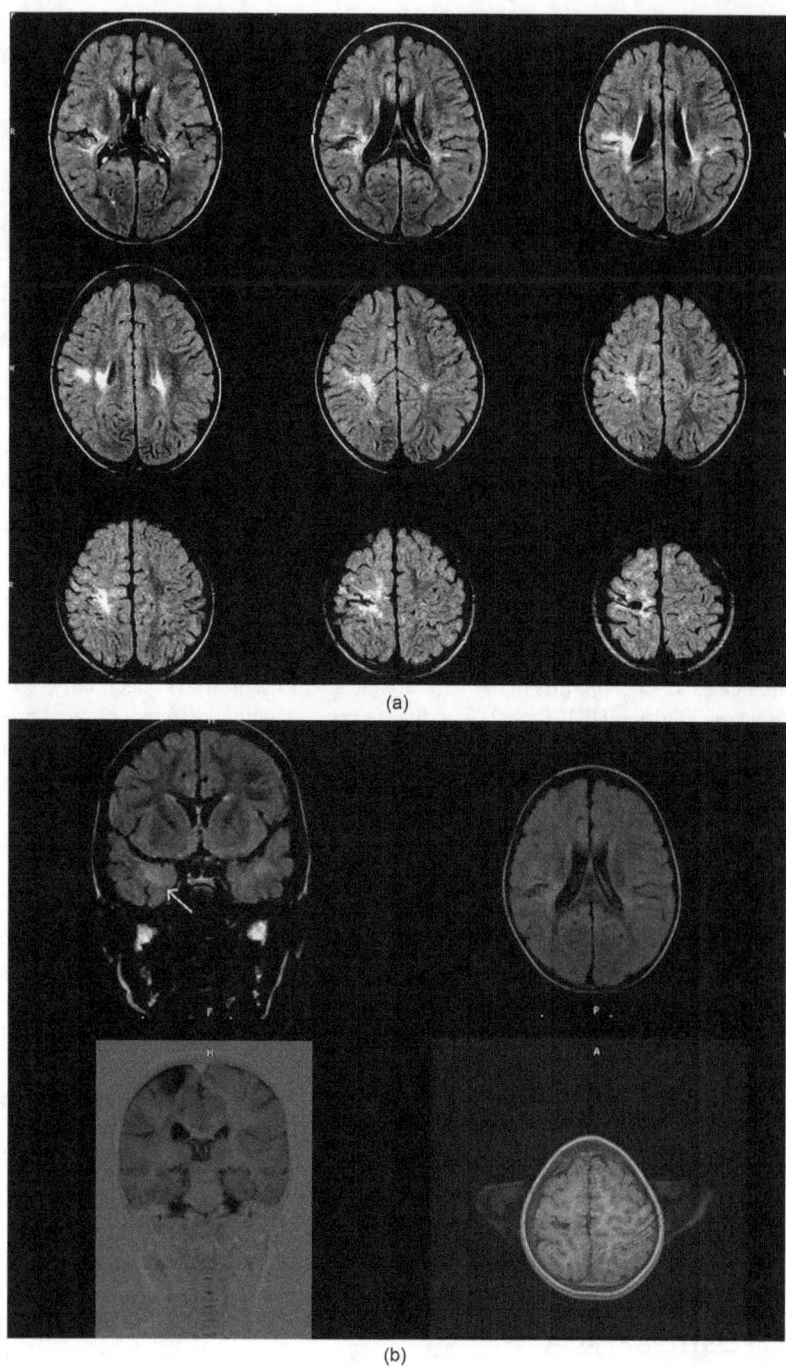

(a)

(b)

FIGURE 24.3 (a and b): MRI depicting right parietal lobe encephalomalacia with peri-ventricular and subcortical white matter signal hyperintensity in the right greater than left temporal lobes.

mild decrease in glucose or a neutrophilic pleocytosis may be seen in the early stages. Hemorrhagic cerebrospinal fluid (CSF) with xanthochromia is a sensitive indicator but is not specific to HSE. PCR of the CSF for herpes virus DNA, a test with both sensitivity and specificity above 90%, has been a significant diagnostic advancement. It is less invasive than the prior gold standard (brain biopsy) and should therefore be carried out in anyone in whom encephalitis is suspected. False negatives may occur very early in the course of the disease; therefore, if the index of suspicion is high, a lumbar puncture should be repeated even after acyclovir has been started.

In HSE, the EEG is abnormal in over 90% of cases. Early changes in HSE consist of focal or lateralized slowing which is maximal over the temporal and/or frontal lobes involved. This is due to the virus predilection for infecting structures involved in the limbic circuitry (mesial temporal structures, isthmus, part of the insula, orbitofrontal cortex, and cingulate gyrus) and is followed by intermittent unilateral or bilateral sharp or slow-wave complexes preceding lateralized periodic discharges (LPDs), or BIPDs, in the temporal regions. LPDs were formerly known as periodic lateralizing epileptiform discharges (PLEDs). The discharges occur every 1–3 seconds.

LPDs are not specific for herpes but reflect acute/subacute focal structural and functional (cortical-subcortical) impairment, whether it is from an infection or an acute infarct. The periodicity is usually seen 2 days to a week after onset but may be seen later and gradually disappears as the patient improves and the disease resolves. If the disease process persists, the complexes become broad, more prolonged suppression is seen after each burst, and in the final stages, there is more diffuse involvement preceding electrocerebral silence.

Hemorrhage seen on computer tomography (CT), primarily in the temporal lobes, is highly suggestive of HSE, but is rarely seen in the early stages of the disease. The CT may be normal early in the course of the illness or may show hypodensities in the temporal lobes with mild mass effect. Patchy enhancement of gyri may also be seen when contrast is used.

MRI is more sensitive and specific in the diagnosis of HSE than CT. The MRI initially reveals gyral edema on T1-weighted images and increased signal on T2 and FLAIR (fluid-attenuated inversion recovery) images in the temporal lobes, orbitofrontal cortex, and cingulate +/− the insula cortex. Petechial hemorrhages may be seen with MRI in the later stages of the disease, but, as with CT, are rarely seen in the early stages. With MRI contrast enhancement, these hemorrhages, usually absent in the early stages, become apparent as the disease progresses. The other limbic structures described above become involved later. As the disease resolves, the long-term neuro-radiological sequelae become apparent with destruction, encephalomalacia, and/or atrophy of portions of the temporal lobes and orbitofrontal lobes primarily, as was seen in the patient described above.

TREATMENT STRATEGY

Hospitalization is a necessity in children in whom encephalitis is suspected. In patients in whom HSE is a part of the differential diagnosis, empiric acyclovir should be started immediately and only discontinued when there is a negative HSV PCR, and an alternative diagnosis is more likely. Treatment for confirmed infections is required for 14–21 days. Acyclovir is not without side-effects: it is potentially nephrotoxic and may cause neutropenia. The dose may need to be adjusted in patients with impaired renal function and frequent blood draws are required.

Seizures are a more common presenting symptom in patients with poor outcome and should be treated aggressively. Clinical seizures may be a treatment and diagnostic dilemma. LPDs often represent the underlying process and have been described in rare cases of "burnt-out" *status epilepticus*. In a patient with prolonged *status* and prior documented subclinical seizures, a therapeutic trial is sometimes carried out.

Benzodiazepines are the evidence-based first-line ASM used to treat prolonged or repetitive seizures. Multiple doses, high doses, or combinations of benzodiazepines with other sedating medications may cause respiratory suppression. Sedation is common with benzodiazepines, which can compromise the ability of the examiner to adequately determine neurological function. Whenever possible, less sedating agents may be initiated if continued treatment is necessary. In cases where oral medications cannot be given, intravenous agents such as IV valproate or IV levetiracetam are available for use in most centers. In patients with persistent seizures, using appropriate ASMs for long-term use is dependent on not only seizure type but also on potential comorbidities.

Treating mood and behavior, obesity or weight loss in poorly functioning and or immobile patients, or bone loss with inducing agents, etc., may influence the physician's choice of ASM. In medically refractory patients, if only focal seizures are seen, resective surgery is an option. Larger palliative procedures such as a functional hemispherotomy can be offered in select patients with focal seizures and significant lateralized injury. In cases where there is bilateral involvement, palliative procedures such as the vagus nerve stimulator, and corpus callosotomy may be offered to reduce morbidity from generalized or focal to bilateral seizure types.

LONG-TERM OUTCOME

In a 12-year prospective study, abnormal EEGs were found in 94% and diagnostic imaging abnormities found in 88% of subjects. Significant neurological sequelae occurred in over 60% of subjects, with 44% of children having persistent seizures. Hsieh et al. revealed a similar outcome, with 14/40 subjects (35%) with poor neurological outcome. Abnormal neuroimaging or abnormal EEG findings were more prevalent in patients with poor outcome. Delayed initiation of acyclovir was another predictor of poor outcome. As stated previously, the limbic structures including the mesial temporal structures are often the neuroanatomical regions of concern, therefore memory and other neuropsychological functions related to limbic circuitry, such as emotion, may be impaired. There are also varying degrees of neurocognitive impairment.

There are emerging data in adult and pediatric patients with HSE showing later development of N-methyl-D-aspartate receptor (NMDAR) antibodies and NMDAR encephalitis although the link is poorly understood. In patients with structural/symptomatical forms of epilepsy, the seizure semiology is determined by the regions maximally involved and by seizure spread. Clinical and electroencephalographic temporal lobe onset seizures are most often seen. Seizures may, however, evolve from one or both hemispheres independently or may present as a more generalized picture, though MRI findings may be focal or multifocal, as seen in the patient described.

CLINICAL PEARLS

- HSV, affecting 2–4 cases per 1,000,000 per year, is the most common cause of encephalitis in the United States.
- Although childhood-acquired HSV may have a wide spectrum of clinical presentations, it has a predilection for the limbic system and the temporal lobes.
- In a patient presenting with new-onset seizures, infectious, inflammatory, and neoplastic processes should be ruled out.
- In HSE, the EEG is abnormal in over 90% of cases.
- Lateralized periodic discharges (formerly known as PLEDs), though not specific for HSE, is the most frequent electroencephalographic finding described in this condition.
- Abnormal neuroimaging, abnormal EEG, and delayed initiation of antiviral therapy (acyclovir) are predictors of poor outcome.

PATHOPHYSIOLOGY/NEUROBIOLOGY OF DISEASE

Of the eight identified human herpes virus family types, HSV 1, frequently associated with orofacial infections, is most often identified in patients with HSE over 6 months of age. Perinatal or congenital HSV infections are often caused by HSV 2. HSV 1 must come into contact with a mucosal surface or broken skin in order to infect the individual; hence, close contact with a person excreting HSV is required. Virions are transported by retrograde flow along axons from the entry point to the nuclei of a limited number of sensory neurons. Viral replication occurs at the site of infection and the dorsal root ganglion.

Distinctive pathological features of HSE include severe inflammation, congestion, hemorrhagic necrosis, and damage or destruction to both gray and white matter, primarily affecting the temporal/medial temporal and orbitofrontal cortex, although other regions may be involved. Approximately a third of cases of HSE are acquired by primary infection and two-thirds occur after a period of latency. The olfactory tract and its close association with the limbic system make it a feasible pathway for HSV to gain access to the CNS. The olfactory route, along with the trigeminal nerve, has been explored in animal models. Viral route of brain access, viral predilection for the temporal lobe and limbic structures, and the cause for viral reactivation are, however, poorly understood in humans.

SUGGESTED REFERENCES

Demaerel P., Wilms G., Robberecht W., Johannik K., Van Hecke P., Carton H., Baert A.L. MRI of herpes simplex encephalitis. *Neuroradiol* 1992;34:490–3.

Elbers J.M., Bitnun A., Richardson S.E., Ford-Jones E.L., Tellier R., Wald R.M., Petric M., Kolski H., Heurter H., MacGregor D. A 12-year prospective study of childhood herpes simplex encephalitis: Is there a broader spectrum of disease? *Pediatrics* 2007;119:e399–407.

Gelisse P., Crespel A., Genton P., Jallon P., Kaplan P. Lateralized periodic discharges: Which patterns are interictal, ictal, or peri-ictal? *Clin Neurophysiol* 2021;132:1593–603.

Hsieh W.B., Chiu N.C., Hu K.C., Ho C.S., Huang F.Y. Outcome of herpes simplex encephalitis in children. *J Microbiol Immunol Infect* 2007;40:34–8.

Lai C.W., Gragasin M.E. Electroencephalography in herpes encephalitis. *J Clin Neurophysiol* 1988;5:87–103.

Nosadini M., Mohammad S., Corazza F., Ruga E.M., Kothur K., Perilongo G., Frigo A.C., Toldo I., Dale R.C., Sartori S. Herpes simplex virus-induced anti-N-methyl-d-aspartate receptor encephalitis: A systematic literature review with analysis of 43 cases. *Dev Med Child Neurol* 2017;59:796–805.

Romero J.R., Kimberlin D.W. Molecular diagnosis of viral infections of the central nervous system. *Clin Lab Med* 2003;23:843–65.

Weil A.A., Glaser C.A., Amad Z., Forghani B. Patients with suspected herpes simplex encephalitis: Rethinking an initial negative polymerase chain reaction result. *Clin Infect Dis* 2002;34:1154–7.

Whitley R.J., Kimberlin D.W. Herpes simplex encephalitis: Children and adolescents. *Semin Pediatr Infect Dis* 2005;16:17–23.

25 Refractory *Status Epilepticus*

Sonali Sen and James J. Riviello, Jr.
Baylor College of Medicine

CONTENTS

CASE PRESENTATION

A 10-year-old boy with a several days' history of fever, malaise, diarrhea, and emesis developed convulsive status epilepticus (CSE) treated with lorazepam, levetiracetam, and phenytoin. Cranial CT was unremarkable, and cerebrospinal fluid (CSF) revealed 6 white blood cells/mm (95% lymphocytes, 5% monocytes), with normal glucose and protein. EEG demonstrated diffuse slowing with occasional temporal spikes. He continued to have frequent seizures described as sudden staring episodes with head and eye deviation to the left and associated with cyanosis. He was intubated and transferred to the ICU where he was treated with a pentobarbital infusion. Pentobarbital was weaned 2 days later, but seizures recurred. Sodium thiopental was given, followed by midazolam. When the seizures persisted, high-dose phenobarbital was used.

DIFFERENTIAL DIAGNOSIS/DIAGNOSTIC APPROACH

This case involves refractory *status epilepticus* (RSE), which is defined as persistent seizure activity despite administration of a benzodiazepine at an appropriate dose followed by a second-line antiseizure medication (ASM). In children, cases of RSE not responding to first-line therapy usually occur secondary to an acute symptomatic SE or an underlying progressive neurological disorder. Psychogenic seizures (or nonepileptic seizures) must also be considered when seizures persist despite treatment but are very unusual in the younger child. Unusual motor movements, an "on/off" pattern of movements, a poor response to treatment, or a lack of metabolic abnormalities, particularly after a long seizure suggest *pseudostatus epilepticus.*

DOI: 10.1201/9781003296478-28

Shorvon has identified the following as causes of RSE:

- Inadequate ASM therapy.
- Failure to start maintenance ASM therapy.
- Failure to reverse ongoing metabolic derangements.
- Failure to identify and treat the underlying cause.
- Failure to identify and treat other medical complications.
- Misdiagnosis, especially of pseudo seizures.

Therefore, when RSE occurs, it is mandatory to exclude underlying etiologies that may require a specific treatment – ASM treatment may suppress seizure activity, but it does not treat the acute precipitating cause.

TREATMENT STRATEGY

As emphasized in Chapter 8, treatment protocols for SE are needed in advance. What happens when first- and second-line therapies fail? Refractory SE (RSE) occurs in 6%–11% of cases. When SE persists, continuous intravenous (CIV) ASMs are typically employed next. Pentobarbital has been used the most, but midazolam, propofol, and more recently ketamine is also commonly administered. The term "barbiturate coma" has been used when barbiturates are given. High-dose phenobarbital and thiopental have also been used.

Pentobarbital has a quick onset and relatively rapid elimination compared with phenobarbital, but hypotension is very common with pentobarbital, compared to high-dose phenobarbital. Midazolam has a shorter half-life and induces less sedation than pentobarbital or phenobarbital. Propofol has a very rapid onset, but hypotension and cardiovascular instability occur, especially with prolonged therapy (the propofol infusion syndrome). As mentioned in Chapter 8, the number and activity of γ-aminobutyric acid type A (GABA$_A$) receptors decrease during prolonged seizures; simultaneously the number and activity of glutamatergic N-methyl-D-aspartate (NMDA) receptors increase. Ketamine, which is an NMDA receptor antagonist, has been proposed to be effective when used early during SE, without adverse effects on hemodynamics. Inhalational anesthetics (e.g., isoflurane) are rarely used (Table 25.1). Published studies have not clearly demonstrated greater efficacy of one treatment over the others.

The Neurocritical Care Society Guidelines recommend an initial 24–48-hour period of seizure cessation prior to weaning the CIV medication. If not successful, treatment should be extended up to 72 hours, and then another wean attempted. If again not successful, we recommend continuing CIV therapy. As in the case above, patients requiring prolonged treatment in patients without a prior history of epilepsy, and without a clear acute cause are defined as having new-onset refractory *status epilepticus* (NORSE). Febrile illness related *status epilepticus* (FIRES) is a subcategory of NORSE, in which a febrile illness occurs 2 weeks to 24 hours prior to the onset of RSE, without any specific infectious organism isolated or even with relatively normal CSF findings. The presumed pathogenesis is a central nervous system (CNS) inflammatory response leading to RSE. In these patients, additional immunomodulatory

TABLE 25.1

Comparison of Different Medications for the Treatment of RSE

Medication	Loading Dose[a]	Infusion Rate[a]	Adverse Effects
Midazolam	0.2 mg/kg Maximum dose: 10 mg	0.1 mg/kg/h If this continues, add 0.2 mg/kg dose and increase rate to 0.2 mg/kg/h If this continues, add another additional dose at 0.2 mg/kg and consider a different agent	Hypotension (usually transient), sedation, respiratory depression, arrhythmia
Pentobarbital	5–10 mg/kg	0.5–1.0 mg/kg/h	Hypotension, decreased myocardial contractility, respiratory depression, infection (especially pneumonia), hepatic dysfunction
Thiopental	4–8 mg/kg	3–5 mg/kg/h	Hypotension, decreased myocardial contractility, respiratory depression, infection (especially pneumonia)
Propofol	1–2 mg/kg	1–5 mg/kg/h	Hypotension, sedation, acidosis, rhabdomyolysis, hypertriglyceridemia
Phenobarbital	20 mg/kg Maximum dose: 1,000 mg	Not infused per hour	Sedation, respiratory depression (less than pentobarbital)
Ketamine	2.5 mg/kg	10 µg/kg/min increase infusion rate by 5–10 µg/kg/min every 10 minutes until 100 µg/kg/min. Additional dose of 1–2 µg/kg/min before each increase	Hypertension, tachycardia; increased or decreased intracranial pressure
Isoflurane	0.5%–3% MAC	Same MAC	Hypotension, decreased myocardial contractility, infection (especially pneumonia), ileus, venous thrombosis

[a] Adjusted to clinical and EEG response.

treatment is recommended. Anakinra, which is an IL-1 receptor antagonist, when used early in the course of FIRES (<2 weeks after onset of RSE) has been associated with decreased seizure frequency, as well as shorter ICU and hospital length of stay. Tocilizumab, an IL-6 receptor antagonist, has also been used but is associated with greater adverse effects.

We continue routine ASMs during CIV therapy. This ensures that therapeutic drug levels are present at the time of the tapering. This is more easily done with the intravenous formulations of ASMs: phenobarbital, phenytoin, valproic acid, levetiracetam, and lacosamide. If pentobarbital is used as a CIV ASM, we typically use phenobarbital. Other ASMs without IV formulations may be administered through a nasogastric tube, but there may be decreased gastrointestinal absorption during CIV therapy, especially with pentobarbital. There is no evidence that any one ASM has better efficacy. The ketogenic diet has also been used in conjunction with traditional ASMs. In a small cohort, the Pediatric *Status Epilepticus* Research Group (PSERG) reported electrographic seizure resolution was observed in 71% of patients within 7 days of initiation of the diet and 78% were able to be weaned off continuous infusions within 2 weeks. Due to its anti-inflammatory effects, early use is recommended in cases of FIRES. Common adverse side effects include gastroparesis and hypertriglyceridemia.

The incidence of side effects increases with the depth and duration of CIV therapy. If repeat cycles are needed, typically a different agent is used. High-dose phenobarbital may have less cardiovascular side effects (such as hypotension) than the other agents, and with chronic high-dosing, respiratory efforts may return. However, phenobarbital has a longer half-life and thus requires a longer time for its elimination.

We use continuous EEG monitoring (CEEG) during CIV therapy, aiming for a burst-suppression period lasting 5–15 seconds. However, controversy exists regarding whether the endpoint of treatment should be clinical or electrographic seizure control *versus* EEG background suppression. The greater the background suppression, the more adverse effects.

LONG-TERM OUTCOME

What is the outcome of RSE? The overall mortality rate is 4%–16%; this varies from the acute to the long-term state, with a 4% acute rate and a 5.4% rate after hospital discharge. The best prognosis occurs if RSE responds to initial suppression and SE does not recur after tapering. Super-refractory *status epilepticus* (SRSE) is defined as SE persisting or recurring after at least 24 hours of appropriate treatment with anesthesia or recurring after withdrawal of anesthesia and requiring anesthetic reintroduction. Such cases have a worse prognosis with a short-term mortality rate of 4%–4.7%.

In our series of 22 children with "severe" RSE treated with prolonged pentobarbital, the mortality and outcome were related to the etiology. The seven deaths occurred in children with either acute symptomatic SE, an underlying progressive encephalopathy, or with a remote symptomatic case with an acute precipitant. The three children in the progressive encephalopathy group consisted of inborn errors of metabolism, two of whom were previously normal, and a febrile illness precipitated the RSE. In the survivors, no child with acute symptomatic RSE returned to baseline neurologic status and all developed severe, drug-resistant epilepsy. PSERG data showed that 50% of patients without a prior history of epilepsy who presented with RSE went on to develop epilepsy and 39% developed a new neurologic deficit.

CLINICAL PEARLS

- Refractory SE is defined as SE that persists despite administration of a benzodiazepine at an appropriate dose followed by a second-line ASM.
- It is mandatory to look for an underlying cause in RSE. The term "metabolic" usually refers to electrolyte disorders, whereas the term "inborn error of metabolism" refers to a primary metabolic or genetic disease.
- FIRES should be considered as a potential cause of RSE and SRSE in patients with preceding febrile illness without clear etiology. Prompt initiation of immunomodulatory therapy as well as ketogenic diet initiation should be considered.
- Aiming therapy to a burst-suppression EEG is controversial. It is not clear if clinical or electrographic seizure suppression has the same efficacy as achieving burst suppression.
- If seizures recur after discontinuing CIV therapy, treat with repeat CIV cycles, but only if a good outcome is possible.
- It is highly unlikely that an acute symptomatic, progressive encephalopathy, or a remote symptomatic super-refractory SE case with an acute precipitant will return to baseline functioning. Therefore, ethical considerations must be employed when making decisions about prolonged treatment.

There are ethical considerations regarding prolonged CIV treatment. The question of treatment duration with respect to outcome is always raised. Mirski et al. reported a good recovery following 53 days of CIV therapy and suggested the following: no time limit when the potential prognosis is good, defined as a young individual with a healthy premorbid state, a self-limited and possibly reversible disease process, and when neuroimaging shows no radiographic lesion that suggests a poor prognosis, such as cortical laminar necrosis. Again, etiology is an important determinant of outcome, and therefore, an extensive evaluation for an underlying cause must be done, especially for infectious or metabolic disorders.

SUGGESTED REFERENCES

Arya R., Peariso K., Gaínza-Lein M., Harvey J., Bergin A., Brenton J.N., Burrows B.T., Glauser T., Goodkin H.P., Lai Y.C., Mikati M.A., Fernández I.S., Tchapyjnikov D., Wilfong A.A., Williams K., Loddenkemper T.; Pediatric Status Epilepticus Research Group (pSERG). Efficacy and safety of ketogenic diet for treatment of pediatric convulsive refractory status epilepticus. *Epilepsy Res* 2018;144:1–6.

Brophy G.M., Bell R., Claassen J., Alldredge B., Bleck T.P., Glauser T., Laroche S.M., Riviello Jr. J.J., Shutter L., Sperling M.R., Treiman D.M., Vespa P.M.; Neurocritical Care Society Status Epilepticus Guideline Writing Committee. Guidelines for the evaluation and management of *status epilepticus*. *Neurocrit Care* 2012;17:3–23.

Claassen J., Hirsch L.J., Emerson R.G., Mayer S.A. Treatment of refractory *status epilepticus* with pentobarbital, propofol, or midazolam: A systematic review. *Epilepsia* 2002;43:146–53.

Gaínza-Lein M., Barcia Aguilar C., Piantino J., Chapman K.E., Sánchez Fernández I., Amengual-Gual M., Anderson A., Appavu B., Arya R., Brenton J.N., Carpenter J.L., Clark J., Farias-Moeller R., Gaillard W.D., Glauser T.A., Goldstein J.L., Goodkin H.P., Huh L., Kahoud R., Kapur K., Lai Y.C., McDonough T.L., Mikati M.A., Morgan L.A., Nayak A., Novotny Jr. E., Ostendorf A.P., Payne E.T., Peariso K., Reece L., Riviello J., Sannagowdara K., Sands T.T., Sheehan T., Tasker R.C., Tchapyjnikov D., Vasquez A., Wainwright M.S., Wilfong A., Williams K., Zhang B., Loddenkemper T.; Pediatric Status Epilepticus Research Group. Factors associated with long-term outcomes in pediatric refractory *status epilepticus*. *Epilepsia* 2021;62:2190–204.

Hirsch L.J., Gaspard N., van Baalen A., Nabbout R., Demeret S., Loddenkemper T., Navarro V., Specchio N., Lagae L., Rossetti A.O., Hocker S., Gofton T.E., Abend N.S., Gilmore E.J., Hahn C., Khosravani H., Rosenow F., Trinka E. Proposed consensus definitions for new-onset refractory *status epilepticus* (NORSE), febrile infection-related epilepsy syndrome (FIRES), and related conditions. *Epilepsia* 2018;59:739–44.

Koh S., Wirrell E., Vezzani A., Nabbout R., Muscal E., Kaliakatsos M., Wickström R., Riviello J.J., Brunklaus A., Payne E., Valentin A., Wells E., Carpenter J.L., Lee K., Lai Y.C., Eschbach K., Press C.A., Gorman M., Stredny C.M., Roche W., Mangum T. Proposal to optimize evaluation and treatment of febrile infection-related epilepsy syndrome (FIRES): A report from FIRES workshop. *Epilepsia Open* 2021;6:62–72.

Lai Y.C., Muscal E., Wells E., Shukla N., Eschbach K., Hyeong Lee K., Kaliakatsos M., Desai N., Wickström R., Viri M., Freri E., Granata T., Nangia S., Dilena R., Brunklaus A., Wainwright M.S., Gorman M.P., Stredny C.M., Asiri A., Hundallah K., Doja A., Payne E., Wirrell E., Koh S., Carpenter J.L., Riviello J. Anakinra usage in febrile infection related epilepsy syndrome: An international cohort. *Ann Clin Transl Neurol* 2020;7:2467–74.

Mirski M.A., Williams M.A., Hanley D.F. Prolonged pentobarbital and phenobarbital coma for refractory generalized *status epilepticus*. *Crit Care Med* 1995;23:400–4.

Ochoa J.G., Dougherty M., Papanastassiou A., Gidal B., Mohamad I., Vossler D.G. Treatment of Super-Refractory *status epilepticus*. *Epilepsy Curr* 2021;21:405–15.

Riviello Jr. J.J., Claassen J., LaRoche S.M., Sperling M.R., Alldredge B., Bleck T.P., Glauser T., Shutter L., Treiman D.M., Vespa P.M., Bell R., Brophy G.M.; Neurocritical Care Society Status Epilepticus Guideline Writing Committee. Treatment of *status epilepticus*: An international survey of experts. *Neurocrit Care* 2013;18:193–200.

Rosati A., De Masi S., Guerrini R. Ketamine for refractory *status epilepticus*: A systematic review. *CNS Drugs* 2018;32:997–1009.

Stredny C.M., Case S., Sansevere A.J., Son M., Henderson L., Gorman M.P. Interleukin-6 blockade with tocilizumab in anakinra-refractory febrile infection-related syndrome (FIRES). *Child Neurol Open* 2020;7. doi: 10.1177/2329048X20979253.

Vossler D.G., Bainbridge J.L., Boggs J.G., Novotny E.J., Loddenkemper T., Faught E., Amengual-Gual M., Fischer S.N., Gloss D.S., Olson M.D., Towne A.R., Naritoku D., Welty T.E. Treatment of refractory convulsive *status epilepticus*: A comprehensive review by the American Epilepsy Society Treatments Committee. *Epilepsy Curr* 2020;20:245–64.

26 Primary Mitochondrial Epilepsies

Russell P. Saneto
Seattle Children's Hospital and University of Washington

CONTENTS

INTRODUCTION

Mitochondrial diseases are a group of heterogeneous disorders that are characterized by altered physiological functioning caused by genetic variants in nuclear DNA (nDNA) and mitochondrial DNA (mtDNA). The induced pathological reductions in mitochondrial energy production give rise to these diseases. One of the hallmarks of mitochondrial disorders is the marked variation in clinical symptoms that arise at varying ages and can involve any single or combination of organs or tissues. Typically, the disease preferentially affects organs with high aerobic metabolism. Primary mitochondrial disorders are often progressive with high mortality and morbidity. Taken as a group, mitochondrial disease represents the most common cause of genetic inborn error of metabolism. The estimated lifetime risk for developing a genetic mitochondrial disease is approximately 1 in 3,200.

The brain with its high energy requirement is one of the most affected organs in mitochondrial disease. Several studies have shown that approximately 35%–60%

DOI: 10.1201/9781003296478-29

of individuals with mitochondrial disease have epilepsy. However, only two of the multiple different types of mitochondrial diseases are defined by the presence of epilepsy; one derived from genetic variants within nDNA (Alpers–Huttenlocher syndrome) and one from variants from mtDNA (myoclonus, epilepsy with ragged-red fibers; MERRF).

ALPERS–HUTTENLOCHER SYNDROME

CASE PRESENTATION

The patient was a 2.5-year-old young girl who was previously healthy but presented with a 2-month history of vomiting with associated complaints of seeing "spiders" walking on the wall. In the hospital, an electroencephalogram (EEG) was performed that demonstrated occipital epileptiform discharges and slowing. She was started on an antiseizure medication (ASM) and sent home. One month later, she presented again to the emergency room with her right hand having nonstop jerking (epilepsia partialis continua), episodes of vomiting, reduced responsiveness, and clumsiness. A repeat EEG demonstrated persistent occipital slowing and discharges (Figure 26.1). Medically induced coma was required to break the status event. During the hospital stay, hallucinations continued episodically. Brain magnetic resonance imaging (MRI) was interpreted as normal, but spectroscopy demonstrated lactate accumulation (Figure 26.2). Due to persistent vomiting, she underwent a small bowel biopsy and antibody

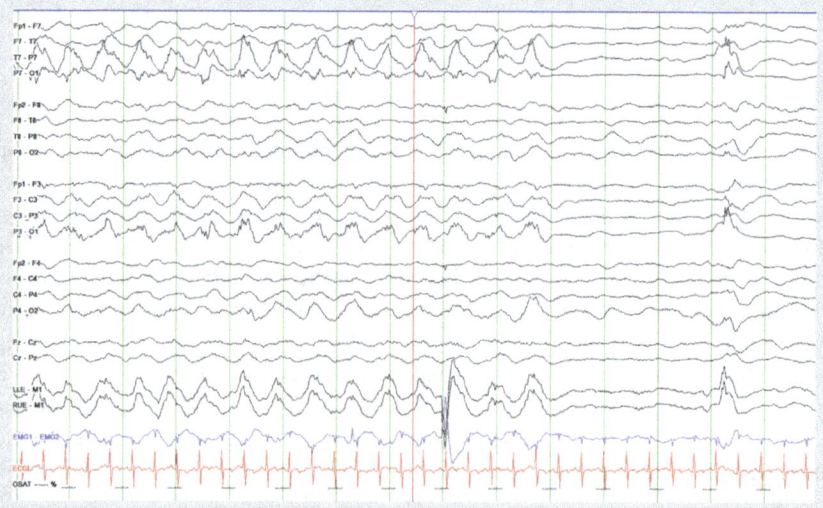

FIGURE 26.1   This EEG epoch shows background slowing with a rhythmic temporo-parieto-occipital delta slowing with overriding faster polyspikes.

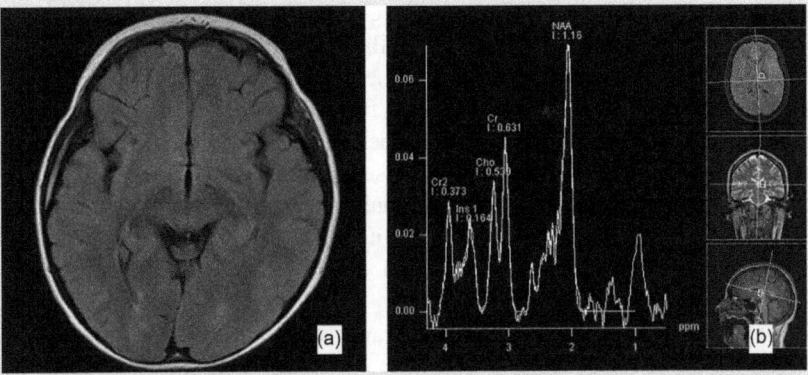

FIGURE 26.2 MRI (panel a) and MRS (panel b) of the case. Panel A demonstrates an axial Fluid Attenuated Inversion Recovery (FLAIR) sequence. This scan demonstrates subtle signal hyperintensity in the posterior head regions. Panel (b) demonstrates the lactate peak at 1.33 parts per million (ppm), taken from a voxel from the left thalamus (arrow).

testing and was found to have celiac disease. She was started on corticosteroid and immunoglobulin treatment. She was discharged on multiple ASMs. Over the next several months she developed limb jerking, mostly in the upper limbs with continued generalized myoclonic and tonic-clonic seizures. The limb jerks continued to increase with multiple EEG studies demonstrating likely segmental myoclonus. Her other seizure types continued. Her development regressed with the loss of most expressive language, and clinically she developed gastrointestinal dysmotility, and frank ataxia. At age of 3.5 years, during an emergency room visit for presumed myoclonic seizures, she was started on valproic acid. Over the course of several months, she developed lethargy with progressive encephalopathy. She was hospitalized and found to have elevated liver transaminases, prolonged clotting indices, elevated ammonia and serum lactate, and fatty liver on ultrasound. Due to liver failure, a liver biopsy was not possible, but genetic testing was pursued. She was found to have bi-allelic pathological variants in the polymerase gamma (POLG) subunit, p. Ala467Thr and p. Gln68X. POLG is the DNA replicase subunit of the mtDNA replicase, the trifunctional protein POL-γ.

DIFFERENTIAL DIAGNOSIS

The differential diagnosis of a patient developing explosive-onset epilepsy in a healthy young child includes a wide range of possibilities such as developmental and epileptic encephalopathies (DEE), monogenetic epilepsies, and somatic *de novo* epilepsy syndromes, and cortical malformations. The lack of tumor or malformation of cortical development on the brain MRI moves the diagnosis toward metabolic/genetic etiologies. The large lactate peak on spectroscopy can point to a metabolic etiology. The occipital dominance of epileptiform discharges suggests a wide range of possibilities, especially with the extensive vomiting. The progressive clinical findings are less compelling for the benign occipital epilepsies of childhood, early (Panayiotopoulos) and late (Gastaut) forms, now referred to as self-limited focal epilepsies in the International League Against Epilepsy (ILAE) classification system. The diagnosis of celiac disease would be compatible with occipital discharges, but the lack of calcifications would draw one away from this diagnosis. Wolf–Hirschhorn syndrome can present with seizures arising from the posterior head regions, but facial features and early global developmental delays are not compatible with the patient.

Gene discovery is rapidly changing the landscape of epilepsy. In a recent study, the overall annual incidence of single-gene epilepsy was found to be 1 per 2,120 live births in children under the age of 3 years. The clinical and biochemical analyte findings in our patient begin to steer diagnosis toward a metabolic-genetic cause. The seizure semiology of myoclonic seizures and segmental myoclonia might point to one of the progressive myoclonic epilepsies (see full discussion in the second case), but the associated findings in this patient of *epilepsia partialis continua*, ongoing lactate elevations, signs of liver failure, rapid developmental neurological regression, and multisystem involvement help to narrow down the diagnosis. Genetic testing demonstrated bi-allelic pathological variants in *POLG* and documented the specific mitochondrial epilepsy syndrome. However, with and without a genetic abnormality, there are a group of findings of biochemical analytes, EEG, MRI, muscle/liver mtDNA levels, electron transport chain enzymatic abnormalities, and liver findings that clinically define *POLG*-induced Alpers–Huttenlocher syndrome.

There is a closely related *POLG*-induced disorder, myocerebrohepatopathy that can be confused with Alpers–Huttenlocher syndrome. In this syndrome, infants usually present with early liver involvement and subsequently develop encephalopathy, hypotonia, renal dysfunction, and rarely seizures. Onset is usually before 7 months of age. Death due to liver failure is before 1 year of age. If the clinician only does genetic testing, a misdiagnosis can occur. However, liver pathology is different from Alpers–Huttenlocher syndrome and if seizures are present, they are minor. The overwhelming finding is the steady progression to liver failure and early death. Clinical acumen with close evaluation of biochemical findings is needed to discern this entity from Alpers–Huttenlocher as pathological *POLG* variants can overlap between the two disorders.

DIAGNOSTIC APPROACH

The age of presentation, normal early development, associated clinical signs and symptoms, and disease course begin to help guide the progression of testing. A classic triad of intractable seizures, developmental regression, and liver dysfunction is the hallmark of the diagnosis. *POLG*-induced Alpers–Huttenlocher syndrome presents between 2 and 5 years of age (range 3 months to 8 years). There is another rare onset peak, seen in females between 17 and 24 years (range 10–27 years). Over 50% of the patients experience the explosive onset of seizures with the EEG showing an occipital predominant slowing with intermixed polyspikes (Figure 26.1).

Onset of seizures heralds the rapid disease progression in most, but not all patients. The posterior dominant abnormal findings can be associated with nausea, vomiting, visual hallucinations, and abnormal eye movements. As the disease progresses, most patients have repeated episodes of status epilepticus, and many have *epilepsia partialis continua*. All develop pharmaco-resistant seizures with multiple seizure types including myoclonic, tonic, tonic-clonic, and nonspecific motor seizures. The myoclonia usually becomes predominant and almost continuous. Concurrent with seizure onset, a progressive global neurocognitive decline is seen. The rapid onset of encephalopathy, location of epileptiform discharges, and biochemical abnormalities separates Alpers–Huttenlocher syndrome from Dravet syndrome and other channelopathies, as well as the progressive myoclonic epilepsies. Early studies suggested that liver failure was due to valproic acid exposure, which was often given due to drug-resistant seizures. However, abnormal liver pathology was consistent with whether valproic acid exposure occurred or not and is distinct from other etiologies of liver failure with this phenotype. Although there is patient-to-patient variation, there is progression to failure.

Clinically, other nonspecific neurological features such as ataxia, migraine headaches, and visual hallucinations become evident due to occipital lobe involvement. The involvement of the calcarine and striate cortices can induce cortical blindness. Cranial nerve dysfunction with abnormal eye movements can occur. Cerebellar involvement can be seen not only with ataxia but also with loss of smooth pursuit eye movements. Nerve conduction testing is usually not performed in young children, but sensory neuropathy is likely. Outside the nervous system, the gastrointestinal system often displays dysmotility, dysphagia, and reflux requiring gastrointestinal tube feedings for nutrition. Pancreatitis can be seen. Cardiomyopathy and arrhythmia abnormalities have been reported.

When a young child develops explosive onset of seizures arising from the occipital region, the standard of care would be to obtain an MRI scan of the brain and metabolic testing for possible etiologies. If seizures become intractable to medications and stagnation or loss of developmental milestones begin to be seen, then further testing should be considered. Liver function testing would be a logical next step if previously not tested. If the latter is indicative of hepatopathy, then genetic sequencing of *POLG* should be undertaken. Bi-allelic pathological variants would close the loop in diagnosing Alpers–Huttenlocher syndrome.

However, if there is suspicion of Alpers–Huttenlocher without genetic testing, the use of the Naviaux criteria can be used to make the diagnosis. The latter criteria are based on multiple system involvement of the disorder, MRI and MRS findings, cortical blindness/optic atrophy, visual-evoked potentials, mtDNA content quantification in liver and muscle, POL-γ enzymatic activity, cerebrospinal lactate and elevated protein, electron transport chain enzymatic abnormality, and/or family history of Alpers–Huttenlocher syndrome.

TREATMENT STRATEGY

Unfortunately, treatment is limited to symptom management. Given the progressive nature of the disorder and devasting associated clinical findings, supportive care, and family education need to be addressed as the family becomes accepting of the diagnosis. Palliative care services should be involved early on, and quality of life needs to be the predominant considerations in care. This illness is relentless and progresses to fatal encephalopathy or liver failure. The various levels of treatment need to be addressed openly with the family. As the disease progresses, placement of a gastrostomy tube for nutrition, tracheostomy, or respiratory supplementation with continuous positive airway pressure or bilevel positive airway pressure-assisted nasal ventilation. The need for multiple services will be appropriate as soon as symptoms develop. An overlooked service is sleep medicine as evidence of central and/or obstructive apnea occurs early in the disorder.

Controlling seizures is important to increase quality of life and prevent associated progression in the brain. However, seizures may be impossible to completely control. At some point, the side effects of the treatment may outweigh the benefit of seizure control. No evidence exists for optimal treatment via randomized placebo-controlled trials. There is some evidence that one of the major pathological reasons for seizures is the loss of gamma-aminobutyric acid (GABA)-containing interneurons, suggesting that those seizure medications increasing the GABA-tone would be, at least in part, effective in controlling seizures. The ASMs lamotrigine, topiramate, and clobazam would be beneficial. Levetiracetam would be helpful with the myoclonic seizures and myoclonia, as would the newer medication brivaracetam. Medications reducing glutamate-mediated excitatory neurotransmission such as parampanel might also help control seizures by normalizing excitatory-inhibitory balance. As the tempo of seizures changes, medication choices usually become narrower. The choices of less sedating medications that are not processed through hepatic metabolism are better. Valproic acid should be avoided at all costs due to the risk of hepatopathy and induction of liver failure.

In early studies, it was found that central folate levels were low in Alpers–Huttenlocher syndrome. We routinely supplement folinic acid to allow transport of folate into the brain. Unfortunately, there are no treatments modifying the course of the illness. Most mitochondrial experts use a combination of vitamin antioxidant supplements – the so-called "mitochondrial cocktail" – to help reduce the oxidative radical formation induced by the disorder. Not all patients report a beneficial change in symptoms. Exercise has been shown to delay disease manifestations in a related mouse model, but thus far has not made its way into the clinic. Target treatment remains unsatisfactory.

LONG-TERM OUTCOME

This disorder is relentless and progressive. Once symptoms start in a child, the average lifespan ranges from 4 to 10 years. Although not clearly established, if our preventative treatments continue to improve and are implemented earlier in the disease course, there may be extended quality of life. Also, the withholding of valproic acid to treat seizures has decreased liver failure and likely extended lifespan. However, death is premature in all cases.

The later onset disease is different in progression and morbidity. Patients meet the Naviaux criteria, but the liver involvement remains limited for a prolonged period. The author follows two patients who are over a decade removed from their diagnosis. There are case reports of patients alive several decades after diagnosis. The small numbers of patients make statements of longevity premature. As more patients in this group are reported, a better estimate of disease severity can be made.

PATHOPHYSIOLOGY/NEUROBIOLOGY OF DISEASE

The exact mechanism of *POLG* pathological variants inducing Alpers–Huttenlocher syndrome is unclear. *POLG* encodes the enzymatically active subunit of the mtDNA heterotrimer POL-γ. The *POLG* protein has 5′-3′ polymerase, 3′-5′ exonuclease, and lyase activity. It acts as a replicase and repair enzyme within the mitochondria. The dysfunctional DNA replicase limits DNA content in the ongoing proliferation of the mitochondrial organelle. In Alpers–Huttenlocher syndrome, the major feature is a significant reduction in mtDNA content and not multiple deletions in mtDNA. Due to the advent of commercial genetic sequencing and DNA measurement, severe depletion of muscle and/or liver mtDNA can be a useful clue to diagnosis. The clinician needs to remember that there are over 20 distinct genes that can induce mtDNA depletion. Also, depending on the stage of disease, mtDNA depletion might be limited. The use of mtDNA content is therefore not sensitive or specific for Alpers–Huttenlocher syndrome.

The exact mechanism of mtDNA depletion remains unclear. The same exact *POLG* pathological variants may cause different diseases. For example, homozygous p. Ala467Thr variants may induce Alpers–Huttenlocher syndrome, juvenile Alpers–Huttenlocher syndrome, ataxia-neuropathy spectrum, and progressive external ophthalmoplegia with and without other system involvement. These various syndromes have different ages of onset ranging from 2 to >40 years of age, overlapping and distinct organ system involvement, and mtDNA depletion or mtDNA multiple deletions. Muscle is the proper tissue to evaluate mtDNA as after birth it is a post-mitotic tissue and so there is less variable content due to possible selection that can occur with proliferation of cells. The older onset patients have multiple mtDNA deletions and no depletion in muscle tissue. How this finding is regulated remains unknown.

Ultimately, the reduced production of energy required for cellular functioning produces cell and organ failure. The minimum energy needs vary between tissues and explains the multisystem and time-related onset of involvement. There are multiple mtDNA synthesized proteins that are necessary for proper mitochondrial function. Of the approximately 1,500 proteins required for mitochondrial functioning, mtDNA only contains 13 polypeptides, 2 ribosomal RNAs, and 22 tRNAs. The compromised replication of mtDNA produces reduced essential mtDNA products, which in turn decreases the amount of available chemical energy in the form of ATP.

CLINICAL PEARLS

- Explosive seizure onset in a normally developing young child with progressive cognitive decline with hepatopathy should raise the suspicion of Alpers–Huttenlocher syndrome.
- Seizures with EEG slowing and epileptiform discharges arising from the posterior head regions that develop into episodes of status epilepticus and/or *epilepsia partialis continua* without MRI structural abnormalities suggestive of tumor or malformation of cortical development should raise suspicion for pursuing genetic testing for *POLG*.
- If there is a suspicion that a patient has Alpers–Huttenlocher syndrome, valproic acid should be absolutely avoided.
- As the disease progresses, multiple medical specialties will need to be involved for symptomatic care and quality of life issues.
- The progressive nature of this disorder requires early involvement of palliative care and ease of information sharing with the family so they can become involved in the early care decisions for their child.

SUGGESTED REFERENCES

Harding B.N. Progressive neurological degeneration of childhood with liver disease (Alpers-Huttenlocher syndrome): A personal review. *J Child Neurol* 1990;5:273–87.

Nguyen K.V., Sharief F.S., Chan S.L., Copeland W.C., Naviaux R.K. Molecular diagnosis of Alpers syndrome. *J Hepatol* 2006;45:108–16.

Rahman S., Copeland W.C. POLG-related disorders and their neurological manifestations. *Nat Rev Neurol* 2019;15:40–52.

Saneto R.P., Cohen B.H., Copeland W.C., Naviaux R.K. Alpers-Huttenlocher syndrome: A review. *Pediatr Neurol* 2013;10:167–78.

Saneto R.P. An update on Alpers-Huttenlocher syndrome: Pathophysiology of disease and rational treatment designs. *Expert Opin Orphan Drugs* 2018;6:741–51.

Wolf N.I., Rahman S., Schmitt B., Taanman J.W., Duncan A.J., Harting I., Wohlrab G., Ebinger F., Rating D., Bast T. *Status epilepticus* in children with Alpers' disease caused by *POLG1* mutations: EEG and MRI features. *Epilepsia* 2009;50:1596–607.

MYOCLONUS, EPILEPSY WITH RAGGED-RED FIBERS

CASE PRESENTATION

The patient began having repetitive jerking at 13 years of age. These movements were described as lightening-like myoclonia, mostly occurring during the day. As time progressed, she also developed myoclonic seizures as well as infrequent generalized tonic-clonic seizures. Her parents also described clumsiness that developed. Clumsiness was attributed to both muscle weakness as well as myoclonia. Initially, it was thought that drop seizures were occurring, but on further testing, most falling episodes were due to ataxia and myoclonia. On neurological exam, she displayed cerebellar ataxia and hypotonia. Once an excellent student, she began to display a progressive decline in cognitive functioning as myoclonia intensified. Over time, she developed optic atrophy, however, other abnormalities were not found. The EEG showed predominantly bursts of atypical, generalized spike-and-wave discharges with a disorganized slow background (Figure 26.3). There were also independent spikes over the left and right hemisphere, and diffuse slow delta bursts. Over several years, the background slowing has been persistent but was not progressive. There were also photomyoclonic responses with photic stimulation on EEG. On repeat EEG, massive body myoclonia was demonstrated (Figure 26.4). Initial MRI of the brain at the time of diagnosis

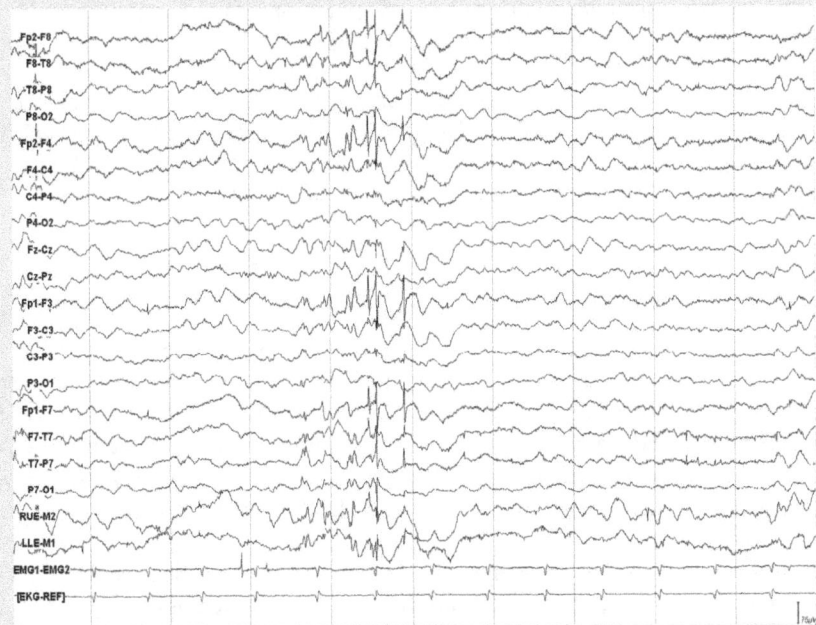

FIGURE 26.3   This EEG epoch shows atypical, generalized spike-and-wave discharges. There is a slow and disorganized background.

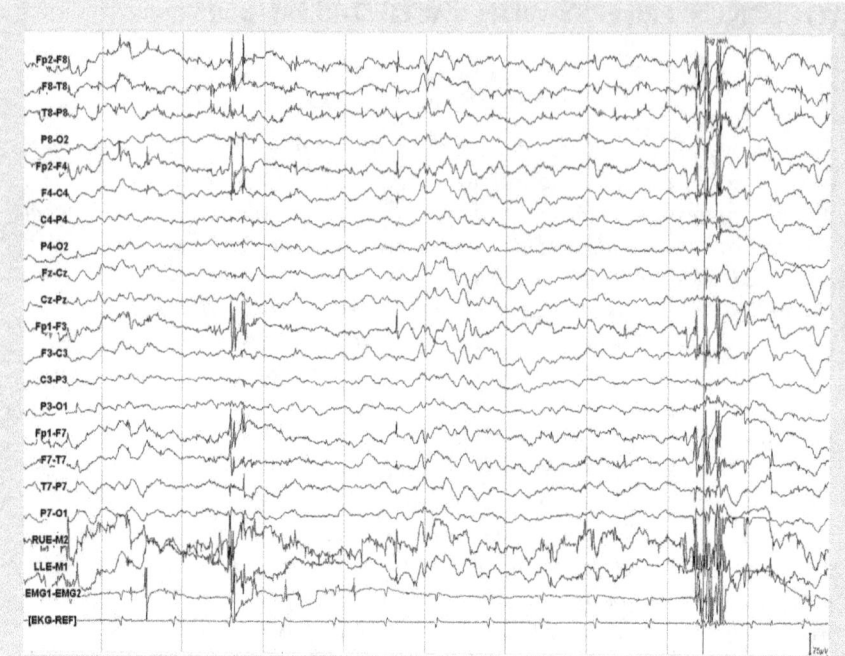

FIGURE 26.4   This EEG epoch demonstrated two events of massive body myoclonia without significant EEG change. There is persistence of the slow and disorganized background with frontally predominant narrow spikes.

was interpreted as normal. A repeat scan a year later was also read as normal. Muscle biopsy showed ragged-red fibers on histological staining. Electron trans-port chain (ETC) enzymology demonstrated normal activity. However, molecular testing identified a mtDNA pathological variant, m.8344 A>G.

DIFFERENTIAL DIAGNOSIS

The differential diagnosis in a child/teenager who develops progressive neurological regression, ataxia, and myoclonic epilepsy include the progressive myoclonic epilepsies. Early in the evaluation process, the hereditary ataxia syndromes would be a consideration if the ataxia component was predominant. However, the presence of myoclonia and myoclonic seizures would be more consistent with the progressive myoclonic epilepsies. There are four main elements of the progressive myoclonic epilepsies:

1. Myoclonic jerks that are segmental, fragmentary, and erratic in region,
2. Epileptic seizures, mainly generalized tonic-clonic and massive myoclonic seizures,
3. Progressive mental deterioration,
4. Variable neurological signs and symptoms, mainly cerebellar, extrapyramidal, and action myoclonus.

Most are genetically determined, and all have a neurologically degenerative course. The signs and symptoms are usually specific or highly suggestive of a particular type of epilepsy. The typical progressive myoclonic epilepsies include: Unverricht-Lundborg disease, MERRF, Lafora body disease, sialidosis type 1, neuronal ceroid lipofuscinoses, juvenile neuronopathic Gaucher disease, dentatorubropallidoluysian atrophy, and juvenile neuroaxonal dystrophy. Most feel that the concept of a definite syndrome of progressive myoclonic epilepsy is archaic, as many epileptic syndromes may have transient episodes of ataxia and/or mental regression and multiple gene etiologies. However, the term progressive myoclonic epilepsy has been maintained in the new guidelines for classification of seizures and syndromes.

We feel the name of myoclonus, epilepsy, with ragged-red fibers is the proper name. Although myoclonic seizures are seen, there are also multiple myoclonus events and therefore the name of the mitochondrial disease reflects these three characteristics. The name of myoclonic epilepsy with ragged-red fibers is often used as well. We prefer to use the former due to the more complete definition of the disorder.

DIAGNOSTIC APPROACH

The age of presentation associated clinical signs and symptoms, clinical course, pattern of inheritance, and ethnic origin of the patient are invaluable in the diagnosis of this group of epilepsies. MERRF has a variable age of onset from 3 years to adulthood. This wide range of onset can be confusing due to other myoclonic epilepsies beginning at various ages, many of which are benign. Usually the clinical history, EEG, and serial neurological examination will help differentiate the various myoclonic epilepsies. There are also other types of mitochondrial disease that express myoclonic seizures, developmental stagnation or regression, and heterogeneous organ involvement.

Based on the clinical presentation and progression of cognitive loss, associated symptoms, and ethnic origin, most of the other progressive myoclonic epilepsies can be potentially diagnosed. Other than the canonical features of myoclonus, generalized seizures, ataxia, ragged-red fibers in muscle, there are frequent other clinical abnormalities noted in MERRF including sensorineural hearing loss, peripheral neuropathy, short stature, exercise intolerance, and optic atrophy. Less frequent clinical signs reported are cardiomyopathy, preexcitation arrhythmia (Wolf-Parkinson-White), pigmentary retinopathy, ophthalmoparesis, pyramidal signs, and multiple lipomas.

Most mitochondrial diseases are multisystem disorders, with those organs requiring the most energy usually demonstrating the presenting phenotype. Myoclonus, generalized seizures, and normal early development are typical in the diagnosis of MERRF. Other mitochondrial diseases due to electron transport chain (ETC) defects and different mitochondrial DNA mutations can present similarly, potentially confounding the correct diagnosis. Screening labs consisting of serum lactate, quantitative serum amino acids, serum acyl carnitine profile, and quantitative urine organic acids should help differentiate possible MERRF from other progressive myoclonic epilepsies, as well as other mitochondrial diseases. Unlike most ETC disorders, the EEG shows a generalized spike/polyspike pattern in MERRF.

Brain MRI and magnetic resonance spectroscopy (MRS) may also help differentiate possible diagnoses. Voxels over the CSF space and the brain showing a lactate peak on MRS would suggest the possibility of a mitochondrial disease. MRI findings can be useful in differentiation of Leigh syndrome and mitochondrial encephalomyopathy, lactic acidosis, and stroke-like episodes (MELAS) from MERRF. Brain MRI in MELAS often demonstrates areas of abnormal T2 signal suggestive of ischemia, while Leigh syndrome is associated with abnormal T2 signal in the brainstem and basal ganglia suggestive of necrosis. If a strong indication of maternal inheritance is present, clinical history is compatible, lactic acid elevations in CSF and serum, and bland findings in other biochemical tests, the investigation of a possible gene mutation in the mtDNA could be pursued at this point.

If the cumulative evidence is indicative but not defining, then proceeding to muscle biopsy for further analysis is suggested. The finding of ragged-red fibers using Gomori trichrome staining would demonstrate the fourth feature of MERRF. Ragged-red fibers in the child and adolescent are very unusual and if present, would be confirmatory given the presence of the other three features. Often there are cytochrome oxidase-negative fibers in both ragged-red fibers as well as non-ragged-red muscle fibers. If ETC enzymology is performed, deficient enzyme activity may or may not be found. It is important that if ETC abnormalities are found and the clinical suspicion is MERRF, ongoing testing should continue. Genetic testing to evaluate for commonly associated mutations should be undertaken to confirm the diagnosis for genetic counseling for other siblings and family members. We have found patients with many phenotypic qualities of MERRF without mitochondrial DNA mutations or ragged-red fibers, who demonstrate ETC deficiencies.

Molecular gene testing would be the next step. If muscle tissue is available, it would be the preferred tissue for examination, but isolated leukocytes can also be used for testing. The most common mitochondrial DNA mutation associated with MERRF is in the gene MT-TK encoding tRNA^{Lys}, m. 8344 A>G. Although over 80% of affected patients have the m. 8344 A>G mutation, another 10% of patients have other point mutations within the MT-TK gene, m. 8356 T>C, m. 8363 G>A, and m. 8361 G>A. There are also other rare mutations in the MT-TK gene as well as other mitochondria-encoded proteins. Mutation in the complex I subunit MT-ND5 has been found to cause an overlap syndrome with MERRF and MELAS phenotype.

TREATMENT STRATEGY

Treatment with conventional ASMs may reduce seizures initially, but seldom produces complete remission as the disease progresses. Those medications that are usually used for myoclonic seizures generally are more efficacious: valproic acid, lamotrigine, zonisamide, levetiracetam, and benzodiazepines. However, medication efficacy tends to be patient specific, and no prospective studies have been performed. In a small study of five patients with mitochondrial disease due to ETC dysfunction, vagus nerve stimulation did not produce a significant reduction in myoclonic seizure frequency. This suggests that placement of the vagus nerve stimulator device be undertaken with caution.

The addition of L-carnitine and coenzyme Q10 has been advocated by some to improve mitochondrial function. However, no prospective studies have been performed to support this assertion. Standard pharmacologic therapy is used to treat other specific organ involvement, such as cardiac symptoms. Currently, there is no treatment for the genetic defect.

LONG-TERM OUTCOME

The outcome in patients with MERRF depends somewhat on heteroplasmy. Heteroplasmy is based on the idea that there are many mitochondria per cell, some of which may contain the mutation while others do not. Those patients having a higher percentage of the mutation likely express the disease earlier in life and have a more progressive course. Heteroplasmy may also account for the variation in disease expression in maternal relatives. Tissue distribution also plays a part in outcome; as more organ systems become involved there is an increased compromise to the quality of life as well as longevity.

PATHOPHYSIOLOGY/NEUROBIOLOGY OF DISEASE

The molecular pathogenesis of mitochondrial tRNA^{Lys} mutations is not completely understood. However, experiments using rho^o cell lines have unveiled important clues. Rho^o cell lines are permanent human cell lines emptied of their mtDNA by exposure to ethidium bromide, then repopulated with mitochondria harboring specific mutations. These transmitochondrial cybrids with a high mutational load have correlated with decreased protein synthesis, and reduced oxygen consumption and respiratory chain function.

The 8344 mutation has been also shown to cause impairment of mitochondrial translation in cultured myoblasts. Polypeptides containing higher numbers of lysine residues are more severely affected by the tRNA^{Lys} mutation, thus suggesting a direct inhibition of protein synthesis. Furthermore, the 8344 mutation has been associated with defects in aminoacylation capacity as well as lower steady-state levels of tRNA^{Lys}. What remains unclear is how these defects orchestrate MERRF pathogenesis.

CLINICAL PEARLS

- Evolving multisystem organ system involvement in a previous normal patient with progressively medically resistant myoclonus should raise the suspicion of MERRF.
- There is no clear correlation between genotype and clinical phenotype for affected individuals, so clinical judgment is of utmost importance.
- If clinical suspicion is MERRF but leukocyte testing is negative, other tissues (muscle) should be used for detection of potential mutations.
- Medications effective against myoclonus, such as benzodiazepines and levetiracetam, form the cornerstone of treatment, but may fail to control seizures as the disease progresses.

SUGGESTED REFERENCES

Berkovic S.F., Cochius J., Andermann E., Andermann F. Progressive myoclonus epilepsies: Clinical and genetic aspects. *Epilepsia* 1993;34(Suppl 3):S19–S30.

DiMauro S., Davidzon G. Mitochondrial DNA and disease. *Ann Med* 2005;37:222–32.

Fukuhara N., Tokiguchi S., Shirakawa K., Tsubaki T. Myoclonus epilepsy associated with ragged-red fibers (mitochondrial abnormalities): Disease entity or a syndrome? Light- and electron-microscopic studies of two cases and review of literature. *J Neurol Sci* 1980;47:117–33.

Hammans S.R., Sweeney M.G., Brockington M., Lennox G.G., Lawton N.F., Kennedy C.R., Morgan-Hughes J.A., Harding A.E. The mitochondrial DNA transfer RNA (Lys)A > G (8344) mutation and the syndrome of myoclonic epilepsy with ragged-red fibers (MERRF): Relationship of clinical phenotype to proportion of mutant mitochondrial DNA. *Brain* 1993;116:617–32.

Shoffner J.M., Lott M.T., Lezza A.M., Seibel P., Ballinger S.W., Wallace D.C. Myoclonic epilepsy and ragged-red fiber disease (MERRF) is associated with a mitochondrial DNA tRNA(Lys) mutation. *Cell* 1990;61:931–7.

27 Tuberous Sclerosis Complex

Aimee F. Luat
Central Michigan University
and
Wayne State University

Harry T. Chugani
NYU School of Medicine

CONTENTS

CASE PRESENTATION

The patient was 2.5 years old when she first presented for further evaluation and management of her intractable seizures. She was an Egyptian girl born at term after an uneventful pregnancy and vaginal delivery. At birth, >3 hypopigmented macules each measuring at least 5 mm were noted. On the day of birth, she began having seizures consisting of eye gaze to one side. Neurologic investigations included lumbar puncture, metabolic studies, electroencephalography (EEG), and brain magnetic resonance imaging (MRI). The MRI showed multiple bilateral cortical tubers. Multiple cardiac rhabdomyomas were noted on echocardiogram. A definite clinical diagnosis of tuberous sclerosis complex (TSC) was made. Her seizures came under control with phenobarbital for 1.5 years and, thereafter, the medication was discontinued. However, her seizures recurred and persisted despite trials of valproic acid, clonazepam, phenobarbital, and lamotrigine. She developed epileptic spasms consisting of sudden and brief flexion of her neck, arms, and legs against her body. These episodes occurred in clusters, especially during drowsiness and upon arousal from sleep. She had global developmental delay and at the age of 2.5 years, she could neither speak single words nor walk independently. There was no *family history of tuberous sclerosis or epilepsy. On physical examination, she was microcephalic with a head circumference of 46 cm (<2nd percentile). More than three hypopigmented macules (≥5 mm in size) were noted on her face and trunk. On neurological examination, she was awake and alert, but could not speak words. She moved her extremities symmetrically but could not walk. Brain MRI was repeated and again showed multiple bilateral cortical tubers (Figure 27.1). A calcified tuber was noted in the right inferior frontal gyrus (white arrow). Multiple calcified subependymal nodules were also noted along the lateral ventricles. Genetic testing confirmed the presence of a TSC2 pathogenic variant. She was started on vigabatrin at 50 mg/kg/day and this was later increased to 80 mg/kg/day. Her seizures were controlled with vigabatrin for the next 1.5 years such that she would have breakthrough seizures only when she was ill. However, her seizures subsequently increased in frequency despite increased doses of vigabatrin and the addition of oxcarbazepine. Due to the medical intractability of her seizures, she was evaluated for epilepsy surgery. Video-EEG captured focal seizures consisting of behavioral arrest, staring and unresponsiveness followed by clusters of epileptic spasms. Ictal EEG showed seizure onset from the right frontal-temporal region. Subclinical seizures coming from the right frontal region were also captured. Interictally, multifocal spike and wave activities were noted. 2-Deoxy-2-[^{18}F] fluoro-D-glucose (FDG) positron emission tomography (PET) scan showed multiple areas of glucose hypometabolism in both the left and right hemispheres (Figure 27.2a). [^{11}C] Methyl-L-tryptophan (AMT) PET scan showed intense uptake only in a right frontal tuber (Figure 27.2b). The child underwent a two-stage epilepsy surgery with extraoperative electrocorticography (ECoG). Numerous clinical as well as electrographic seizures of right frontal onset were captured. She underwent a right frontal lobectomy guided by ECoG and the AMT-PET. Pathology showed multiple areas of dysplastic*

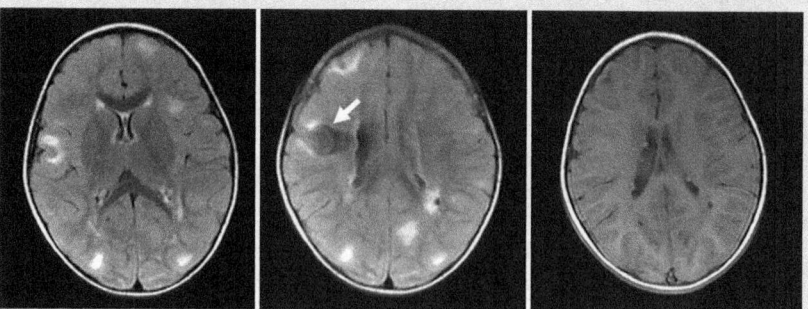

FIGURE 27.1 Fluid attenuated inversion recovery (FLAIR) pulse sequence MRI showed multiple and extensive areas of high signal intensity in both the left and right cerebral hemispheres consistent with multiple cortical and subcortical tubers. A calcified tuber located in the right inferior frontal gyrus (arrow) can be noted showing low signal intensity on FLAIR.

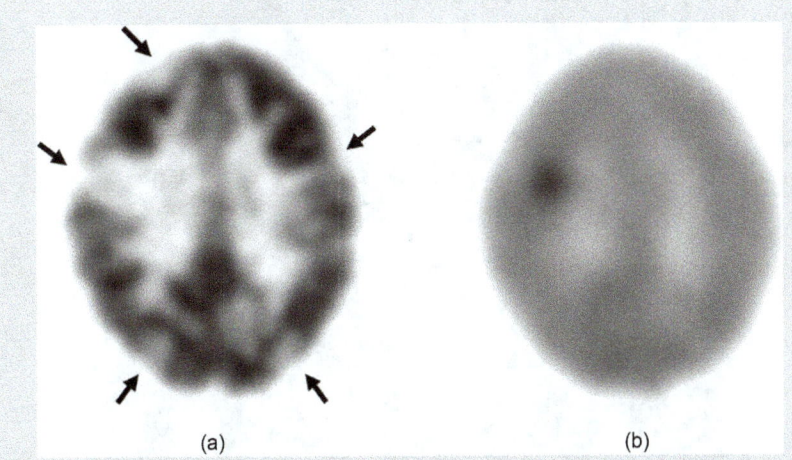

(a)   (b)

FIGURE 27.2 (a) 2-Deoxy-2-[18F] fluoro-D-glucose (FDG) positron emission tomography scan (PET) scan showed multiple areas of glucose hypometabolism (black arrows) in both the left and right hemispheres. (b) [^{11}C] Methyl-L-tryptophan (AMT) PET scan showed intense uptake in a right frontal tuber.

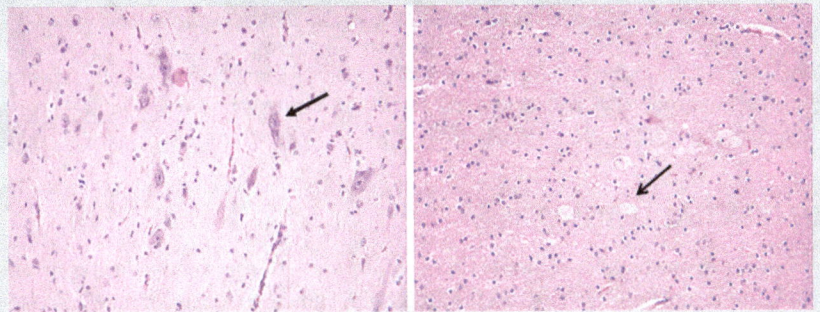

FIGURE 27.3 Histopathology of the resected right frontal cortex using hematoxylin and eosin stain (H&E) showing the presence of giant cells (left arrow) and balloon cells (right arrow).

cortex with loss of normal laminar architecture. Increased fibrillarity of the neuropil was also noted. Dysplastic cells including balloon cells and cyto-megalic neurons were noted (Figure 27.3). Currently, she is 21 years old and has been seizure free for over 10 years but requires antiseizure medications (ASMs) as her EEG remains abnormal. She has developed multiple enlarging renal angiomyolipomas (Figure 27.4), which are currently being treated with everolimus.

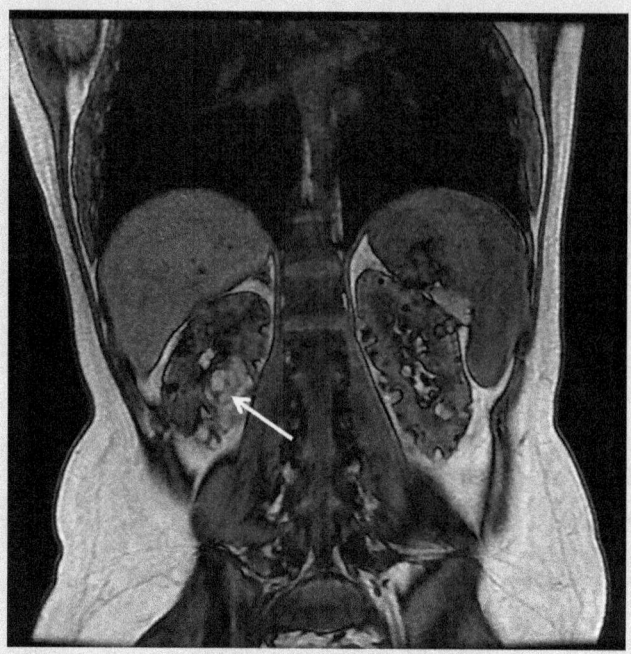

FIGURE 27.4   Coronal T2-weighted abdominal MRI demonstrating our patient's renal angiomyolipomas with the largest noted on the right (white arrow).

DIFFERENTIAL DIAGNOSIS

The causes of intractable epilepsy in children are heterogeneous. In the newborn period, intractable epilepsy is rarely idiopathic. Hence, extensive neurologic investigations should be performed in order to establish and treat the underlying cause. In neonates, a broad range of systemic and central nervous system disorders should be considered, including hypoxic-ischemic encephalopathy, intracranial hemorrhage, infection, metabolic and genetic disorders, and cerebral malformations. TSC has rarely been reported as a cause of neonatal seizures. The frequent absence of the traditional stigmata of TSC in neonates may account for its underdiagnosis in this age group. Therefore, a high index of suspicion for TSC in every neonate who presents with idiopathic intractable seizures is necessary. Based on the current diagnostic criteria (Table 27.1), identification of a pathogenic variant in the *TSC1* or *TSC2* gene is sufficient to give a definite diagnosis of TSC regardless of the clinical findings.

The diagnosis of our patient was straightforward with the typical clinical findings of TSC – namely, the presence of multiple hypopigmented macules, cardiac rhabdomyomas, and multiple cortical tubers. It should be noted that the onset of either focal seizures or epileptic spasms in infants with hypomelanotic macules, as in our case, strongly suggests the diagnosis of TSC.

DIAGNOSTIC APPROACH

TSC is characterized by the development of hamartomas in multiple organs of the body including the skin, brain, kidneys, heart, and eyes. The 1998 diagnostic criteria were revised in 1999, 2013, and most recently in 2021 (Table 27.1). Diagnosing TSC in newborns can be difficult since the skin and visceral lesions may not be apparent at this age. The use of a Wood's (ultraviolet) lamp may allow for the detection of small or subtle skin lesions. The use of genetic testing (sequencing methods, i.e., epilepsy panels and whole exome sequencing) in infants with early-life epilepsies has also increased the recognition of TSC irrespective of their clinical features. In our patient, the diagnosis was clear since the clinical features of TSC were readily apparent. When TSC is diagnosed, regardless of age, brain, and abdominal MRI, detailed and complete skin and eye exam as well age-appropriate cardiac evaluation is recommended. Parents and caregivers should be counseled on how to recognize epileptic spasms and focal seizures. Baseline routine EEG with recording during sleep is recommended and a follow-up long-term EEG may be needed if abnormal. TSC-associated neuropsychiatric disorders

---

TABLE 27.1

Revised Clinical Diagnostic Criteria for Tuberous Sclerosis Complex (TSC)

Major Features	Minor Features
Hypomelanotic macules (≥ 3; at least 5mm diameter)	"Confetti" skin lesions
Angiofibroma (≥ 3) or fibrous cephalic plaque	Dental enamel pits (≥ 3)
Ungual fibroma (≥ 2)	Intraoral fibromas (≥ 2)
Shagreen patch	Retinal achromic patch
Multiple retinal hamartomas	Multiple renal cysts
Multiple cortical tuber and/or radial migration lines	Nonrenal hamartomas
Subependymal nodule (≥ 2)	Sclerotic bone lesions
Subependymal giant cell astrocytoma	
Cardiac rhabdomyoma	
Lymphangiomyomatosis (LAM)	
Angiomyolipomas ≥ 2	

Source: Adapted from Northrup et al. (2021).

Definite TSC: 2 major or 1 major with 2 minor features.

Possible TSC: either 1 major or ≥ 2 minor features.

Genetic diagnosis: A pathogenic variant in TSC1 or TSC2 is diagnostic of TSC (most TSC-causing variants are sequence variants that clearly prevent TSC1 or TSC2 protein production. Some variants compatible with protein production [e.g., some missense changes] are well established as disease-causing; other variant types should be considered with caution).

A combination of the 2 major clinical features LAM and angiomyolipomas without other features does not meet criteria for a definite diagnosis.

(TAND) checklist should also be administered to identify neuropsychiatric issues that need to be addressed. Genetic testing for the causative genes of tuberous sclerosis, *TSC1* and *TSC2* is recommended for genetic counseling or when the diagnosis is suspected or in question and cannot be confirmed clinically, such as in ambiguous cases.

TREATMENT STRATEGY

Epilepsy in TSC is often resistant to ASMs and may have a negative impact on the child's neurocognitive development; hence, there is some urgency in achieving seizure control. Reduced gamma-aminobutyric acid (GABA)ergic neurotransmission has been hypothesized as the basis behind the efficacy of vigabatrin in the treatment of epilepsy in TSC. Vigabatrin is a structural analog of GABA and produces its antiseizure effect by irreversibly inhibiting GABA transaminase (GABA-T), the degradative enzyme for GABA, thus significantly increasing GABA levels (i.e., inhibition) in brain. Recent studies suggest that in mouse models of TSC, vigabatrin also inhibits the mechanistic or mammalian target of rapamycin (mTOR) pathway, the dysregulated pathway in TSC. Vigabatrin has an efficacy rate of 95% in TSC-associated epileptic spasms. However, potential adverse effects include irreversible concentric visual field loss and brain MRI signal abnormalities (particularly in the basal ganglia).

For the past decade, advances in TSC research led to major improvements in its management including the use of presymptomatic vigabatrin therapy prior to the onset of clinical seizures, the use of mTOR inhibitors and purified cannabidiol in TSC-associated epilepsy. However, despite the availability of unique mechanistic-based treatments, drug refractory epilepsy continues to occur in 60% of TSC cases (in contrast to 30% in the general epilepsy population). In such cases, resective epilepsy surgery may provide a good therapeutic option especially if a single tuber is acting as the epileptic focus, as exemplified in our case. Epilepsy surgery in TSC can be a challenge because the suspected epileptogenic tuber can be difficult to identify amidst multiple bilateral lesions. Conventional MRI and EEG often show multifocal abnormalities. Likewise, the FDG-PET scan also shows multifocal areas of hypometabolism without specifically indicating the epileptogenic region. AMT ([^{11}C] methyl-L-tryptophan) is an analog of tryptophan, and AMT-PET can be used to measure brain serotonin synthesis capacity noninvasively in humans. The use of AMT-PET scanning has proven to be a useful tool in differentiating between epileptogenic and nonepileptogenic tubers and has improved epilepsy surgery outcomes in TSC.

In our case, AMT-PET showed intense uptake concordant with the ictal EEG onset zone thereby strengthening the localization of the potential epileptogenic zone. The precise mapping of the epileptogenic zone was aided by ECoG, and cessation of the patient's seizures after surgical resection of the right frontal lobe confirmed the accuracy of AMT-PET. Other treatment approaches, such as ketogenic diet and neurostimulation, may also be effective and are generally well tolerated. These alternative treatments should be strongly considered in those patients who are not appropriate surgical candidates.

EPILEPSY IN TUBEROUS SCLEROSIS COMPLEX

Epilepsy is the most common neurological feature of TSC, occurring in 80% to over 90% of cases, often commencing in the first year of life. Epileptic spasms and focal seizures are the most common seizure types. TSC is an important cause of epileptic spasms accounting for between 10% and 25% of cases. Our patient initially had focal seizures followed by the development of spasms with co-existent focal-onset seizures.

Epileptic spasms in TSC have distinctive clinical and EEG features. Each episode is usually associated with focal or lateralizing features such as tonic eye deviation, head turning, or nystagmus. Infants with epileptic spasms due to TSC exhibit a particular awake interictal EEG characterized by multifocal asynchronous spike discharges and irregular slow activity that increases and becomes generalized during non-rapid eye movement (REM) sleep. Hypsarrhythmia often appears later in the course or may not appear at all. The ictal EEG in TSC may start with a focal discharge of spikes and polyspikes in the region of the epileptogenic tuber, followed by generalized irregular slow-wave and background attenuation. Our patient's ictal EEG demonstrated the phenomenon of focal seizures and epileptic spasms as a single ictal event supporting the notion that cortical "triggering" mechanisms may be the underlying basis in the pathogenesis of epileptic spasms in certain groups of children.

Recent studies suggest that in infants with TSC, the development of interictal epileptiform discharges can predict the development of clinical seizures in 75% of cases and preventative therapy with vigabatrin may improve the neurological prognosis, both in terms of seizures and cognitive development. Furthermore, the safety and efficacy of everolimus and cannabidiol in significantly reducing seizures in TSC have been demonstrated in randomized clinical trials which led to its FDA approval in 2018 and 2020, respectively.

LONG-TERM OUTCOME

Patients with TSC have a high prevalence of cognitive and behavioral difficulties, including autism. Epileptic spasms and early intractable epilepsy may increase this risk, and side effects of polytherapy with ASMs may also blunt cognition. Many patients may respond to medical management with ASMs; however, up to 60% of patients with early-onset seizures may prove medically refractory. Epilepsy surgery may render more than 50% of appropriately selected patients seizure free, as in our case. In addition to neurological issues, renal involvement including renal angiomyolipoma is a major cause of morbidity and mortality in TSC, highlighting the importance of a multidisciplinary approach for each individual affected by this disorder.

PATHOPHYSIOLOGY/NEUROBIOLOGY OF THE DISEASE

TSC is caused by pathogenic inactivation of *TSC1* (hamartin) or *TSC2* (tuberin) genes located in chromosome 9q34 and chromosome 16p13.3, respectively. *TSC2* pathogenic variants account for most sporadic cases while pathogenic variants in either gene can be seen in familial (autosomal dominant) cases. Somatic mosaicism may also occur and can explain cases with very mild phenotype or with only a single

CLINICAL PEARLS

- Tuberous sclerosis should be considered in infants and children with seizures, particularly epileptic spasms.
- The understanding of the molecular pathogenesis of TSC led to clinical trials involving the use of mTOR inhibitors in TSC-associated clinical manifestations and its subsequent FDA approval in the treatment of seizures, SEGAs, and renal angiomyolipomas.
- Advances in TSC research has significantly changed the management of TSC-associated epilepsy, including the use of presymptomatic vigabatrin therapy prior to the onset of clinical seizures and the use of purified cannabidiol as adjunctive therapy.
- In a subgroup of TSC patients whose seizures remain medically intractable, resection of the epileptogenic tuber may provide long-lasting seizure freedom and "rescue" cognitive deterioration.

manifestation of TSC (e.g., a single cortical tuber). A negative genetic testing is seen in 10%–15% of TSC patients.

Under normal conditions, hamartin and tuberin bind with the 3rd protein, TBC1D7, to form a complex that inhibits the mTOR pathway, the central regulator of cellular growth, size, and proliferation. When either *TSC1* or *TSC2* is inactivated, mTOR pathway upregulation occurs with consequent abnormal cellular growth and proliferation in various organ systems. This molecular insight led to the evaluation of mTOR inhibitors for TSC in clinical trials and its subsequent U.S. Food and Drug Administration (FDA) approval for TSC-associated manifestations including seizures, subependymal giant cell astrocytoma (SEGA), and renal angiomyolipoma. In the brain, neuronal abnormalities including cortical tubers are seen, which can explain many of the neurologic manifestations of the disease. TSC is considered a prototype "mTORopathy" which characterizes a group of brain developmental disorders that includes cortical dysplasia and hemimegalencephaly. Pathologically, cortical tubers show cytomegaly and balloon cells, as noted in our case. The tumorigenesis in several TSC lesions can be explained by Knudson's two-hit hypothesis, in which a germline mutation in one allele of *TSC1* or *TSC2* gene is followed by a somatic mutation in the other allele, leading to derangement in cell growth and hamartoma formation. This has been demonstrated in the development of SEGAs and renal angiomyolipoma.

SUGGESTED REFERENCES

Bissler J.J., Kingswood J.C., Radzikowska E., Zonnenberg B.A., Frost M., Belousova E., Sauter M., Nonomura N., Brakemeier S., de Vries P.J., Whittemore V.H., Chen D., Sahmoud T., Shah G., Lincy J., Lebwohl D., Budde K. Everolimus for angiomyolipoma associated with tuberous sclerosis complex or sporadic lymphangioleiomyomatosis (EXIST-2): A multicenter, randomized, double-blind, placebo-controlled trial. *Lancet* 2013;381: 817–24.

Caban C., Khan N., Hasbani D.M., Crino P.B. Genetics of tuberous sclerosis complex: Implications for clinical practice. *Appl Clin Genet* 2016;10: 1–8.

Chugani H.T., Luat A.F., Kumar A., Govindan R., Pawlik K., Asano E. α-[11C]-Methyl-L-tryptophan–PET in 191 patients with tuberous sclerosis complex. *Neurology* 2013;81: 674–80.

De Ridder J., Verhelle B., Vervisch J., Lemmens K., Kotulska K., Moavero R., Curatolo P., Weschke B., Riney K., Feucht M., Krsek P., Nabbout R., Jansen A.C., Wojdan K., Domanska-Pakieła D., Kaczorowska-Frontczak M., Hertzberg C., Ferrier C.H., Samueli S., Benova B., Aronica E., Kwiatkowski D.J., Jansen F.E., Jóźwiak S., Lagae L.; EPISTOP consortium. Early epileptiform EEG activity in infants with tuberous sclerosis complex predict epilepsy and neurodevelopmental outcomes (2021). *Epilepsia* 2021;62: 1208–19.

Franz D.N., Belousova E., Sparagana S., Bebin E.M., Frost M., Kuperman R., Witt O., Kohrman M.H., Flamini J.R., Wu J.Y., Curatolo P., de Vries P.J., Whittemore V.H., Thiele E.A., Ford J.P., Shah G., Cauwel H., Lebwohl D., Sahmoud T., Jozwiak S. Efficacy and safety of everolimus for subependymal giant cell astrocytomas associated with tuberous sclerosis complex (EXIST-1): A multicenter, randomized, placebo-controlled phase 3 trial. *Lancet* 2013;381: 125–32.

French J.A., Lawson J.A., Yapici Z., Ikeda H., Polster T., Nabbout R., Curatolo P., de Vries P.J., Dlugos D.J., Berkowitz N., Voi M., Peyrard S., Pelov D., Franz D.N. Adjunctive everolimus therapy for treatment-resistant focal-onset seizures associated with tuberous sclerosis (EXIST-3): A phase 3, randomised, double-blind, placebo-controlled study. *Lancet* 2016;388: 2153–63.

Kotulska K., Kwiatkowski D.J., Curatolo P., Weschke B., Riney K., Jansen F., Feucht M., Krsek P., Nabbout R., Jansen A.C., Wojdan K., Sijko K., Głowacka-Walas J., Borkowska J., Sadowski K., Domańska-Pakieła D., Moavero R., Hertzberg C., Hulshof H., Scholl T., Benova B., Aronica E., de Ridder J., Lagae L., Jóźwiak S.; EPISTOP Investigators. Prevention of epilepsy in infants with tuberous sclerosis complex in the EPISTOP Trial. *Ann Neurol* 2021;89: 304–14.

Krueger D.A., Care M.M., Agricola K., Tudor C., Mays M., Franz D.N. Everolimus long-term safety and efficacy in subependymal giant cell astrocytoma. *Neurology* 2013;80: 574–80.

Krueger D.A., Wilfong A.A., Holland-Bouley K., Anderson A.E., Agricola K., Tudor C., Mays M., Lopez C.M., Kim M.O., Franz D.N. Everolimus treatment of refractory epilepsy in tuberous sclerosis complex. *Ann Neurol* 2013;74: 679–87.

Krueger D.A., Wilfong A.A., Mays M., Talley C.M., Agricola K., Tudor C., Capal J., Holland-Bouley K., Franz D.N. Long-term treatment of epilepsy with everolimus in tuberous sclerosis. *Neurology* 2016;87: 2408–15.

Northrup H., Aronow M.E., Bebin E.M., Bissler J., Darling T.N., de Vries P.J., Frost M.D., Fuchs Z., Gosnell E.S., Gupta N., Jansen A.C., Jóźwiak S., Kingswood J.C., Knilans T.K., McCormack F.X., Pounders A., Roberds S.L., Rodriguez-Buritica D.F., Roth J., Sampson J.R., Sparagana S., Thiele E.A., Weiner H.L., Wheless J.W., Towbin A.J., Krueger D.A.; International Tuberous Sclerosis Complex Consensus Group. Updated international tuberous sclerosis complex diagnostic criteria and surveillance and management recommendations. *Pediatr Neurol* 2021;123: 50–66.

Thiele E.A., Bebin E.M., Bhathal H., Jansen F.E., Kotulska K., Lawson J.A., O'Callaghan F.J., Wong M., Sahebkar F., Checketts D., Knappertz V.; GWPCARE6 Study Group. Add-on cannabidiol treatment for drug-resistant seizures in tuberous sclerosis complex: A placebo-controlled randomized clinical trial. *JAMA Neurol* 2021;78: 285–92.

28 Sturge–Weber Syndrome

Sabrina Tavella-Burka
Cleveland Clinic

Ajay Gupta
Neurological Institute Cleveland Clinic

CONTENTS

CASE PRESENTATION

A 9-month-old male, a product of nonconsanguineous marriage, was seen for management of drug-resistant epilepsy. Pregnancy was unremarkable except for maternal supraventricular tachycardia (previous history of similar episodes). A left facial nevus was noted at birth. At the age of 6 weeks, parents noticed episodes of whole-body stiffness, arching, and upward eye-rolling followed by vomiting. He would become limp and lethargic for several minutes after the spell. Gastroesophageal reflux was suspected but medical management proved unsuccessful. At the age of 4 months, a nocturnal episode of irritability, pallor, and vomiting lasting several hours was followed by right-sided hemiplegia, for which he was hospitalized. Ischemic stroke was suspected; however, an acute noncontrast brain computed tomography (CT) scan was normal. The right-sided hemiplegia gradually recovered over 4–6 weeks without residual weakness. Subsequently, parents noted new episodes of behavioral arrest, body stiffness, dusky color, unresponsiveness, and right foot jerking for 1–2 minutes. He would become limp and lethargic and have right arm weakness for several minutes after each spell. The spells occurred approximately once a day. Once every 2 weeks, this type of seizure would evolve into a generalized motor seizure. His seizures were treated with phenobarbital, phenytoin, oxcarbazepine, and clonazepam without any success.

DOI: 10.1201/9781003296478-31

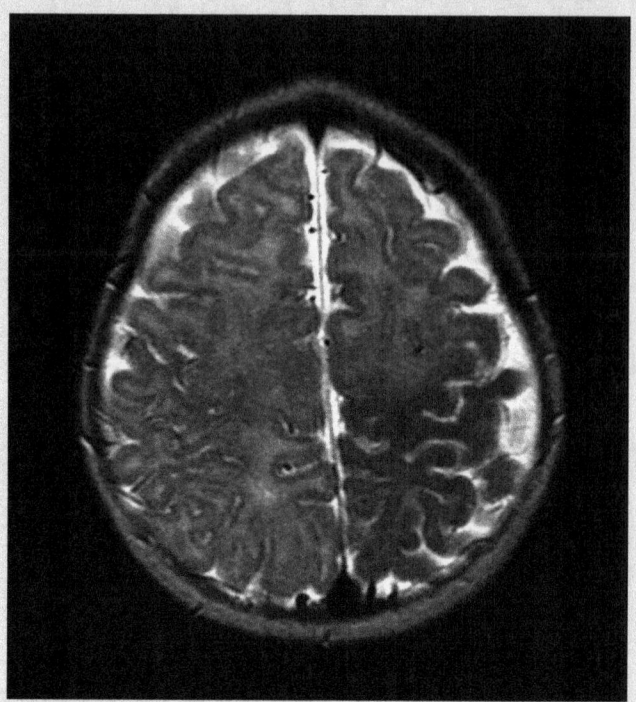

FIGURE 28.1 T2-weighted brain MRI of the patient showing volume loss in the left parietal and occipital region involving both gray and white matter.

At 8 months of age, his parents noticed left-hand preference and concerns for developmental delay were raised. Physical examination was remarkable for port-wine nevus in the trigeminal V1 distribution involving the left upper eyelid and medial canthus. Dexterity was impaired and weakness was noted in the right hand and arm, especially when he tried to approach or transfer the object from the left hand, suggesting moderate right hemiparesis. Muscle tone, bulk, and strength and reflexes were symmetrical on both sides. Video-electroencephalogram (EEG) monitoring revealed interictal sharp waves in the left parieto-occipital region with continuous slowing and decreased background rhythm in the left hemisphere. Ictal EEG showed onset from the left parieto-occipital region during a typical focal seizure ending in a right hemiclonic seizure. Brain magnetic resonance imaging (MRI) scan (Figure 28.1) showed typical findings of Sturge–Weber syndrome (SWS). Brain fluorodeoxyglucose-positron-emission tomography (FDG-PET) showed hypermetabolism in the left posterior quadrant suggesting increased FDG uptake due to a nearly continuous burst of interictal spiking. Ophthalmologic examination revealed a likely right visual field deficit by confrontation testing, and intraocular pressure and fundus examination were normal. After a

*discussion of risks, benefits, and alternatives, the patient underwent func-
tional hemispherectomy at age of 9 months. There was no further recurrence
of seizures and antiseizure medications (ASMs) were discontinued 10 months
after the surgery. At 5 years follow-up, the patient remains seizure free and
has a mild developmental delay. He is ambulatory with his right hand being
weak and spastic.*

DIFFERENTIAL DIAGNOSIS

The important differential diagnostic entity to consider is a facial venous angioma
without any cerebral angiomatosis. There are other rare congenital vascular disorders involving brain and skin. Klippel–Trénaunay syndrome classically presents as
a triad of varicosities, bone or soft-tissue hypertrophy, and cutaneous hemangiomas.
Wyburn–Mason syndrome is a congenital neurocutaneous entity comprised of ipsilateral arteriovenous malformations of the midbrain, vascular abnormalities affecting the visual pathway and facial nevi. PHACE syndrome comprises posterior fossa
brain malformations, hemangiomas, arterial anomalies, coarctation of the aorta, cardiac defects, and eye abnormalities.

DIAGNOSTIC APPROACH

The clinical features are variable, but the association of neurological deficits and
port-wine stain of the face suggest SWS. Sturge–Weber Syndrome occurs sporadically in all races that results from a mutation in *GNAQ* (chromosome 9q21.2). The
prevalence is estimated to be one per 50,000. The dermatological lesion of a facial
port-wine stain (PWS) is usually present at birth and consists of a flat lesion of variable size, involving the upper eyelid and forehead. The size of the cutaneous angioma
does not predict the size of intracranial angioma. It is unilateral in 70% of cases, usually ipsilateral to the brain involvement. Even when the facial angioma is bilateral,
the pial angioma tends to be unilateral or asymmetric in most patients. Children with
a high risk of neurological involvement in PWS phenotypes include the hemifacial,
median, and forehead phenotype, involving the frontonasal embryonic prominence.
The characteristic neurological and radiographic features of SWS may rarely be
present without cutaneous angioma. Only 10%–20% of children with a port-wine
nevus of the forehead have a leptomeningeal angioma. Typically, SWS involves the
occipital and posterior parietal lobes, but it can affect the entire ipsilateral cerebral
hemisphere, other cranial regions, and even both cerebral hemispheres extensively.
Bilateral brain lesions occur in 15% of children.

Seizures are the most common neurological presentation and occur in 72%–80%
of children with SWS. The age range of seizure onset varies between birth and
23 years, with a median age of 6 months. The risk of developing seizures is highest
in the first 2 years of life and occurs earlier in patients with bilateral disease. The
most common type of seizure is a focal-onset seizure, usually with a hemitonic or
hemiclonic semiology. Bilateral tonic-clonic seizures are commonly seen, usually

later in childhood and adolescents. There is also an increased incidence of prolonged seizures or *status epilepticus* in SWS patients. Fever and infection or a trivial head trauma may trigger the onset of seizures in many children.

Seizures frequently accompany stroke-like episodes. Onset of a motor deficit may precede a cluster of prolonged seizures rather than seizures followed by Todd's paralysis; however, this distinction is difficult to make in children. Fixed hemiparesis contralateral to the facial angioma eventually occurs in 50% of children. It often appears after a focal-onset seizure and progresses in severity in a stuttering fashion after subsequent seizures. Transient episodes of hemiplegia, not related to clinical or EEG evidence of seizure activity may also occur. Some patients have associated migraine-like headache, attention deficit disorder, and cognitive impairment. Glaucoma occurs in 30%–70% of cases and usually develops before the age of 10 years. Almost every patient with SWS-associated glaucoma has a PWS that crosses the facial midline and involves the nose and upper eyelids. These areas are derived from the frontonasal prominence embryological precursor. There may be an associated vascular abnormality in the conjunctiva, sclera, retina, and choroid. There is also an increased incidence of retinal detachment secondary to hemorrhage from choroidal vessels. Eye involvement may result in acute or chronic visual loss that may not be readily apparent in young child without an evaluation by an ophthalmologist.

The new 2021 consensus statement for the management and treatment of SWS notes that for children born with a high-risk PWS without seizures or neurological symptoms, routine brain MRI is not recommended unless presymptomatic treatment is being considered. In symptomatic children with suspected SWS, MRI should include pre- and postcontrast sequences for better visualization, including special sequences for visualization of calcium and the transmedullary venous system. The imaging may show enhancement of the leptomeningeal angioma, enlarged transmedullary veins, choroid plexus hypertrophy, white matter abnormalities, patchy parenchymal gliosis, calcification, neuronal loss, and gliosis. However, the brain MRI may only show subtle or no abnormalities in young infants who are subsequently diagnosed with SWS. CT scanning of the brain, although routinely not done, may show cortical calcifications, typically described as "tram track" or "gyriform" appearance (Figure 28.2). Calcification may be absent or minimal in neonates and infants. Functional imaging with FDG-PET often demonstrates cortical hypometabolism. Another MR technique, diffusion tensor imaging (DTI), often demonstrates abnormal water diffusion suggesting a lack of integrity of the white matter underneath the leptomeningeal angioma. The EEG frequently shows ipsilateral slowing to the cerebral involvement with or without spike-and-sharp-wave discharges. Quantitative EEG (qEEG) may provide an objective measure of EEG asymmetry that correlates with clinical status and brain asymmetry seen on MRI.

TREATMENT STRATEGY

Seizures may be difficult to control with ASMs. Broad-spectrum ASMs effective against focal seizures may prove helpful. There is currently no FDA-approved ASM for SWS. Mammalian target of rapamycin (mTOR) inhibitors such as sirolimus have been investigated for treatment in SWS. One small pilot study showed that low-dose

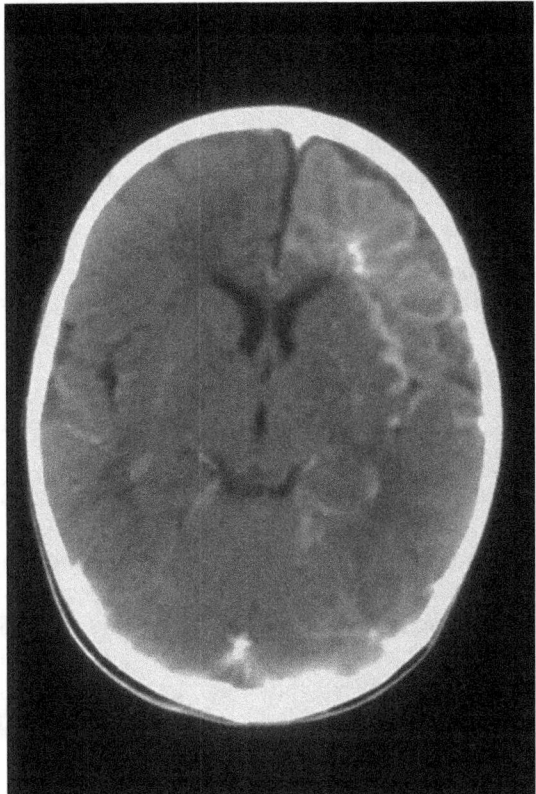

FIGURE 28.2 Contrast-enhanced head CT of a patient with SWS showing left frontal calcification and left side leptomeningeal angioma enhancement. Calficications may not be appreciated on the routine brain MRI and can appear later in life.

sirolimus is safe and led to improvement in cognitive impairment and in processing speed in patients with a history of stroke-like episodes. There is ongoing research exploring strategies for prevention or disease-modification of epileptogenesis before seizure onset, as this approach has recently been shown to be effective in the treatment of TSC individuals.

In some patients, the disease is progressive and there is a view that early resective surgery may be effective in halting the progression. It is not possible to predict who will develop drug-resistant epilepsy. Surgery should be considered when seizures are refractory to medical treatment. Visually guided complete excision of the angiomatous cortex with or without the guidance of electrocorticography is the primary surgical procedure for epilepsy surgery. Hemispherectomy is considered in children with extensive unilateral brain involvement and a fixed hemiparesis.

The ketogenic diet or vagus nerve stimulation may provide alternative treatment options for refractory patients, particularly in those with bilateral ictal onset zones. Aspirin 3–5 mg/kg/day is often recommended with SWS as primary prevention or secondary prevention after the first stroke-like episode, but the literature is mixed about its utility since there have been no controlled trials. A well-hydrated state at all times, and especially during illnesses and *status epilepticus* episodes, may be important to promote cerebral venous drainage and avoid secondary hypoxic brain injury from venous stasis.

Laser therapy is the recommended intervention for cutaneous PWS and multiple treatments are often required to significantly lighten the lesions. The PWS may grow and thicken as the child grows. Medical and surgical treatment of glaucoma includes beta-blockers, carbonic anhydrase inhibitors, ophthalmic drops, and surgery. Regular evaluation by an ophthalmologist is recommended, particularly for patients with choroidal lesions.

LONG-TERM OUTCOME

The clinical progression of SWS is characterized by a stuttering course, with periodic worsening and episodes of status epilepticus and stroke-like episodes. There is an elevated risk for neurologic complications in widespread or bi-hemispheric disease. Seizures occurring before 2 years of age increase the risk of intellectual disability and refractory epilepsy. Some patients continue to have daily seizures after the initial deterioration despite various ASMs, whereas others have long seizure-free intervals. The timing of surgery is important. The majority (70%–80%) of patients may be seizure-free or significantly improved (i.e., >75%–90% seizure reduction) after surgery, and early surgery may improve developmental outcomes in refractory patients. The completeness of resection or disconnection of diseased tissue is a crucial factor in achieving epilepsy control.

CLINICAL PEARLS

- SWS patients with early-onset and frequent seizures usually have a more severe clinical course. SWS may show progressive clinical deterioration with drug-resistant epilepsy, neurological deficits, and cognitive regression.
- Epilepsy surgery is an effective treatment for patients with drug-resistant epilepsy. Epilepsy surgery should be considered early in the course of the disease.
- When a child is born with a facial PWS involving upper and lower eyelids, contrast-enhanced brain MRI should be considered.
- Eye involvement may result in acute and chronic visual loss; therefore, ophthalmic examination and follow-up examination by an expert is crucial to prevent loss of vision.
- Future advancements in the prevention or modification of epileptogenesis before seizure onset in SWS may result from the current investigations attempting to elucidate the mechanisms of SWS disease progression.

PATHOPHYSIOLOGY/NEUROBIOLOGY OF DISEASE

SWS is a sporadic disease due to a somatic activating mutation in *GNAQ*. During the sixth week of intrauterine life, the primitive embryonal vascular plexus develops around the cephalic portion of the neural tube and under the ectoderm in the region destined to be the facial skin. In SWS, it is hypothesized that the vascular plexus fails to regress, as it should in the embryo in the ninth week, resulting in angiomatosis of related tissues. The intracranial lesion is thought to be due to proliferation of lepto-meningeal vessels in the subarachnoid space that causes shunting of blood away from the brain tissue. This shunting results in decreased blood flow, decreased venous return, and focal hypoxia leading to cellular death. This is seen radiographically as gliosis, volume loss, and calcification.

SUGGESTED REFERENCES

Bourgeois M., Crimmins D.W., de Oliveira R.S., Arzimanoglou A., Garnett M., Roujeau T., Di Rocco F., Sainte-Rose C. Surgical treatment of epilepsy in Sturge-Weber syndrome in children. *J Neuosurg* 2007;106(Suppl 1):S20–S8.

Di Rocco C., Tamburrini G. Sturge-Weber syndrome. *Childs Nerv Syst* 2006;22:909–21.

Hatfield L.A., Crone N.E., Kossoff E.H., Ewen J.B., Pyzik P.L., Lin D.D., Kelley T.M., Comi A.M. Quantitative EEG asymmetry correlates with clinical severity in unilateral Sturge-Weber syndrome. *Epilepsia* 2007;48:191–5.

Sabeti S., Ball K.L., Bhattacharya S.K., Bitrian E., Blieden L.S., Brandt J.D., Burkhart C., Chugani H.T., Falcheck S.J., Jain B.G., Juhasz C., Loeb J.A., Luat A., Pinto A., Segal E., Salvin J., Kelly K.M. Consensus statement for the management and treatment of Sturge-Weber syndrome: Neurology, neuroimaging, and ophthalmology recommendations. *Pediatr Neurol* 2021;121:59–66.

Smegal L.F., Sebold A.J., Hammill A.M., Juhasz C., Lo W.D., Miles D.K., Wilfong A.A., Levin A.V., Fisher B., Ball K.L., Pinto A.L., Comi A.M. Multicenter research data of epilepsy management in patients with stuge-weber syndrome. *Pediatr Neurol* 2021;119:3–10.

Thomas-Sohl K.A., Vaslow D.F., Maria B.L. Sturge-Weber syndrome: A review. *Pediatr Neurol* 2004;30:303–10.

Zallmann M., Leventer R.J., Mackay M.T., Ditchfield M., Bekhor P.S., Su J.C. Screening for Sturge-Weber syndrome: A state-of-the-art review. *Pediatr Dermatol* 2018;35:30–42.

Section IV

The Child

29 Self-Limited Epilepsy with Centrotemporal Spikes (Benign Rolandic Epilepsy)

Olivia Kim-McManus
UC San Diego School of Medicine

CONTENTS

CASE PRESENTATION

A previously healthy, developmentally normal 8-year-old boy presented with a new-onset seizure out of sleep shortly after going to bed. Parents heard a strange sound, immediately went to his room, and found him having full body jerking and stiffening, excessive drooling, and urinary incontinence. Duration was about 2 minutes, although the onset of the seizure was not witnessed. His neurological evaluation included a routine EEG which revealed independent right and left centrotemporal spikes, seen with increased predominance during sleep. MRI of the brain was normal. The diagnosis of self-limited epilepsy with centrotemporal spikes (SeLECTS) was made based on clinical history and EEG findings. Family was hesitant to start daily prophylaxis with an anti-seizure medication (ASM). However, the patient had focal unilateral facial twitching with drooling and dysarthric speech without alteration in awareness several days later, consistent with focal seizures, which parents had not previously observed. He then reported that these focal seizures had happened several times in the past few months prior to his bilateral tonic-clonic seizure out of sleep. Family agreed to start levetiracetam. The patient did not have any further seizures and was weaned off his ASM 2 years later after his follow-up EEG revealed normal brain activity.

DOI: 10.1201/9781003296478-33

DIFFERENTIAL DIAGNOSIS

Seizure semiology of focal seizures in SeLECTS, previously referred to as benign Rolandic epilepsy and childhood epilepsy with centrotemporal spikes, typically consists of arousals out of sleep with oropharyngeal manifestations, unilateral facial sensorimotor symptoms, at times with unilateral facial and limb clonic movements, impairment of awareness, and speech arrest, sometimes with secondarily generalized tonic-clonic activity and urinary or bowel incontinence (~50%). Postictal focal motor deficits (i.e., Todd's paresis) may occur and this phenomenon is characterized by transient unilateral extremity weakness and decreased muscle tone. Less commonly, daytime seizures may also occur, during which awareness is frequently preserved with aphasia and focal sensorimotor manifestations involving the face and limb.

Focal seizures with similar seizure semiologies can be seen in the setting of focal structural abnormalities such as congenital brain malformations, stroke, and tumors. Nonlesional focal epilepsies can also present as such, depending on seizure onset zone, often including unilateral centrotemporal or insular regions. An important differentiating feature in SeLECTS includes alternating right or left-sided sensorimotor involvement, as opposed to unilateral features typically seen with other focal epilepsies.

An exception is epilepsy of infancy with migrating focal seizures, a severe early-onset epileptic encephalopathy secondary to genetic etiologies such as pathogenic *SCN2A* or *KCNT1* mutations, in which independent hemispheric-onset seizures can be seen. Additional clinical history including age of seizure onset and neurocognitive development would be important features to easily differentiate between such pediatric epilepsy syndromes and SeLECTS.

As focal seizures in SeLECTS often occur out of sleep, differential diagnoses for abnormal sleep arousals include non-rapid eye movement sleep parasomnias such as night terrors or confusional arousals during which there is alteration of awareness with confusion, at times with autonomic changes consisting of tachycardia and mydriasis, with no patient recollection of nocturnal events. REM sleep parasomnias are also included, as well as sleep enuresis and REM sleep behavior disorder with abnormal vocalizations or movements out of sleep and skeletal muscle dysfunction in the form of atonia. Frontal lobe epilepsies such as sleep-related hypermotor epilepsy, associated with neuronal nicotinic acetylcholine receptor dysfunction, also present with stereotyped nocturnal arousals, although these are usually characterized by stereotyped hyperkinetic movements with tonic or dystonic posturing not seen in SeLECTS.

DIAGNOSTIC APPROACH

SeLECTS is the most common and well-characterized focal childhood epilepsy syndrome, accounting for ~10%–20% of all childhood-onset epilepsies. Age of onset, seizure semiology, neurodevelopmental baseline, and neurodiagnostic workup in the form of EEG will help guide diagnosis and clinical management. Typically, seizure onset is around 5–8 years of age, with rare but reported occurrences before age 2 years.

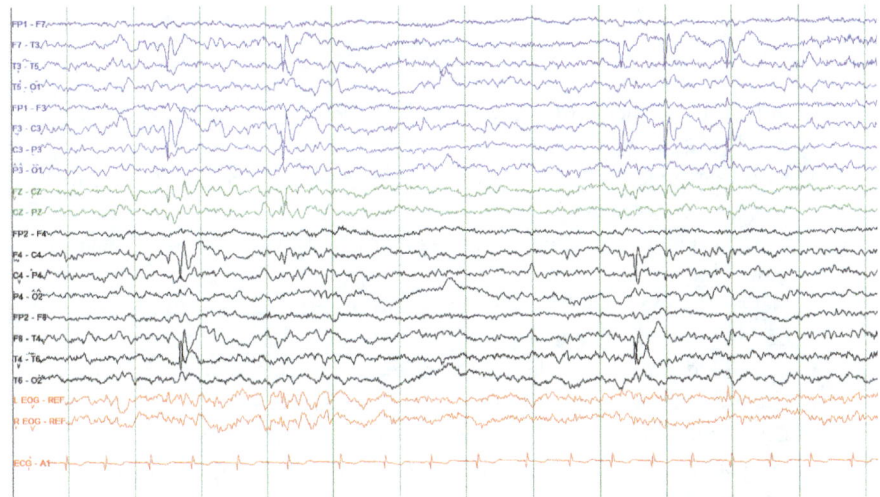

FIGURE 29.1   EEG showing bilateral sharp–slow waves in the centrotemporal regions of a child with self-limited epilepsy with centrotemporal spikes.

Seizures often remit within 2–5 years of onset, typically by 14–16 years of age. Usual clinical manifestations include unilateral facial sensorimotor and oropharyngeal symptoms (tongue, throat, unilateral lower face numbness and paresthesias; focal tongue or unilateral lower face twitching), speech arrest with an inability to speak due to sensorimotor deficits, and hypersalivation.

EEG will provide diagnostic confirmation with independent synchronous and asynchronous, broad, diphasic, focal right and left centrotemporal spike discharges with shifting predominance over the left and right hemispheres, often with a transverse horizontal dipole. These focal epileptiform discharges are further activated by drowsiness and sleep. In rarer atypical cases, there may be a high burden of epileptiform discharges during sleep meeting criteria for developmental epileptic encephalopathy with spike-and-wave activation in sleep, with a spike-wave index of >85% in NREM sleep which is associated with cognitive difficulties involving learning and language.

A brain MRI should be obtained for atypical presentations in which only unilateral centrotemporal epileptiform discharges are seen, which may suggest other focal epilepsies with underlying structural brain abnormalities. Genetic epilepsy panels may be obtained as known genetic associations for hereditary predisposition for SeLECTS include mutations in *GRIN2A*, *ELP4*, *RBFOX1/3*, less frequently, GABA$_A$ receptor variants, *KCNQ2/3*, and *DEPDC5*.

TREATMENT STRATEGY & LONG-TERM OUTCOME

Previously, children with SeLECTS were not prescribed daily ASMs given the paucity of seizure activity. However, there is increasing evidence for neuropsychological deficits in children with SeLECTS, regardless of the seizure frequency, particularly

CLINICAL PEARLS

- SeLECTS is the most common and well-characterized focal childhood epilepsy syndrome.
- Children typically present with seizures around 5 years of age with resolution of seizures by adolescence.
- Classic seizure semiology and characteristic EEG findings will help guide diagnosis.
- Neuroimaging is indicated if there are atypical EEG features concerning other focal epilepsies.
- Comorbid neuropsychological manifestations with learning difficulties are often seen, regardless of seizure frequency.
- Daily medications for seizure prophylaxis are increasingly recommended for seizure control and improved neuropsychological performance.

in the realms of expressive and receptive language, reading difficulties due to visuospatial impairments, as well as behavioral concerns, related to the predominance of interictal epileptiform activity contributing to disrupted normal neural networks. Thus, children are increasingly treated with daily ASMs for focal seizures in SeLECTS. Standard treatments include levetiracetam, oxcarbazepine, carbamazepine, and less commonly, valproic acid or lamotrigine. Rarer cases with electrical status epilepticus in slow-wave sleep (ESES) may require corticosteroids or high-dose benzodiazepines. Overall prognosis is that SeLECTS is very favorable with seizure remission usually by adolescence and major resolution of neurocognitive difficulties.

SUGGESTED READING

Aricò M., Arigliani E., Giannotti F., Romani M. ADHD and ADHD-related neural networks in benign epilepsy with centrotemporal spikes: A systematic review. *Epilepsy Behav* 2020;112: 107448.

Ross E.E., Stoyell S.M., Kramer M.A., Berg A.T., Chu C.J. The natural history of seizures and neuropsychiatric symptoms in childhood epilepsy with centrotemporal spikes (CECTS). *Epilepsy Behav* 2020;103: 106437.

Zanaboni M.P., Varesio C., Pasca L., Foti A., Totaro M., Celario M., Provenzi L., De Giorgis V. Systematic review of executive functions in children with self-limited epilepsy with centrotemporal spikes. *Epilepsy Behav* 2021;123: 108254.

30 Self-Limited Epilepsy with Autonomic Seizures (Panayiotopoulos Syndrome)

Korwyn Williams
Phoenix Children's Hospital

CONTENTS

CASE PRESENTATION

A 5-year-old girl without a significant past medical history and normal development was brought by her family to the Emergency Department for altered mental status. She had awoken that morning complaining of stomach upset and vomited three times. She then repeatedly asked the same question. After the unusual behavior began, the parents brought her to the hospital. On review of systems, her mother thought she looked pale and her eyes appeared dilated. They denied fever, ill contacts, or access to medications or household chemicals. Her development was normal, and she had no risk factors for epilepsy. Her family history was unremarkable. She was mildly tachycardic and appeared pale but was not ill-appearing or diaphoretic. She answered questions with inappropriate responses and did not cooperate fully with the exam. Her pupils were dilated, but reactive. During the course of the interview, the patient's eyes deviated to the right and soon her right arm exhibited clonic activity. She was given lorazepam which aborted the seizure. The patient appeared sleepy afterward. Computed tomography of the head was unremarkable. Other studies, including cerebrospinal fluid analysis, proved to be normal. An electroencephalogram (EEG) was notable for intermittent

DOI: 10.1201/9781003296478-34

slowing over the left central region and independent epileptiform discharges during a sleep over the left centrotemporal and occipital regions, but no electrographic seizures. On further questioning, the parents recalled a similar episode 3 months prior, where she awoke from sleep complaining of stomach upset. She appeared pale, retched, and then vomited. She seemed "out of it" for several minutes, which they attributed to the vomiting. They also recalled that she complained frequently of stomach upset. A diagnosis of autonomic seizures was entertained. The patient returned to baseline in a few hours. Her exam at that time was now unremarkable. The family was prescribed a benzodiazepine as a rescue medication, but not started on daily antiseizure medication (ASM) at the time. She had no further episodes for the subsequent 3 years, before being lost to follow-up.

DIFFERENTIAL DIAGNOSIS

In this age group, ingestions/toxidromes, metabolic disturbances, and central nervous system or gastrointestinal infectious etiologies should be considered. However, the absence of signs of infection (e.g., fever, meningismus, and diarrhea) and the quick resolution following definitive seizure treatment make them less likely. The normal head CT makes a stroke unlikely. Absent a history of headaches and given the age, migraine variants would also be unlikely.

While autonomic findings can occur in almost any type of seizure, the patient's symptoms of retching, emesis (seen in 75% with this syndrome), pupillary dilatation, and pallor are striking and consistent with an autonomic seizure. Given her age, self-limited epilepsy with autonomic seizures (SeLEAS), formerly known as Panayiotopoulos syndrome or early-onset childhood occipital epilepsy, is the most likely diagnosis. It was initially described in 1989 as nocturnal seizures characterized by tonic eye deviation and vomiting, which would occasionally evolve into a bilateral tonic-clonic seizure. When initially described, occipital epileptiform abnormalities were commonly associated with the condition.

The International League Against Epilepsy's Task Force on Nosology and Definitions published a position paper in 2022, laying out the features of this epilepsy syndrome. SeLEAS is more commonly seen in those between 3 and 6 years of age but has been reported in patients between 1 and 14 years old. There is no sex predilection or concerning antecedent perinatal or developmental concerns, although febrile seizures are reported in less than 20%. Autonomic symptoms are required for the diagnosis; in addition to those already described, malaise, headache, flushing, drooling, incontinence, and syncope. While alertness can be preserved initially, altered awareness often supervenes, and the diagnosis becomes even more apparent in the >50% who ultimately demonstrate versive head or eye movements, hemiclonic, and/or focal to bilateral tonic-clonic activity. The seizures themselves can last more than 30 minutes, making this the most common cause of pediatric nonconvulsive *status epilepticus* after febrile seizures. Most occur from sleep. The seizures are infrequent; nearly 80% of the patients have 5 or less seizures, with a quarter experiencing only 1 seizure.

Childhood occipital visual epilepsy (formerly known as Gastaut syndrome, or late-onset benign childhood seizures with occipital spikes) deserves a brief mention in contradistinction to SeLEAS. Its peak onset is 7–9 years of age. The seizures usually last only a few minutes and always begin with striking visual hallucinations or amaurosis. These patients might complain of an ictal or postictal migraine. They too may evolve like SeLEAS into bilateral tonic-clonic seizures. However, the onset of visual symptomology is strikingly different.

DIAGNOSTIC APPROACH

The cornerstone of the evaluation is the history, but the EEG provides limited support. The most common finding is occipital epileptiform discharges (synchronous or unilateral), which are seen in three-quarters of the patients. However, sequential studies have shown migration to centrotemporal and frontopolar regions. Rarely, the EEG can be normal. Sleep activates the discharges significantly and may be the only time epileptiform discharges are seen. Ictal discharges have been reported from the occipital, frontal, and temporal regions, but seizure manifestations can be subtle (in one case, the only ictal change was tachycardia for 10 minutes before eye deviation and convulsive activity occurred).

While a genetic basis for SeLEAS is suspected from the higher prevalence of febrile seizures in first-degree relatives, SeLEAS is a diagnosis that is most firmly established in hindsight. As such, imaging is not always required. However, recurrent seizures, atypical presentations, or focal background slowing should prompt neuroimaging, as autonomic seizures could be structural, metabolic, or genetic in nature. Genetic testing has not revealed a consistent abnormality, although there are case reports of *SCN1A* pathogenic variants. At this time, there is no indication to perform genetic testing.

TREATMENT STRATEGIES

Since the seizures in this syndrome are infrequent and uncommon, these patients are usually not placed on a daily ASM. However, if the seizures are frequent or concerning, carbamazepine, valproic acid, and topiramate among others have been used. In one large series, almost 90% were seizure free after treatment, but approximately 5% continued to have seizures despite treatment. For those who present with *status epilepticus*, providing an abortive benzodiazepine is reasonable.

LONG-TERM OUTCOME

The prognosis for this condition is generally favorable. Only one-third of patients will experience a second seizure. The seizures are infrequent and almost always remit within 6 years (most within 3 years) of the first seizure. Notably, the epileptiform abnormalities may persist after seizures have remitted. The overall neurodevelopmental trajectory is normal, as is expected for a self-limited epilepsy of childhood, but there are only limited studies in this population. About 20% of these children can develop seizures during late childhood and adolescence, typically Rolandic seizures or absence seizures, which almost always remit as well.

CLINICAL PEARLS

- Self-limited epilepsy with autonomic seizures (SeLEAS) is an age-defined benign epilepsy of childhood with a peak incidence between 3 and 6 years of age, previously known as Panayiotopoulos syndrome.
- The seizures are autonomic in nature, with the most common signs being pallor and recurrent ictal vomiting but can be variable. Later in the course of the seizure, awareness may become impaired, eye deviation may be seen, and evolution to bilateral tonic-clonic activity can occur.
- The seizures are typically long (at least 5 minutes) and a significant number may present in nonconvulsive status epilepticus.
- The EEG can show multifocal or even extra-occipital epileptiform discharges.
- Neuroimaging and genetic testing are not necessary, in the appropriate clinical context.
- ASM therapy is often not necessary, and the long-term prognosis is very good for eventual seizure remission.

NEUROBIOLOGY/PATHOPHYSIOLOGY OF DISEASE

The neurobiological correlation between the epileptiform discharges and the semiology is unknown. Autonomic centers typically are midline deep structures of the brain, so the basis of the epileptiform discharges leading to autonomic seizures is unclear. In addition, seizures in the same patient may lead to different autonomic symptoms, suggesting that epileptic propagation can follow different pathways. Small case series have localized various autonomic phenomena (i.e., ictal bradycardia, asystole, and ictal pallor) using video-EEG monitoring to temporal lobe seizures.

SUGGESTED REFERENCES

Caraballo R., Cersosimo R., Fejerman N. Panayiotopoulos syndrome: A prospective study of 192 patients. *Epilepsia* 2007;48:1054–61.

Ferrie C.D., Caraballo R., Covanis A., Demirbilek V., Dervent A., Fejerman N., Fusco L., Grünewald R.A., Kanazawa O., Koutroumanidis M., Lada C., Livingston J.H., Nicotra A., Oguni H., Martinovic Z., Nordli D.R. Jr., Parisi P., Scott R.C., Specchio N., Verrotti A., Vigevano F., Walker M.C., Watanabe K., Ferrie C.D., Caraballo R., Covanis A., Demirbilek V., Dervent A., Kivity S., Koutroumanidis M., Martinovic Z., Oguni H., Verrotti A., Vigevano F., Watanabe K., Yalcin D., Yoshinaga H. Panayiotopoulos syndrome: A consensus view. *Dev Med Child Neurol* 2006;48:236–40.

Panayiotopoulos C.P. Benign nocturnal childhood occipital epilepsy: A new syndrome with nocturnal seizures, tonic deviation of the eyes, and vomiting. *J Child Neurol* 1989;4:43–9.

Specchio N., Wirrell E.C., Scheffer I.E., Nabbout R., Riney K., Samia P., Guerreiro M., Gwer S., Zuberi S.M., Wilmshurst J.M., Yozawitz E., Pressler R., Hirsch E., Wiebe S., Cross H.J., Perucca E., Moshé S.L., Tinuper P., Auvin S. International League Against Epilepsy classification and definition of epilepsy syndromes with onset in childhood: Position paper by the ILAE Task Force on nosology and definitions. *Epilepsia* 2022;63:1398–442.

Tedrus G.M.A.S., Fonseca L.C. Autonomic seizures and autonomic status epilepticus in early onset benign childhood occipital epilepsy. *Arq Neuropsiquiatr* 2006;64:723–6.

Yoshinaga H., Panayiotopoulos C.P. Autonomic status epilepticus in Panayiotopoulos syndrome and other childhood and adult epilepsies: A consensus view. *Epilepsia* 2007;48:1165–72.

31 Childhood Occipital Visual Epilepsy

Maria Augusta Montenegro
UC San Diego School of Medicine

CONTENTS

CASE PRESENTATION

A 6-year-old girl was first seen at the emergency department after presenting with a first generalized tonic-clonic seizure. The patient reported seeing several colorful balls for 1 or 2 minutes in the prior week. During the postictal period, the girl complained of a throbbing headache associated with photophobia, nausea, and vomiting. Neurological examination and brain MRI were normal. EEG showed very frequent right occipital sharp-and-slow waves that disappeared after eye opening (Figure 31.1). Hyperventilation and intermittent photic stimulation did not trigger additional epileptic discharges or seizures. Oxcarbazepine was started but the patient still experienced a few additional seizures in the ensuing months. These were characterized by elementary visual hallucinations (colorful balls) for 1 or 2 minutes (Figure 31.2). After an increase in oxcarbazepine dosage, the patient became seizure free. During the follow-up period, she had a few episodes of migraine headache that responded well to ibuprofen. The patient was weaned off her antiseizure medication 2 years later and remained seizure free since then.

DOI: 10.1201/9781003296478-35

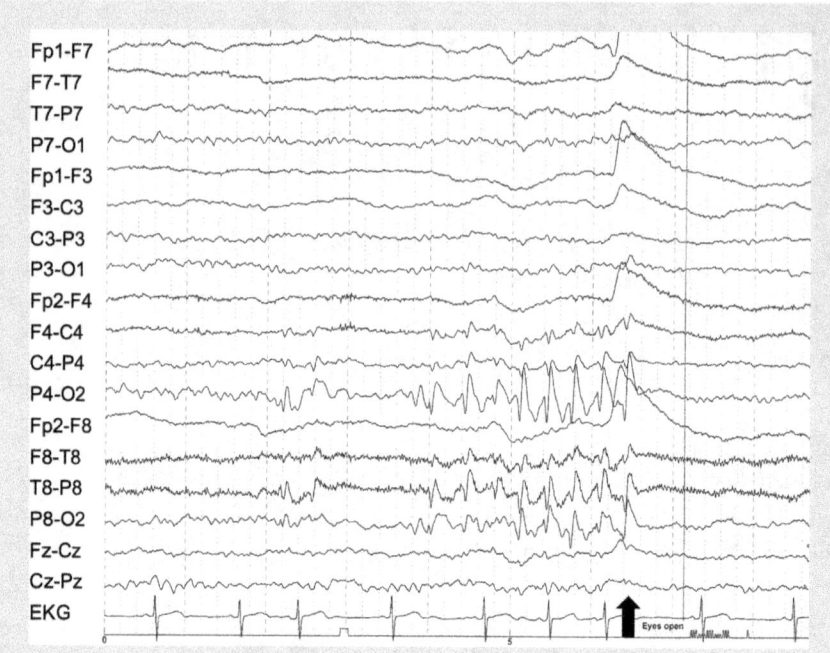

FIGURE 31.1   EEG during wakefulness showing normal background and very frequent sharp-and-slow waves in the right occipital head region. Note that when the patient opens her eye (arrow) the epileptiform discharges disappear (fixation-off phenomenon).

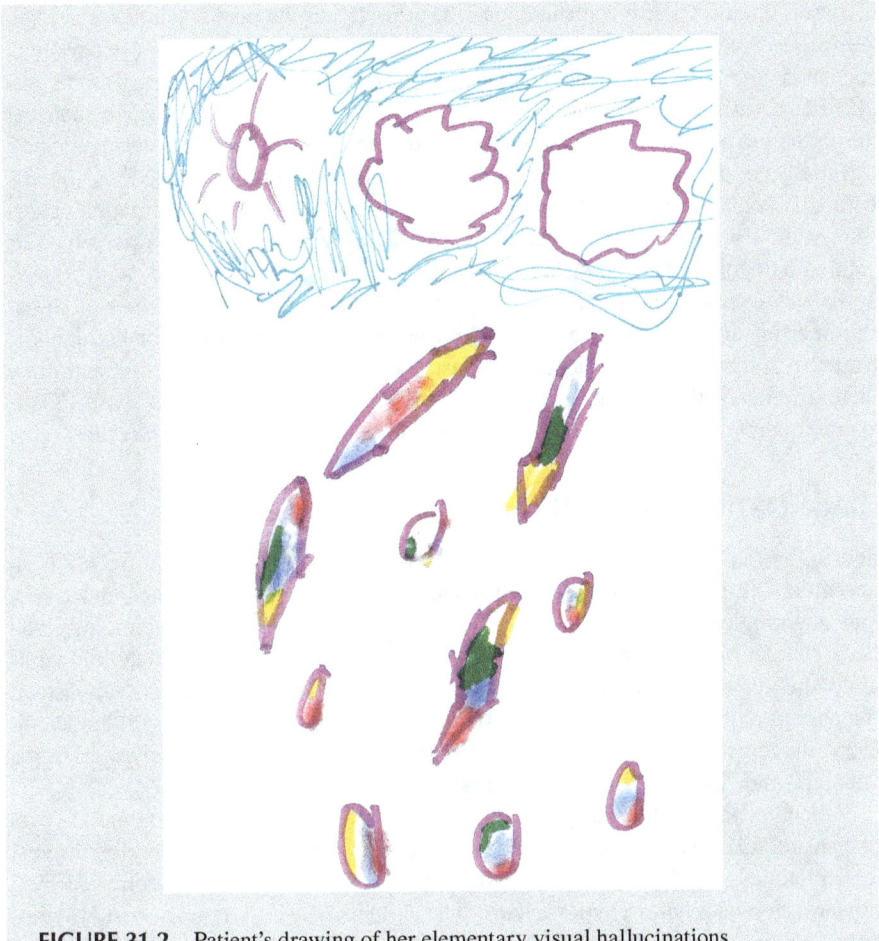

FIGURE 31.2 Patient's drawing of her elementary visual hallucinations.

DIFFERENTIAL DIAGNOSIS

Childhood occipital visual epilepsy (COVE) has four main differential diagnostic considerations: (1) occipital lobe epilepsy due to a structural brain lesion, (2) photosensitive occipital lobe epilepsy, (3) self-limited epilepsy with autonomic seizures (Panayiotopoulos syndrome), and (4) migraine (with aura or acephalgic).

The first goal is to establish whether there is a structural lesion in the occipital lobe. This is easily done by ordering a brain MRI. Once this has been excluded, a careful description of seizure semiology is important to differentiate COVE from other types of self-limited epilepsies. Photosensitive occipital lobe epilepsy also affects children with normal neurological development and is characterized by elementary visual hallucinations like the ones seen in COVE, followed by head version. The key finding that helps to differentiate it from COVE is that seizures are triggered by intermittent photic stimulation.

In self-limited epilepsy with autonomic seizures (Panayiotopoulos syndrome) the seizure arises from sleep and are characterized by impairment of awareness, eye deviation, and autonomic features (especially ictal vomiting). The main confounding factor is that the EEG can also show occipital spike-and-slow waves with fixation-off phenomenon, but the discharges are usually multifocal, with predominance in the posterior head regions.

Finally, migraine with visual aura and acephalgic migraine (visual symptoms without associated headache) can be differentiated by the visual hallucination's characteristics. Epilepsy "aura" develops within a few seconds, which is perceived as colored balls or circles and lasts from seconds to 2 minutes. Migraine "aura" develops slowly over several minutes and lasts for up to an hour, which is black or shiny/shimmering in appearance, and the child describes linear, zigzag, or hemianopic features. Sometimes the child cannot describe the visual symptoms, but can draw them, usually with impressive details (Figure 31.2). Note that patients with COVE also frequently have migraines, and one diagnosis does not preclude the other.

DIAGNOSTIC APPROACH

Self-limited epilepsies of childhood are characterized by a normal brain MRI, an unremarkable perinatal history with normal developmental milestones and a normal neurological examination. The diagnosis is based on seizure semiology and EEG characteristics. COVE is a type of self-limited epilepsy previously known as idiopathic (or benign) occipital epilepsy, or childhood occipital epilepsy of Gastaut. Because psychosocial and learning difficulties can be associated with childhood epilepsy, the term self-limited is currently used to substitute the previously used terms "benign" and "idiopathic" as descriptors of childhood epilepsies.

Patients with COVE usually present with their first seizure between 6 and 15 years of age, and seizures are characterized by elementary visual symptoms (colored spots, ictal blindness, etc.) for a few seconds to a few minutes. It can be followed by a bilateral clonic (or hemi-clonic) seizure. The child usually describes the visual symptoms as colored small bright lights at the center of the visual field. Headache with migraine-like characteristics often occurs in the postictal period.

Seizure semiology and EEG findings are two of the most important diagnostic findings. The EEG shows normal background activity associated with very frequent bilateral spike-and-slow waves in the occipital head region; however, unilateral discharges may also occur. Fixation-off phenomena (i.e., epileptiform abnormality disappears with eye opening) is often seen and is a valuable tool for its diagnosis. Hyperventilation and photic stimulation do not have any impact on the recording. Neuroimaging is important to rule out a structural lesion in the occipital lobe.

TREATMENT STRATEGY

Treatment with an antiseizure medication (ASM) should be offered because if untreated most patients will have additional focal seizures and occasional bilateral tonic-clonic seizures. Oxcarbazepine, levetiracetam, and carbamazepine are considered first-line options and can usually be tapered off after a minimum of 2 years of seizure freedom. In contrast to other self-limited epilepsies, COVE may require

> ### CLINICAL PEARLS
>
> - Fixation-off phenomena (i.e., epileptiform abnormality disappears with eye opening) is a valuable tool for the diagnosis of COVE.
> - Brain MRI should be performed to rule out a structural lesion in the occipital region.
> - Migraine headache is frequently associated with COVE and should be addressed as part of the treatment.
> - The prognosis is good but not as favorable as the ones seen in other types of self-limited epilepsies. Some patients may need higher doses of ASM to become completely seizure free.

higher doses of an ASM, and some patients will need a trial with a second ASM (either alone or in combination) before becoming seizure free.

LONG TERM OUTCOME

The overall prognosis is good, but it is not as favorable as the one seen in patients with self-limited epilepsy with centrotemporal spikes. Most patients with COVE will become seizure free after introduction of ASM, but patients may still experience focal seizures and occasional bilateral tonic-clonic seizures. These patients may need higher doses of ASM to become completely seizure free.

Migraine frequently occurs in patients with COVE (not just during the postictal period); however, some families (and even neurologists) may not be aware of this issue because treatment is usually focused on seizure control, and less so with respect to comorbidities. Actively addressing the occurrence of migraine headaches and their treatment may greatly improve the child's quality of life.

Poor academic performance is associated with some forms of self-limited childhood epilepsy. Learning should be assessed at 6 years of age (or at diagnosis) and repeated annually. Also, active screening for learning difficulties should be performed after changing or increasing ASM dosing.

SUGGESTED REFERENCES

Auvin S., Wirrell E., Donald K.A., Berl M., Hartmann H., Valente K.D., Van Bogaert P., Cross J.H., Osawa M., Kanemura H., Aihara M., Guerreiro M.M., Samia P., Vinayan K.P., Smith M.L., Carmant L., Kerr M., Hermann B., Dunn D., Wilmshurst J.M. Systematic review of the screening, diagnosis, and management of ADHD in children with epilepsy. Consensus paper of the Task Force on Comorbidities of the ILAE Pediatric Commission. *Epilepsia* 2018;59:1867–80.

Berg A.T., Berkovic S.F., Brodie M.J., Brodie M.J., Buchhalter J., Cross J.H., van Emde Boas W., Engel J., French J., Glauser T.A., Mathern G.W., Moshé S.L., Nordli D., Plouin P., Scheffer I.E. Revised terminology and concepts for organization of seizure and epilepsies: Report of the ILAE Commission on Classification and Terminology, 2005–2009. *Epilepsia* 2010;51:676–85.

Caraballo R.H., Cersosimo R.O., Fejerman N. Childhood occipital epilepsy of Gastaut: A study of 33 patients. *Epilepsia* 2007;49:288–97.

Caraballo R., Koutroumanidis M., Panayiotopoulos C.P., Fejerman N. Idiopathic childhood occipital epilepsy of Gastaut: A review and differentiation from migraine and other epilepsies. *J Child Neurol* 2009;24:1536–42.

Gastaut H. A new type of epilepsy: Benign partial epilepsy of childhood with occipital spike-waves. *Clin Electroencephal* 1982;13:13–22.

Panayiotopoulos C.P. Inhibitory effect of central vision on occipital lobe seizures. *Neurology* 1981;31:1330–3.

Specchio R., Wirrell E.C., Scheffer I.E., Nabbout R., Riney K., Samia P., Nabbout R., Riney K., Samia P., Guerreiro M., Gwer S., Zuberi S.M., Wilmshurst J.M., Yozawitz E., Pressler R., Hirsch E., Wiebe S., Cross H.J., Perucca E., Moshé S.L., Tinuper P., Auvin S. International League Against Epilepsy classification and definition of epilepsy syndromes with onset in childhood: Position paper by the ILAE Task Force on nosology and definitions. *Epilepsia* 2022;63:1398–442.

32 Photosensitive Occipital Lobe Epilepsy

Maria Augusta Montenegro
UC San Diego School of Medicine

CONTENTS

CASE PRESENTATION

A 12-year-old boy was first seen at an emergency department due to seizures characterized by elementary visual hallucinations (bright lights) followed by involuntary lateral head and eye versions, without impairment of awareness. The family recalled that one similar episode occurred in the prior few weeks, but they did not seek medical attention. Each event lasted less than 2 minutes in length, and both events occurred while playing a video game. There was no history of other clinical episodes of concern. He was the product of an uneventful pregnancy and delivery without any history of brain insults (trauma or infection). Neurological examination and brain MRI were normal. EEG showed a normal background and interictal occipital spike-and-wave discharges. During intermittent photic stimulation, there was a photoparoxysmal response in the occipital head regions. Hyperventilation did not trigger additional epileptiform discharges or seizures. The diagnosis of photosensitive occipital lobe epilepsy (POLE) was made, and he was started on oxcarbazepine. After 2 years of treatment, the patient was weaned off antiseizure medication (ASM) and has remained seizure free since then (Figure 32.1).

DOI: 10.1201/9781003296478-36

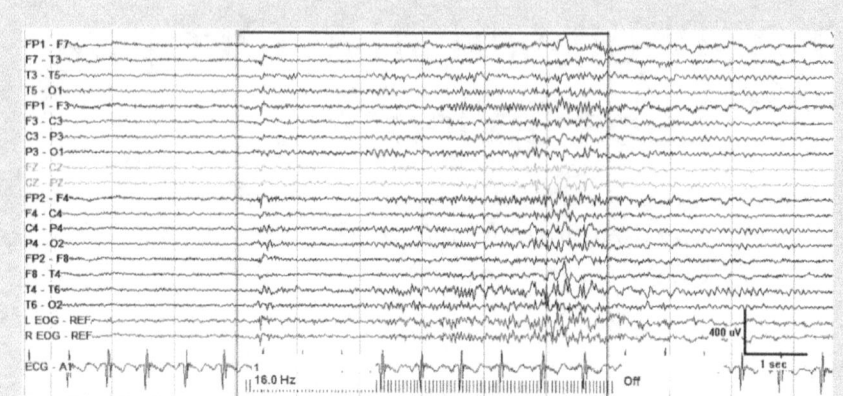

FIGURE 32.1   EEG during wakefulness showing photoparoxysmal response characterized by temporo-parieto-occipital spike–wave (greater over the right hemisphere) triggered by 16Hz intermittent photic stimulation.

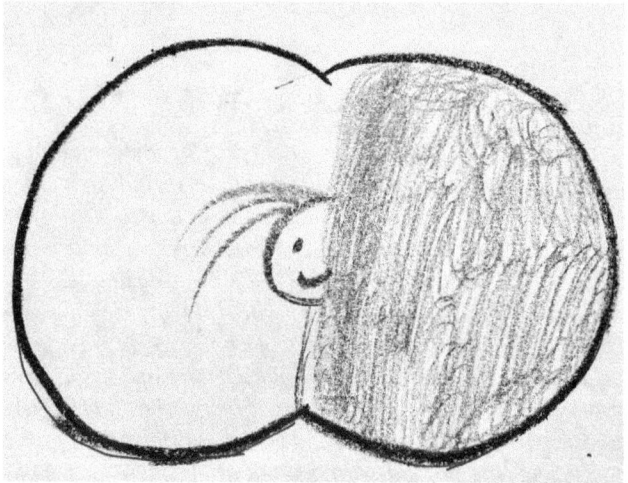

FIGURE 32.2   Migraine "aura". This is a drawing from a child that could not explain in detail the characteristics of her migraine "aura". The drawing shows in detail that she experienced hemianopsia.

DIFFERENTIAL DIAGNOSIS

Migraine with visual aura and acephalgic migraine (visual symptoms without associated headache) can be differentiated by the visual hallucination's characteristics. Migraine "aura" develops slowly over several minutes and lasts for up to an hour, which is black or shiny, and the child describes linear, zigzag phenomena, or hemianopsia (Figure 32.2). In contrast, epilepsy "aura" develops within a few seconds, which is characterized by colored spots, blurring, or ictal blindness and lasts for seconds up to 1 or 2 minutes. Sometimes the child cannot describe the visual symptoms, but can often draw them, usually with impressive details.

Once the diagnosis of epilepsy has been established, a structural lesion in the occipital lobe should be ruled out by neuroimaging. If the brain MRI is normal, the most common differential diagnosis is childhood occipital visual epilepsy (COVE).

COVE is a type of self-limited epilepsy previously known as idiopathic (or benign) occipital epilepsy, or childhood occipital epilepsy of Gastaut. Patients with COVE usually present with their first seizure between 6 and 15 years of age, and seizures are characterized by elementary visual symptoms (colored spots, ictal blindness, etc.) lasting a few seconds to a few minutes. It can be followed by a bilateral clonic (or hemiclonic) seizure.

Most children with POLE or COVE describe the visual symptoms as bright colored lights in the center of the visual field. The visual symptoms of COVE and POLE are very similar and should not be used as a reliable feature to establish the differential diagnosis. EEG provides the highest yield for diagnosis because only POLE has occipital spike-and-wave or polyspike-and-wave complexes triggered by intermittent photic stimulation.

DIAGNOSTIC APPROACH

POLE affects children and adolescents with normal neurological development and the diagnosis is based on clinical history and EEG findings. Seizures are characterized by elementary visual hallucinations (colored spots, ictal blindness, or blurring vision), followed by head and eye versions. Most patients do not have impairment of awareness, but there may be some degree of unresponsiveness. The key finding that helps to differentiate it from COVE is that seizures are triggered by intermittent photic stimulation.

POLE is considered a form of reflex epilepsy, a form of epilepsy that can be triggered by a specific stimulus. Photosensitive epilepsies are the most common form of reflex epilepsy, and although POLE is a type of focal epilepsy, visually-induced seizures (by intermittent photic stimulation) are a frequent characteristic of genetic generalized epilepsies or GGE (idiopathic generalized epilepsies). Therefore, it is not surprising that patients with POLE frequently have a positive family history of GGE.

Some patients with POLE also have seizures that are not induced by photic stimulation, but it is common to find a history of seizures while watching TV or playing video games. The EEG shows a normal background and occipital spikes or spike-and-wave discharges in the occipital head region during intermittent photic stimulation. Centrotemporal and/or generalized epileptic discharges can also occur. In addition, sleep can activate the discharges.

TREATMENT STRATEGY

Treatment with an ASM should be offered because if untreated most patients will have additional seizures. Seizures are often controlled with monotherapy, but occasional seizures might occur if the patient is exposed to intermittent photic stimulation. As

CLINICAL PEARLS

- Seizures are characterized by elementary visual hallucinations (colored spots or blurring), followed by head version.
- EEG shows a normal background and occipital spikes or spike-and-wave discharges at the occipital region during intermittent photic stimulation. Centrotemporal and/or generalized epileptic discharges can also occur.
- Most patients will become seizure free after starting an ASM.

with most self-limited epilepsies, standard treatments include levetiracetam, oxcarbazepine, carbamazepine, and less commonly, valproic acid or lamotrigine.

LONG-TERM OUTCOME

The prognosis is very favorable, and most patients with POLE will become seizure free after initiation of an ASM. However, there are reports of patients with POLE in which the epilepsy evolved to GGE at older ages.

Poor academic performance is associated with some forms of childhood epilepsy. Learning should be assessed at 6 years of age (or at diagnosis) and repeated annually. Also, active screening for learning difficulties should be performed after changing or increasing the dose of the ASM.

PATHOPHYSIOLOGY/NEUROBIOLOGY OF DISEASE

Although there is not a specific gene associated with POLE, nor a commercially available genetic test to establish its diagnosis, there are robust data suggesting that it has a genetic etiology. One-third of the patients have a positive family history of epilepsy, with family members presenting with GGE or self-limited epilepsy with centrotemporal spikes (SeLECTS).

SUGGESTED REFERENCES

Bonini F., Egeo G., Fattouch J., Fanella M., Morano A., Giallonardo A.T., di Bonaventura C. Natural evolution from idiopathic photosensitive occipital lobe epilepsy to idiopathic generalized epilepsy in an untreated young patient. *Brain Dev* 2014;36:346–50.

Guerrini R., Dravet C., Genton P., Bureau M., Bonanni P., Ferrari A.R., Roger J. Idiopathic photosensitive occipital lobe epilepsy. *Epilepsia* 1995;36:883–91.

Specchio N., Wirrell E.C., Scheffer I.E., Nabbout R., Riney K., Samia P., Guerreiro M., Gwer S., Zuberi S.M., Wilmshurst J.M., Yozawitz E., Pressler R., Hirsch E., Wiebe S., Cross H.J., Perucca E., Moshé S.L., Tinuper P., Auvin S. International league against epilepsy classification and definition of epilepsy syndromes with onset in childhood: Position paper by the ILAE Task Force on nosology and definitions. *Epilepsia* 2022;63:1398–442.

33 Childhood Absence Epilepsy

Stéphane Auvin
Université Paris-Cité & Institut Universitaire de France (IUF)

CONTENTS

CASE PRESENTATION

Parents brought in their previously healthy son for evaluation due to "strange spells" reported by his teacher. Recently, the parents noted at the dinner table that their son paused when he was telling a story. He had mild ptosis with slight rhythmic blinking and mouthing movements that did not abate when they called him. This unresponsiveness lasted approximately 10 seconds, after which he returned abruptly to normal, but had no recollection of his parents' efforts to communicate with him. The parents called their pediatrician who arranged for an EEG. The EEG demonstrated frequent generalized 3 Hz spike-and-slow-wave discharges during awake and sleep states, and that could also be induced by hyperventilation (HV). The patient was unable to repeat words said to him during longer periods of 3Hz discharges. Motor automatisms were evident during these lengthier episodes.

DIFFERENTIAL DIAGNOSIS

Even though CAE should be a straightforward diagnosis, some children experience delays in receiving proper medical attention due to the subtle and non-alarming nature of their presentation. Attention deficit hyperactivity disorder (ADHD) may be misdiagnosed in children with absence epilepsy and vice-versa. ADHD occurs in about 30% of children with CAE. There are very few studies evaluating the clinical features enabling rapid distinction between ADHD and absence epilepsy. Three features have been suggested as supporting nonepileptic staring rather than absence seizures: (1) lack of interruption of play; (2) events are more commonly noted by a

DOI: 10.1201/9781003296478-37

professional rather than a parent; and (3) episodes are interruptible by external stimuli, such as touch. Most importantly, hyperventilation induces absence seizures in most children with untreated CAE. When the clinical and electroencephalographic picture is classic, formulating a differential diagnosis is not required. In this case, there is no indication to perform a brain MRI or additional laboratory testing. Nonresponse to treatment, and *a fortiori* the presence of drug resistance, mandates a reexamination of the syndromic and etiological diagnosis.

In case of early-onset (i.e., before 3–4 years of age) episodes suggesting CAE, a lumbar puncture should be considered, especially to look for cerebrospinal fluid (CSF) and simultaneous serum glucose levels with a CSF/serum ratio of <0.6. In this situation, approximately 10% of patients may have an underlying defect in the glucose transporter type 1 (GLUT-1), resulting in the GLUT1 deficiency syndrome. If this diagnosis is suspected, testing for a potential mutation in the SLC2A1 gene should be conducted. This is essential as the initial treatment of choice (i.e., the ketogenic diet) should be initiated promptly to mitigate adverse neurodevelopmental outcomes.

There are also other epilepsy syndromes occurring in children or adolescents with typical absence seizures. Typical absence seizures can be observed in juvenile absence epilepsy (JAE) and juvenile myoclonic epilepsy (JME). Both these latter syndromes are seen in older children (after 8–10 years of age). In JAE, the frequency of absence seizures is often lower than in CAE. Furthermore, absence episodes in JAE are more often associated with generalized tonic-clonic seizures at the time of diagnosis (shortly after the onset of absence seizures). In JME, patients present with generalized myoclonic seizures and generalized tonic-clonic seizures.

DIAGNOSTIC APPROACH

The proper diagnosis can be readily made by having the patient hyperventilate in the outpatient office setting. The induction of a state of unresponsiveness, cessation or slowing of hyperventilation, the appearance of minor automatisms, and the almost immediate return of consciousness without a post-ictal state collectively are consistent with a typical absence seizure. An EEG will confirm that these clinical events are typical absence seizures by documenting generalized 3 Hz rhythmic spike-and-slow-waves discharges. The EEG recording will also serve to confirm the lack of other EEG abnormalities (Figure 33.1). Photosensitivity is unusual in patients with CAE.

The diagnosis of CAE can be further confirmed through the clinical history. At the time of diagnosis, typical absence seizures are the only seizure type. Moreover, although a history of febrile seizures is not uncommon, any other seizure type at time of diagnosis (e.g., focal, myolonic, or tonic seizures) rule out the diagnosis of CAE.

The International League Against Epilepsy (ILAE) has recently updated the syndrome definition and diagnostic criteria. Table 33.1 summarizes the main characteristics of CAE.

In most cases, there is no major diagnostic challenge distinguishing between CAE and JAE. However, the age range of these two syndromes overlaps to some extent. But there are usually distinctive features. The prognosis of and the treatment

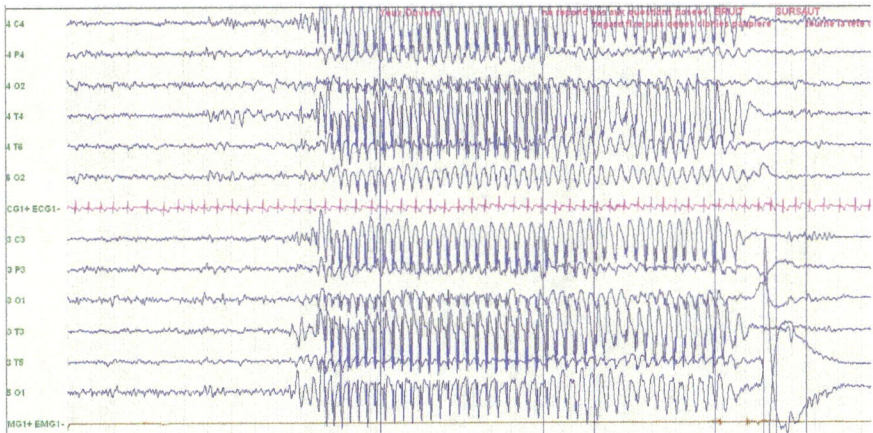

FIGURE 33.1   This representative EEG shows the spontaneous emergence of a 3.5 Hz frontally dominant generalized spike-and-slow-wave discharge lasting 12–14 seconds and having a slightly asymmetric onset but becoming symmetrical within 0.5 seconds. The patient had slight movements of the eyelids but was not responsive during the discharge.

approach for these two epilepsy syndromes are different. JAE usually presents later than age 9 years but there are rare CAE patients presenting that late and occasional JAE patients presenting earlier. Further, JAE patients very often exhibit generalized tonic-clonic seizures. Given the above, only in very few instances would it be difficult clearly distinguish between CAE from JAE at the time of diagnosis.

TREATMENT STRATEGY

Since 2010, there has been a strong evidence-based approach for the treatment of CAE. A randomized, double-blind study comparing three antiseizure medications (ASMs) for CAE was conducted: ethosuximide, lamotrigine, and valproate. The primary endpoint was the disappearance of seizures after 16 weeks and a secondary endpoint was the presence of an attention deficit. 453 children were included in this study: 148 in the valproate group, 156 in the ethosuximide group, and 149 in the lamotrigine group. At the end of 16 weeks, valproate and ethosuximide had similar absence-free rates (58% and 53%, NS). These rates were better than those observed with lamotrigine (29%) (increased to 12 mg/kg/day in 16 weeks). There was no difference between these groups in terms of discontinuation of treatment due to side effects. Attentional deficits were present in 49% of children treated with valproate, whereas they were observed in only 33% of children receiving ethosuximide ($p = 0.03$). Moreover, a 12-month follow-up study of these same patients found a higher rate of discontinuation of treatment due to side effects in the valproate group, as well as a more pronounced level of attention problems.

A prospective cohort study confirmed ethosuximide as first-line treatment. This was a follow-up study of patients with CAE carried out to assess the outcome at 5 years (seizure free and untreated). 59 patients were included: 41 and

TABLE 33.1

ILAE Diagnostic Criteria for Childhood Absence Epilepsy

	Mandatory	Alerts	Exclusionary
Seizures	Typical absence seizures	GTCS prior to or during the period of frequent absence seizures Staring spells with typical duration >30 seconds or with post-ictal confusion or fatigue Absences occurring <daily in an untreated patient	Any of the following seizure types: • Prominent myoclonic seizures • Prominent eyelid myoclonia • Myoclonic-absence seizures • Atonic seizures • Tonic seizures • Atypical absence seizures • Focal impaired awareness seizures
EEG	Paroxysms of 3 Hz (2.5–4 Hz) GSW at the start of the absence (may have been obtained historically)	Consistently unilateral focal spikes Lack of HV activated 2.5–4 Hz GSW in untreated patient who performs HV well for 3 minutes or longer Recording a typical staring spell without EEG correlate in a child with a history of 2.5–4 Hz GSW Persistent slowing of the EEG background in the absence of sedating medication	Diffuse background slowing
Age at onset		2–3 or 11–13 years at onset	<2 or >13 years
Development at onset		Mild intellectual disability	Moderate to profound intellectual disability
Neurological exam		Potentially relevant neurological examination abnormalities, excluding incidental findings (see text)	
Comorbidities			Cognitive stagnation or decline
Imaging		Potentially relevant abnormal neuroimaging, excluding incidental findings (see the text)	
Other studies – genetic, etc.			Low CSF glucose and/or *SLC2A1* pathogenic variant (testing not needed in most cases but strongly recommended in children with onset <3 years, with microcephaly and/or intellectual disability)

Abbreviations: GTCS, generalized tonic-clonic seizures; GSW, generalized spike-and-slow-wave; HV, hyperventilation; CSF, cerebrospinal fluid.

18 were treated with ethosuximide and valproate as first line, respectively. The response to initial treatment was identical (59% for ethosuximide and 56% for valproate). Multivariate analysis of seizure-free patients showed that ethosuximide was associated with a better rate of complete remission (hazard ratio 2.5 (CI95:1.1–6.0)). Similarly, the long-term remission rate was higher in patients who received ethosuximide.

Based on these two studies, the use of ethosuximide as a first-line treatment for CAE is recommended. Valproate should be considered next if ethosuximide does not provide full control of absence seizures. Decisions regarding when medications can be weaned off are often difficult to make. A conservative approach is to wait a minimum of 2 years after diagnosis, as few studies support the view that 1 year of treatment may be sufficient. It may be helpful to repeat an EEG study (with hyperventilation) while the patient is still on medication. Additionally, if the patient remains seizure free after a medication taper, one might consider checking another EEG to confirm seizure freedom.

LONG-TERM OUTCOME

The outcome of CAE is usually favorable with cessation of seizures without long-term treatment with ASMs. It should be noted; however, that children with CAE have a greater incidence of attention deficit hyperactivity disorder (ADHD) than the general childhood population (30% vs. 10%, respectively). Approximately 10% of children with CAE evolve to other epilepsy syndromes. Negative prognostic factors include atypical early (<4 years) or late (>10 years) onset, early refractory clinical course, and the presence of photosensitivity.

CLINICAL PEARLS

- CAE can often be reliably diagnosed with a simple 2–3-minute office hyperventilation trial. Having the child repeatedly blow air against a suspended piece of paper (to keep it from dropping) or a pinwheel is more effective than non-directed hyperventilation.
- The automatisms occurring with CAE may appear complex. A premature (and incorrect) diagnosis of focal-onset seizures might lead to the wrong choice of an ASM.
- An EEG recording with hyperventilation will enable electroclinical confirmation of a typical absence seizure.
- Ethosuximide is the first-line treatment for CAE.
- ADHD is a frequent comorbidity. All children with CAE should be screened for ADHD as soon as they have been appropriately treated.
- Carbamazepine, oxcarbazepine, gabapentin, tiagabine, pregabalin, and vigabatrin may precipitate both absence and myoclonic seizures. Therefore, they are contraindicated in CAE.

PATHOPHYSIOLOGY/NEUROBIOLOGY OF DISEASE

The pathophysiology of absence seizures has been linked to augmented oscillatory thalamic-cortical rhythms involving layer VI neocortex and thalamic relay neurons, and the interaction of GABAergic neurons in the nucleus reticularis thalami (NRT). An important molecular target of ASMs effective against absence seizures is the low-threshold T-type voltage gated calcium channel. The pathophysiology of absence seizures differs from other epilepsies which may, in part, explain the unique efficacy of ethosuximide in this syndrome. Although multiple genetic abnormalities have been linked to CAE, no specific diagnostic genetic tests have yet been developed for this disorder.

SUGGESTED REFERENCES

Auvin S. Advancing pharmacologic treatment options for pharmacologic treatment options for children with epilepsy. *Expert Opin Pharmacother* 2016;17:1475–82.

Auvin S., Wirrell E., Donald K.A., Berl M., Hartmann H., Valente K.D., Van Bogaert P., Cross J.H., Osawa M., Kanemura H., Aihara M., Guerreiro M.M, Samia P., Vinayan K.P., Smith M.L., Carmant L., Kerr M., Hermann B., Dunn D., Wilmshurst J.M. Systematic review of the screening, diagnosis, and management of ADHD in children with epilepsy. Consensus paper of the Task Force on Comorbidities of the ILAE Pediatric Commission. *Epilepsia* 2018;59:1867–80.

Elmali A.D., Auvin S., Bast T., Rubboli G., Koutroumanidis M. How to diagnose and classify idiopathic (genetic) generalized epilepsies. *Epileptic Disord* 2020;22:399–420.

Glauser T.A., Cnaan A., Shinnar S., Hirtz D.G., Dlugos D., Masur D., Clark P.O., Capparelli E.V., Adamson P.C.; Childhood Absence Epilepsy Study Group. Ethosuximide, valproic acid, and lamotrigine in childhood absence epilepsy. *N Engl J Med* 2010;362(9):790–9.

Hirsch E., French J., Scheffer I.E., Bogacz A., Alsaadi T., Sperling M.R., Abdulla F., Zuberi S.M., Trinka E., Specchio N., Somerville E., Samia P., Riney K., Nabbout R., Jain S., Wilmshurst J.M., Auvin S., Wiebe S., Perucca E., Moshé S.L., Tinuper P., Wirrell E.C. ILAE definition of the Idiopathic Generalized Epilepsy Syndromes: Position statement by the ILAE Task Force on Nosology and Definitions. *Epilepsia* 2022;63:1475–99.

34 Epilepsy with Myoclonic Absences

Anita M. Devlin
North Children's Hospital and Newcastle University, UK

CONTENTS

CASE PRESENTATION

The patient is a 6-year-old who caused concern at school when, in the preceding 2 months, he was noticed to have "funny movements". He had required special assistance with schoolwork early on. Despite great effort, he struggled and became frustrated, while classmates accomplished things easily. Sometimes this resulted in angry outbursts and at other times he would exhibit acting out behaviors such as disturbing other children or making faces repeatedly. The "funny movements" had started when the class was preparing for the end-of-school-year tests. The movements consisted of repeated jerks of both arms which progressively elevated his arms while at the same time, his head jerked backward. This occurred several times a day and episodes lasted approximately 20 seconds during which time he did not respond to his name or efforts to arrest this activity. Stephen reverted to normal quickly afterward and carried on. One teacher initially thought that this activity was behavioral and was related to stress and another thought that the movements looked like tics. However, one evening Stephen was standing in the kitchen talking to his mother when he stopped talking, experienced an event and was incontinent of urine. His mother recognized that this was not behavioral and arranged an appointment with a pediatrician who, after documenting a full history and examination, ordered an electroencephalogram (EEG) study. The EEG showed a slightly slow background for age and captured an episode of jerking of the upper limbs which gradually elevated his arms giving a ratcheting

DOI: 10.1201/9781003296478-38

appearance, associated with jerking of his head, staring and unresponsiveness for 20 seconds. The events were associated with regular 3 Hz generalized spike-and-wave discharges on the EEG, with muscle contractions time-locked at the same frequency recorded by EMG electrodes on the deltoid muscles. He was treated with multiple combinations of anti-seizure medications (ASMs) which included sodium valproate, ethosuximide, lamotrigine, levetiracetam, and clobazam. Unfortunately, the myoclonic absence seizures continued, and 12 months later he experienced his first generalized tonic-clonic seizure. The cognitive gap between him and his peers gradually widened and he required more educational support.

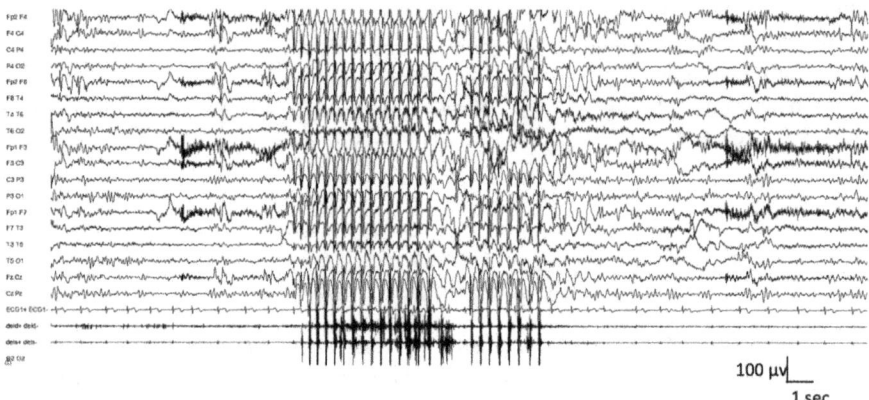

100 μV
1 sec

FIGURE 34.1   Ictal polygraphic electroencephalographic recording in an 8-year-old child with epilepsy with myoclonic absences, showing a paroxysmal generalized 3-Hz spike-and-wave discharge. Electromyographic channels (right and left deltoids) show bilateral myoclonic jerks synchronous with epileptiform abnormalities, and between jerks, there is a sustained increase in muscle tone. (Reproduced from Specchio et al. (2022); with permission.)

DIFFERENTIAL DIAGNOSIS

Epilepsy with myoclonic absence is a rare childhood epilepsy syndrome and although the exact incidence is unknown, it has been reported to account for 0.5%–1% of all epilepsies in a specialty center. Males are more commonly affected (70%) and the most common age of onset is approximately 7 years (range of 1–12 years). The birth history is usually normal but 50% of patients have developmental impairment at presentation and this rises to 70% with increasing age. Neurological examination is usually normal.

Absence seizures are accompanied by rhythmic jerks of the upper limbs which occur at the same frequency and are time-locked to the 3–3.5 Hz spike and wave on the EEG (Figure 34.1). Attacks can be provoked by hyperventilation. There is progressive abduction of the arms which is most often bilateral and symmetric but can be asymmetric and the patient may bend forward but typically does not fall. The jerks may involve the head and legs and there may also be perioral myoclonia and urinary incontinence.

Seizures have an abrupt onset and offset and last 10–60 seconds multiple times daily and awareness can vary from complete loss of awareness to retained awareness. Myoclonic absences are the only seizure type in 33% of patients but generalized tonic-clonic seizures can precede the myoclonic absences or occur subsequently in 45%. Myoclonic absence *status epilepticus* is rare. The emergence of other seizure types (clonic, tonic, atonic) can indicate a less favorable prognosis.

The differential diagnosis includes childhood absence epilepsy (CAE), epilepsy with eyelid myoclonia (EEM), and Lennox–Gastaut syndrome (LGS) – especially when myoclonic absences are accompanied by other seizure types. However, true myoclonic absences, as described above, are a distinct seizure type and are not seen in CAE, LGS or EEM. In CAE, absence seizures are accompanied by 3 Hz spike-and-wave discharges on EEG which can be provoked by hyperventilation. Oral and motor automatisms occur in the majority (86%), with eyelid and perioral myoclonia in 76%. Although subtle myoclonic jerks may be seen, they are of low amplitude without rhythmicity and without stepwise abduction of the arms. This distinction is important and has prognostic significance.

EEM is another rare epilepsy syndrome characterized by episodes of eyelid myoclonia. These consist of brief (<6 seconds), repetitive, and often rhythmic 3–6 Hz myoclonic jerks of the eyelids, with a simultaneous upward deviation of the eyeballs and extension of the head with or without impaired awareness. The EEG is significantly different compared to EMA in that EEM shows interictal, bursts of fast (3–6 Hz) irregular generalized polyspike-and-wave complexes with a characteristic response to eye closure and intermittent photic stimulation which shows fast (3–6 Hz) generalized polyspikes or polyspike-and-wave complexes that are mandatory for the diagnosis. In EMA, photic stimulation provokes a response in only 14% of individuals with generalized spike-and-wave EEG changes or by eliciting seizures with 3–3.5 Hz spike-and-wave discharges.

LGS is a developmental and epileptic encephalopathy (DEE), which is characterized by the onset of multiple types of drug-resistant seizures with onset between 18 months and 8 years. One of the seizure types must be tonic seizures and although EMA may evolve to include multiple seizure types including tonic seizures. Tonic seizures are not present at onset and are not a defining seizure type of EMA. Approximately 1/3 of children diagnosed with LGS will have experienced an epilepsy syndrome or seizures previously, which is not the case with EMA. Those with LGS often experience frequent atypical absence seizures (<2.5 Hz spike and wave on EEG) with impaired awareness and up to 75% will experience nonconvulsive *status* characterised by ongoing atypical absence seizures associated with erratic, generalized, or multifocal myoclonic and atonic components, and intermittent brief tonic seizures.

DIAGNOSTIC APPROACH

The diagnostic gold standard is capturing a seizure on EEG with simultaneous EMG and video recording. This can be aided by hyperventilation which can provoke generalized spike-and-wave discharges and may also trigger myoclonic absence seizures. The EEG background is typically normal and the occipital intermittent rhythmic delta activity seen in CAE is not present. Interictal 3 Hz generalized spike-and-wave and polyspike-and-wave abnormalities can occur. Ictal EEG shows regular 3 Hz generalized spike-and-wave discharges that are time-locked with the myoclonic jerks that are most often bilateral and symmetrical. However, an ictal EEG is not required for the diagnosis as long as the attacks have been witnessed by someone with expertise in the diagnosis of epilepsy in children.

Cranial MRI scanning should be performed where possible, particularly if there are positive neurological examination findings, as neuroimaging is abnormal in 17% of cases. Comparative genomic hybridization (also called the CGH array) and whole exome or whole genome sequencing should also be performed where available as EMA has been reported in association with inv dup(15) genotype, trisomy 12p, Angelman syndrome, as well as variants in *SYNGAP1*, *SLC2A1*, and *SCN1A* (Dravet syndrome). However, these cases all exhibited significant learning disability, so this investigation is particularly relevant in that context.

TREATMENT STRATEGY

In rare epilepsy syndromes, there are often no RCTs and the available treatment efficacy data are retrospective. Such data suggest that if myoclonic absences are the only seizure type, ethosuximide can be considered first-line treatment, recognizing that it will not prevent generalized tonic-clonic seizures. Should ethosuximide be ineffective or should generalized tonic-clonic seizures emerge, lamotrigine can be considered as an add-on or substitute treatment. Lamotrigine is generally associated with fewer unwanted side effects than sodium valproate which, in addition, is not recommended for women able to have children. However, lamotrigine is slightly less effective than valproic acid.

Single or combination treatment with these three medications is the most common approach. However, if seizures are not controlled, additional treatments such as levetiracetam, clobazam, clonazepam, topiramate, and zonisamide can be attempted as none have been shown to worsen absence seizures. Combination therapy is often required, and seizures are often resistant to treatment with only 33% patients becoming seizure free at 12 months in one study. When drug resistance occurs it is important not to impair learning and quality of life with polypharmacy that is little or no more effective than fewer medications. ASMs that should be avoided include phenobarbital, phenytoin, carbamazepine, oxcarbazepine, and vigabatrin. The ketogenic diet is a treatment option after the 3rd appropriately chosen ASM, and vagus nerve stimulator implantation can also be considered in drug-resistant cases.

LONG-TERM OUTCOME

Myoclonic absences are the only seizure type throughout in approximately 1/3 of cases however, generalized tonic-clonic seizures occur in 45% but are rare (maybe once per year) in half of the cases. Seizure remission occurs in approximately 40% of patients and in the remainder myoclonic absences ± generalized tonic-clonic seizures persist. The prognosis is more favorable if myoclonic absences are the only seizure type and are controlled by medication. Learning disability is evident in half of cases at presentation, but this increases with increasing age and is ultimately seen in 70%. Cognitive deterioration may be seen in those whose seizures are treatment-resistant and, in some cases, there can be evolution to a more severe form of epilepsy such as Lennox–Gastaut syndrome.

PATHOPHYSIOLOGY/NEUROBIOLOGY OF DISEASE

Etiologic factors can be identified in 35% of cases including prematurity, perinatal injury, cerebral palsy, and chromosomal/genetic factors as previously described. A recent International League Against Epilepsy (ILAE) publication suggests that abnormal neuroimaging with an identified causative lesion precludes the classification of the epilepsy as epilepsy with myoclonic absences. In those without an identifiable

CLINICAL PEARLS

- EMA can be diagnosed in the office consultation if attacks are witnessed by someone familiar with this syndrome who recognizes the unique semiology. Review of videos of seizures provided by the parents/caregivers can also facilitate the diagnosis. Seizures can often be provoked in the office by hyperventilation (e.g., by blowing on a pinwheel). This is particularly relevant in situations with limited access to EEG.
- Typical absences associated with myoclonias restricted to muscles in the face and neck are not associated with a poor prognosis.
- Carbamazepine, oxcarbazepine, gabapentin, tiagabine, pregabalin, vigabatrin, phenytoin, and phenobarbitone may exacerbate seizures in patients with absences.
- Consider ketogenic dietary therapy in those with EMA who do not respond to the third appropriately chosen ASM.
- Drug resistance is common in EMA and it is important to implement ASMs to the fewest medications required to obtain the optimum antiseizure effect to avoid side effects and additional impairments caused by polypharmacy.
- Children presenting with myoclonic seizures under the age of 5 years require assessment by a pediatric neurologist. Myoclonus with "developmental delay" or developmental stagnation can be a presenting feature of neuronal ceroid lipofuscinosis (Batten disease) which was previously an untreatable and fatal neurodegenerative disorder. Enzyme replacement therapy is now available but early treatment is critical to the outcome.

etiology, a family history of generalized seizures is found in 20% although a history of febrile seizures is rare. Most cases are likely to follow complex inheritance – meaning that they have a polygenic basis with or without environmental triggers and have shared genetic etiologies with the genetic generalized epilepsies.

Recent electrical recordings and imaging of large neuronal networks with single-cell resolution have revealed that cortical mechanisms, rather than an exclusively thalamic rhythmogenesis, are involved in ictogenesis and the resulting spike-wave discharges at specific frequencies. This evidence also supports previous findings on the essential role of basal ganglia networks in absence seizures, in particular the ictal increase in firing of substantia nigra GABAergic neurons.

SUGGESTED REFERENCES

Berg A.T., Levy S.R., Testa F.M. Evolution and course of early life developmental encephalopathic epilepsies: Focus on Lennox-Gastaut syndrome. *Epilepsia* 2018;59:2096–105.

Bureau M., Tassinari C.A. Epilepsy with myoclonic absences. *Brain Dev* 2005;27:178–84.

Crunelli V., Lőrincz M.L., McCafferty C., Lambert R.C., Leresche N., Di Giovanni G., David F. Clinical and experimental insight into pathophysiology, comorbidity and therapy of absence seizures. *Brain* 2020;143:2341–68.

Genton P., Bureau M. Epilepsy with myoclonic absences. *CNS Drugs* 2006;20:911–6.

Hiraide T., Hattori A., Ieda D., Hori I., Saitoh S., Nakashima M., Saitsu H. De novo variants in SETD1B cause intellectual disability, autism spectrum disorder, and epilepsy with myoclonic absences. *Epilepsia Open* 2019;4:476–481.

Hirsch E., French J., Scheffer I.E., Bogacz A., Alsaadi T., Sperling M.R., Abdulla F., Zuberi S.M., Trinka E., Specchio N., Somerville E., Samia P., Riney K., Nabbout R., Jain S., Wilmshurst J.M., Auvin S., Wiebe S., Perucca E., Moshé S.L., Tinuper P., Wirrell E.C. ILAE definition of the idiopathic generalized epilepsy syndromes: Position statement by the ILAE Task Force on Nosology and Definitions. *Epilepsia* 2022;63:1475–99.

Maurizio Elia R.G., Musumeci S.A., Bonanni P., Gambardella A., Aguglia U. Myoclonic absence-like seizures and chromosome abnormality syndromes. *Epilepsia* 2005;39:660–3.

Specchio N., Wirrell E.C., Scheffer I.E., Nabbout R., Riney K., Samia P., Guerreiro M., Gwer S., Zuberi S.M., Wilmshurst J.M., Yozawitz E., Pressler R., Hirsch E., Wiebe S., Cross H.J., Perucca E., Moshé S.L., Tinuper P., Auvin S. International League Against Epilepsy classification and definition of epilepsy syndromes with onset in childhood: Position paper by the ILAE Task Force on Nosology and Definitions. *Epilepsia* 2022;63:1398–442.

Zanzmera P., Menon R.N., Karkare K., Soni H., Jagtap S., Radhakrishnan A. Epilepsy with myoclonic absences: Electroclinical characteristics in a distinctive pediatric epilepsy phenotype. *Epilepsy Behav* 2016;64(Pt A):242–7.

35 Lennox–Gastaut Syndrome

Jong M. Rho
UC San Diego School of Medicine

CONTENTS

CASE PRESENTATION

This is a nearly 3-year-old boy who was completely well until 6 months ago when he experienced two brief (<2 minutes) generalized convulsions 1 month apart, both associated with fever. Although these were diagnosed as simple febrile seizures, he was referred to a pediatric neurologist who ordered a routine 1.5T brain MRI scan. This study was interpreted as normal. However, the outpatient EEG study revealed generalized background slowing and generalized atypical spike-wave discharges occurring at a frequency of 2.0– 2.5 Hz and generalized polyspikes during sleep (Figures 35.1 and 35.2). A follow-up 24-hour video-EEG study captured multiple generalized myoclonic and tonic seizures, both associated with generalized spike-wave discharges followed by voltage suppression. No focal or lateralizing features were noted. This patient was placed on valproic acid monotherapy. Despite serum levels (in the 100–120 range), he continued to have frequent seizures, and then developed "drop" seizures that became progressively more frequent. Further medication trials with topiramate, zonisamide, levetiracetam, and clonazepam were unsuccessful, and he was ultimately placed on the ketogenic diet. His generalized myoclonic seizures improved substantially, but he was still experiencing several drop seizures per day. Notably, his speech and attention became slowly impaired, and he developed difficulty walking with mild ataxia. A high-resolution (3T) brain MRI was interpreted as normal, and a comprehensive metabolic/genetic work-up (including genetic testing for severe myoclonic epilepsy of infancy) failed to reveal an etiology. As his

---

DOI: 10.1201/9781003296478-39

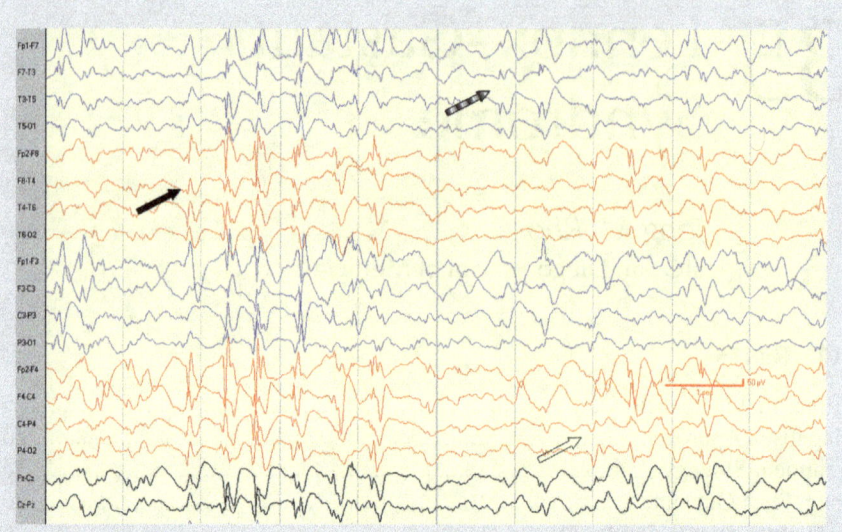

FIGURE 35.1 Generalized 2–2.5 Hz slow spike–wave complexes (solid arrow) and spikes lateralized to the left and right hemispheres (dashed and open arrow, respectively).

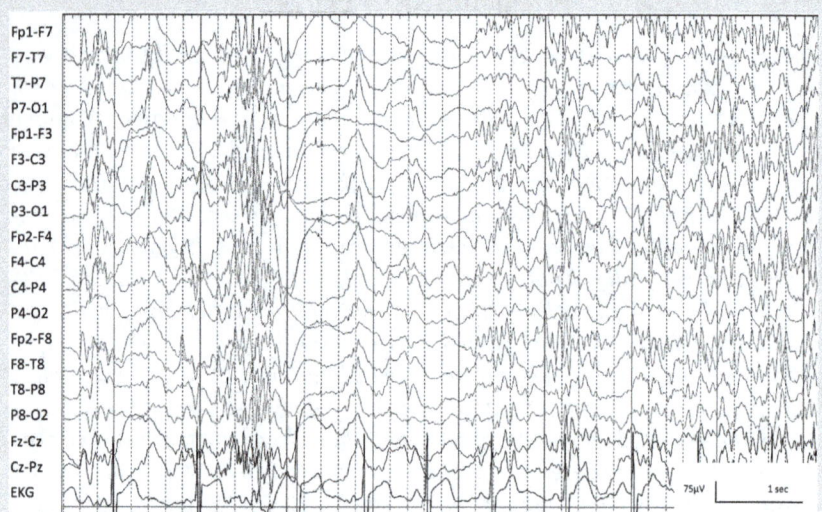

FIGURE 35.2 Sleep EEG showing generalized paroxysmal fast activity (generalized sharp waves around 10Hz).

neurological condition steadily worsened, he underwent an anterior two-thirds corpus callosotomy as a palliative procedure, to which he responded favorably. Although he experienced a transient left foot drop after surgery, his speech returned slowly (but not fully), and within a month he was able to put three words together again. The ketogenic diet was weaned off, and he was left on a regimen of zonisamide and levetiracetam. His gait and ataxia improved, and he was having only 1–2 "drop" seizures per day, but none of the myoclonic or tonic seizures.

DIFFERENTIAL DIAGNOSIS

Lennox–Gastaut syndrome (LGS) first appeared in the medical literature in 1969, even though important clinical and EEG features in this subgroup of epileptic patients had been noted as early as 1939. This syndrome comprises a clinical triad consisting of (1) diffusely slow spike-wave discharges (occurring at a frequency of 1.5–2.5 Hz), (2) psychomotor delay, and (3) multiple electroclinical seizure types refractory to medical therapy (including generalized tonic, atonic, atypical absence, myoclonic, tonic-clonic, and even focal-onset seizures).

The hallmark seizure type is the generalized tonic seizure which most often occurs while falling asleep. In most cases, LGS manifests between 2 and 8 years of age, represents 3%–10% of all pediatric epilepsies, and in this condition, males are more frequently affected than girls. A structural/metabolic etiology (usually a remote brain injury acquired during the perinatal period or early infancy) can be identified in proximately 2/3 of the patients. Further, it is not uncommon for LGS to be preceded by a history of infantile spasms.

The major differential diagnostic consideration is epilepsy with myoclonic-atonic seizures (aka, Doose syndrome) which appears between 2 and 5 years of age, often with generalized tonic-clonic (GTC) seizures. The affected child, however, is developmentally normal prior to onset of seizures, but developmental decline can occur if they are not controlled adequately. Within several months of onset, the characteristic drop attacks occur, along with atypical absence seizures.

Another consideration is Dravet syndrome which has an earlier onset, often in the first year of life, and is characterized by prolonged GTC seizures associated with fever, and later myoclonic, focal, and (rarely) tonic seizures. The EEG is normal at onset, but after a few months often shows generalized, focal, or multifocal epileptiform discharges. There are no polyspikes during NREM sleep.

There is also the developmental epileptic encephalopathy with spike-and-wave activation in sleep (D/EE-SWAS) which can result in speech/language regression, slow spike-wave discharges, as well as atonic and atypical absence seizures. However, tonic seizures do not occur in D/EE-SWAS. Finally, epileptic spasms – i.e., spasms that persist beyond infancy - can also produce drop attacks. Careful video-EEG monitoring of episodes can help distinguish between LGS and these other rare entities. If the clinician obtains a generic history of "drop attacks" without other ancillary data (most importantly, the EEG), then other diagnostic considerations would include syncope (neurogenic or cardiogenic), cataplexy (seen in narcoleptic patients), and hyperekplexia (or "startle disease"). It is important to note, however, that there are several epileptic syndromes and epileptic encephalopathies that share some but not all clinical and/or EEG features of LGS. And many LGS patients may lack all of the characteristic features, especially during the early stages of disease evolution.

DIAGNOSTIC APPROACH

There are two general goals of the diagnostic approach toward LGS. The first is to establish a clear diagnosis of the syndrome, and the second is to determine its specific etiology. The single most important diagnostic tool is the EEG, and as is often the case, long-term video-EEG monitoring to accurately define specific seizure types and specific EEG abnormalities (both ictal and interictal).

The next most useful diagnostic test is the brain MRI, since a variety of structural lesions can produce LGS; these include destructive pathologies such as meningitis/ encephalitis, hypoxic-ischemic injury, stroke, trauma, as well as developmental anomalies such as tuberous sclerosis complex and disorders of neuronal migration (e.g., focal cortical dysplasia). A head CT scan can be valuable in demonstrating the presence of calcifications which can be seen in conditions such as congenital CMV infection.

Multiple genes have been described in association with LGS; therefore, specialized genetic testing should be considered in patients without a clearly established etiology, especially those with normal neuroimaging. Depending on other features of the physical and neurological examinations, specific metabolic and/or degenerative disorders affecting the central nervous system should be considered, including biochemical assays and biopsies. It should be noted that upward of 30% of LGS patients have no evidence of pre-existing brain damage, despite the fact that approximately one-third of LGS patients have a prior history of infantile spasms.

TREATMENT STRATEGY

By and large, the treatment of LGS has been challenging and disappointing. The optimum treatment for LGS remains unclear, and no study to date provides solid evidence of any single drug to be highly effective. However, given the multiplicity of seizure types seen in LGS, and the fact that certain drugs such as carbamazepine and phenytoin can exacerbate generalized spike-wave epilepsies, it is generally recommended that broad-spectrum (i.e., effective against both focal and generalized seizure types) antiseizure medications (ASMs) be utilized.

Valproic acid has traditionally been the drug of choice as it can provide beneficial effects against all seizure types, but caution is advised when using valproic acid in young patients (especially those under 2 years of age) on polypharmacy (as this substantially increases the risk of hepatotoxicity). Other newer broad-spectrum ASMs include topiramate, lamotrigine, and felbamate, which have been shown to be effective in double-blind, placebo-controlled trials. However, felbamate is associated with a high incidence of serious side effects such as aplastic anemia/pancytopenia and hepatic failure.

While there are numerous additional uncontrolled studies of other medications being effective for patients with LGS (including zonisamide, clonazepam, nitrazepam, vigabatrin, prednisone, IVIG, etc.), the reported benefits have been variable, limited, or short lived. More recently clobazam, rufinamide, cannabidiol, and fenfluramine have been approved for seizures associated with LGS and may ultimately provide long-term benefits for some patients. Nonpharmacological options, such as the ketogenic diet, vagus nerve stimulation, and corpus callosotomy (especially for the atonic seizures) have been shown to be beneficial to varying degrees. In practice, the majority of children with LGS need combination therapy, with both ASMs and nonpharmacological options. Each patient should be considered individually, with a careful assessment of potential benefits of the chosen therapy weighed against the risks of adverse effects.

LONG-TERM OUTCOME

Long-term prognosis of LGS is generally poor, as medically intractable seizures persist in over 90% of patients, and recurrent episodes of status epilepticus are not uncommon. Not only do patients experience significant neurocognitive impairment, they are also exposed to a 3%–7% risk of mortality (often coming from accidents, and as such, protective helmets are often advised for patients with drop attacks).

Studies have demonstrated a steady worsening of IQ, behavioral, and psychiatric symptoms. Without significant improvement from medical and/or surgical treatment strategies, LGS can be appropriately considered a progressive epileptic encephalopathy. Unlike infantile spasms, where the majority (>80%) of patients outgrow their seizures (but often followed later in life by other seizure types), patients with LGS may evolve to a more refractory form of epilepsy, i.e., epileptic spasms, or continue to exhibit electroclinical features of LGS well into adulthood.

PATHOPHYSIOLOGY/NEUROBIOLOGY OF DISEASE

While the mechanisms underlying the electroclinical expression of LGS remain unclear, there is a unique age dependence on the onset, which invokes disturbances

CLINICAL PEARLS

- A strong clinical index of suspicion can be made on the basis of a thorough medical history. LGS is an early childhood epileptic encephalopathy consisting of multiple seizure types, especially tonic seizures during sleep.
- A diagnosis can be made on the basis of long-term video-EEG monitoring.
- While LGS patients are defined as treatment-resistant, there are a number of effective nonpharmacological options, including the ketogenic diet, vagus nerve stimulation, and corpus callosotomy. Additionally, immunomodulation with IVIG or steroids can be helpful in some patients.
- Most successful treatment strategies appear to involve combination therapies which may provide complementary benefits.

in normal maturational processes. The fact that many diverse etiologies can produce the same clinical syndromes suggests a final common mechanistic pathway that may be activated in genetically susceptible individuals. In terms of pathological substrates, both frontal lobes and subcortical structures such as the thalamus have been implicated.

SUGGESTED REFERENCES

Asadi-Pooya A.A. Lennox-Gastaut syndrome: A comprehensive review. *Neurol Sci* 2018;39(3):403–14.

Brigo F., Jones K., Eltze C., Matricardi S. Anti-seizure medications for Lennox-Gastaut syndrome. *Cochrane Database Syst Rev* 2021;4(4):CD003277.

Cross J.H., Auvin S., Falip M., Striano P., Arzimanoglou A. Expert opinion on the management of Lennox-Gastaut syndrome: Treatment algorithms and practical considerations. *Front Neurol* 2017;8:505.

Keator C.G. Epilepsy surgery is a viable treatment for Lennox Gastaut syndrome. *Semin Pediatr Neurol* 2021;38:100894.

Montouris G., Aboumatar S., Burdette D., Kothare S., Kuzniecky R., Rosenfeld W., Chung S. Expert opinion: Proposed diagnostic and treatment algorithms for Lennox-Gastaut syndrome in adult patients. *Epilepsy Behav* 2020;110:107146.

Sharawat I.K., Panda P.K., Sihag R.K., Panda P., Dawman L. Efficacy and safety of corpus callosotomy and ketogenic diet in children with Lennox Gastaut syndrome: A systematic review and meta-analysis. *Childs Nerv Syst* 2021;37(8):2557–66.

Strzelczyk A., Schubert-Bast S. Expanding the treatment landscape for Lennox-Gastaut syndrome: Current and future strategies. *CNS Drugs* 2021;35(1):61–83.

Zhang L., Wang J., Wang C. Efficacy and safety of antiseizure medication for Lennox-Gastaut syndrome: A systematic review and network meta-analysis. *Dev Med Child Neurol* 2022;64(3):305–13.

36 Epilepsy with Myoclonic-Atonic Seizures (Doose Syndrome)

A.G. Christina Bergqvist
University of Pennsylvania

CONTENTS

CASE PRESENTATION

A 3-year-old boy with a normal birth, developmental and past medical history. At age three, he had his first generalized tonic-clonic (GTC) seizure during a viral illness with a high fever. He was given a diagnosis of febrile seizures. In the following months, he had five GTCs without fever and was evaluated by a neurologist. He was given a diagnosis of focal epilepsy and he was started on oxcarbazepine which exacerbated the GTCs. A workup including an MRI of his brain and a metabolic screen (plasma amino acids, urine organic acids, lactate and pyruvate, acylcarnitine esters) was normal. An initial EEG showed biparietal theta but no epileptiform discharges (Figure 36.1). He was switched to valproic acid.

Over the following year, he developed multiple seizure types – myoclonic (MS), myoclonic-atonic seizures (MAS) with clinical semiology of shoulder jerks followed by head or whole-body drops. He had two bouts of nonconvulsive status epilepticus, and prolonged absences. There was a family history of febrile seizures, but no one with epilepsy, and a sister with high-functioning autism. He had an expanded genetic work up, chromosomes, epilepsy panel, and whole exome sequencing, which did not reveal any definitive mutations known to cause epilepsy. The EEG developed generalized bifrontally maximal 3–3.5 Hz spike-wave discharges. During periods of increased seizure activity, the spike-and-slow waves were in the 2–3 Hz range. One video-EEG monitoring session

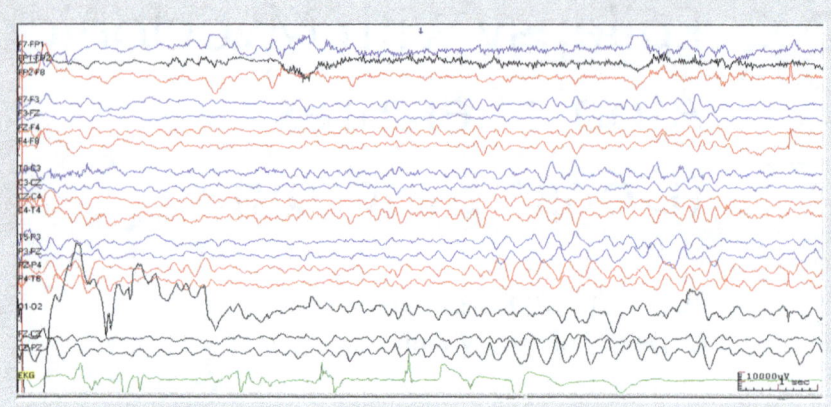

FIGURE 36.1   EEG showing biparietal theta activity.

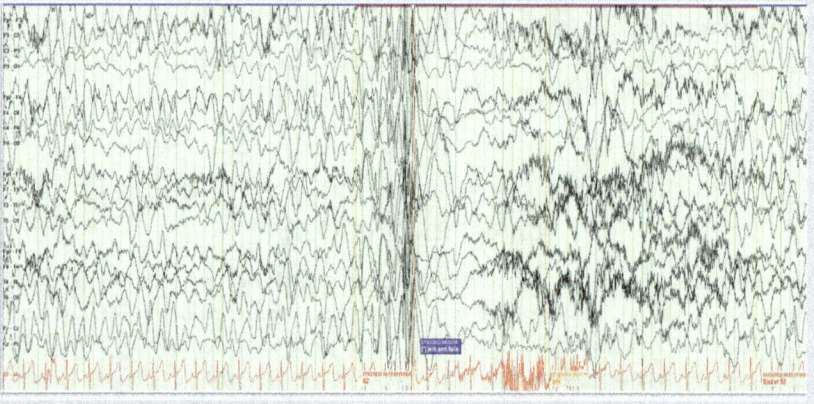

FIGURE 36.2   EEG showing generalized polyspike-and-slow wave discharges during a myoclonic-atonic seizure.

captured the child's GTC and MAS with generalized discharges at seizure onset (Figure 36.2). An ophthalmology evaluation of his retina was normal.

Medical treatment trials continued: valproic acid was pushed to 125 mg/dL as monotherapy, clobazam was added which reduced the GTCs but resulted in hyperactivity and drooling, and lamotrigine was pushed to a level of 14 mg/dL with brief improvement in his seizure control. Similarly, zonisamide improved the myoclonic seizures briefly but they later returned. GTC seizures continued daily, and absences and MAS were seen throughout the day. Cannabidiol was tried but caused fatigue and worsened his seizures, so it was discontinued. Up to this point, he had been a normally developing child, but now his language regressed to where he was speaking in one or two-word sentences or pointing.

He would spend most of his day sitting surrounded by pillows to avoid falls and head injuries. His motor function was affected, and he had a wide-based ataxic gate. At age 4 years, he was started on the 4:1 ketogenic diet (KD). Within 1 week of KD therapy, his MS and MAS abated. Within 9 months the GTC and absences had stopped. Within 12 months of KD treatment, he has successfully weaned off all his medications, and his language, cognition, and motor function returned to normal. After almost 5 years of KD therapy, he was successfully weaned onto regular food without the recurrence of his seizures. He is currently 22 years old, a college graduate, and in his first job working as an accountant.

DIFFERENTIAL DIAGNOSIS

This child has a diagnosis of epilepsy with myoclonic-atonic seizures (EMAS), aka myoclonic astatic epilepsy (MAE), or Doose syndrome after the initial reporting author. Doose syndrome is classified as a generalized epilepsy, which develops in normal children between the ages of 6 months and 6 years, with maximal onset around age 2–3 years. It is more common in boys than in girls by a 2:1 ratio. It is characterized by multiple seizure types of predominantly MS, MAS, GTC, absences, and myoclonic absences seizures.

Myoclonic-atonic seizures are the characteristic seizure type in this syndrome and typically consist of symmetric myoclonic jerks of the upper extremities, followed by atonia causing a head drop or a whole body fall if standing. Generalized tonic-clonic seizures usually herald the syndrome, and every child with EMAS will develop MAS. Rarely nocturnal generalized tonic seizures may develop. The differential diagnosis includes myoclonic epilepsies of infancy, Dravet syndrome, Lennox Gastaut syndrome (LGS), and any of the progressive myoclonic epilepsies. The differentiation between these disorders can be difficult and is based on developmental status prior to seizures, age of onset, seizure types, and EEG patterns, as well as the absence of metabolic findings, and a normal brain MRI.

LGS is the most significant differential diagnosis. There are several features that should help distinguish Doose syndrome from LGS. Children with LGS do not have a normal developmental history before the onset of seizures. Tonic seizures predominate and they also have focal seizures with secondary generalization when documented on video-EEG. Atypical absences are prominent with LGS, but these are not seen with Doose syndrome. Children with LGS may also have focal discharges and activation of generalized discharges during slow-wave sleep which is not a characteristic of Doose syndrome. LGS is classically associated with slow spike-and-wave activity on EEG, while children with Doose syndrome have faster generalized discharges that can become slow during the severe phase of the epilepsy.

Dravet syndrome is a mixed epilepsy with both focal and generalized seizures and can be differentiated from Doose syndrome by earlier onset of seizures (more typically in the first year of life, and often associated with fever or illness). While myoclonic seizures predominate in the first years of life, they do not have MAS. Both disorders have GTCs, but hemi-convulsive seizures are only seen with Dravet syndrome. A cause for the Dravet phenotype is very likely to be found with epilepsy panel testing, with 80% having a defect in the voltage-gated sodium channel (*SCN1A*) or *PCDH-19* genes and 20% having defects in other known genes with phenotypic overlap. Less than 14% of children with the Doose syndrome phenotype have a genetic defect identified. The cognitive outcome is almost universally negative in Dravet syndrome while approximately 2/3 of the children with Doose have "normal" cognitive function once their seizures abate.

Occasionally progressive encephalopathies (ex. mitochondrial disorders, late-infantile neuronal ceroid lipofuscinosis) may mimic the clinical course, but in general, for these conditions, myoclonic seizures predominate. These disorders may also be distinguished through biochemical and genetic testing with whole exome or mitochondrial genetic analysis.

DIAGNOSTIC APPROACH

A thorough history focusing on the development and the seizure types as they emerge is essential to making the correct diagnosis. Video-EEG monitoring is essential for diagnosis as it can document specific seizure types. Initial EEGs are often normal or may show a characteristic bicentral or parietal theta before the epileptiform discharges emerge (Figure 36.1). Generalized 3 Hz or irregular polyspike-and-wave discharges then evolve. Myoclonic seizures are associated with a burst of 2–4 Hz spike-and-wave or polyspike-and-wave activity and involve symmetric myoclonus, most often the proximal upper extremities. Focal discharges on initial EEG are an exclusion criterion.

Children with Doose syndrome often become encephalopathic when their seizures become frequent and/or severe. Progressive encephalopathies and myoclonic seizures due to inborn errors of metabolism should be ruled out by metabolic screenings (serum lactate and pyruvate, plasma amino acids, urine organic acids, acylcarnitine esters) and epilepsy genetic testing such as epilepsy panels. Brain MRI/MRS imaging is normal in Doose and remains so during their disease course.

TREATMENT STRATEGY

The optimal treatment for Doose syndrome is not known. There has been no randomized clinical trial comparing all our current treatment options. Treatment is therefore extrapolated from our knowledge of treating genetic generalized epilepsies. Many children with Doose syndrome are initially erroneously treated with oxcarbazepine or carbamazepine (initial diagnosis thought to be focal-onset epilepsy) which will worsen the seizures. Antiseizure medications (ASMs) that have shown promise in small clinical case series include valproic acid, ethosuximide, topiramate, lamotrigine, and levetiracetam, felbamate, cannabidiol, zonisamide, and steroids. These ASMs are often combined with benzodiazepines, although side effects and tolerance may limit their utility.

The ketogenic diet (KD), a high fat, adequate protein, and very low carbohydrate diet that mimics the metabolic changes that occur with fasting have shown promising efficacy in the Doose syndrome population, offering up to 50% seizure freedom. Lower ratio KDs such as modified Atkins diet, have also shown an ability to reduce seizures in Doose but may take a bit longer to work compared to the higher ratio diets. Ketogenic diets are often used as a last resort at many epilepsy centers but should be implemented sooner in these children and offered as second therapy if possible. While studies have demonstrated the beneficial effects of vagus nerve stimulation against atonic seizures, no studies have directly addressed its utility in Doose syndrome. Corpus callosotomy and other epilepsy surgeries are not indicated.

LONG-TERM OUTCOME

Long-term prognosis in the Doose group is variable and ranges from seizure freedom with normal development to severe retardation and continued refractory seizures. In the largest series of children with Doose syndrome, it was reported that about half the children older than 7 years became seizure-free for at least 2 years or more in follow-up. Others have found slightly higher remission rates in the range of about two-thirds. Seizure recurrence years after initial remission has been reported but is rare. If seizures recur, they are usually easily controlled with a single ASM. A relationship between poor control of seizures and cognitive deterioration has been hypothesized but not proven.

PATHOPHYSIOLOGY/NEUROBIOLOGY OF DISEASE

The etiology for Doose syndrome is unknown but a genetic mechanism is suspected. The male predominance and high incidence of a family history of epilepsy or febrile seizures support the genetic hypothesis. Many series report 30%–50% family history of febrile seizures or epilepsy. Relationships to the GEFS+ genes, *SLC2A1* and *SLC6A1*, have been suggested from the analysis of small datasets but have not been confirmed with more extensive testing. It is likely that the Doose syndrome phenotype results from several genetic abnormalities, and that both modifier genes and environmental factors, may play additional roles.

CLINICAL PEARLS

- Doose syndrome is a diagnosis of exclusion and should be supported by proper documentation of the initial normal developmental history, seizure type and evolution, EEG findings, absence of structural changes on MRI, normal metabolic screen, and genetic testing.
- Treatment should be aggressive and initially include use of ASMs used for generalized epilepsy.
- Ketogenic diets should be considered early in the treatment of these children and offered to the family once the Doose syndrome diagnosis is made.
- Prognosis for Doose syndrome is variable with about one-half of patients eventually achieving seizure freedom and 2/3 near normal intelligence.

SUGGESTED REFERENCES

Doose H. Myoclonic-astatic epilepsy. *Epilepsy Res Suppl* 1992;6:163–8.

Kelley S.H., Kossoff E.H. Doose syndrome (myoclonic-astatic epilepsy): 40 years of progress. *Dev Med Child Neurol* 2010;52:988–93.

Kilaru S., Bergqvist A.G. Current treatment of myoclonic astatic epilepsy: Clinical experience at the Children's Hospital of Philadelphia. *Epilepsia* 2007;48:1–5.

Nickels K., Thibert R., Rau S., Demarest S., Wirrell E., Kossoff E.H., Joshi C., Nangia S., Shellhaas R.; Pediatric Epilepsy Research Consortium. How do we diagnose and treat epilepsy with myoclonic atonic seizures (Doose syndrome)? Results of the Pediatric Epilepsy Research Consortium Survey. *Epilepsy Res* 2018;144:14–9.

Oguni H. Epilepsy with myoclonic-atonic seizures, also known as Doose syndrome: Modification of the diagnostic criteria. *Eur J Paediatr Neurol* 2022;36:37–50.

Tang S., Addis L., Smith A., Smith A., Topp S.D., Pendziwiat M., Mei D., Parker A., Agrawal S., Hughes E., Lascelles K., Williams R.E., Fallon P., Robinson R., Cross H.J., Hedderly T., Eltze C., Kerr T., Desurkar A., Hussain N., Kinali M., Bagnasco I., Vassallo G., Whitehouse W., Goyal S., Absoud M.; EuroEPINOMICS-RES Consortium, Møller R.S., Helbig I., Weber Y.G., Marini C., Guerrini R., Simpson M.A., Pal D.K. Phenotypic and genetic spectrum of epilepsy with myoclonic atonic seizures. *Epilepsia* 2020;61:996–1007.

37 Landau-Kleffner Syndrome

Frank M. C. Besag
London NHS Foundation UK
UCL, London, UK
KCL, London, UK

CONTENTS

CASE PRESENTATION

An 8-year-old aphasic girl presented with a history of normal development until 3 years of age when she was evaluated for "incoherent speech". An adenotonsillectomy was performed, and grommets were inserted but her speech continued to deteriorate and by 5 years of age, it was unintelligible. An audiogram was normal. Speech therapy resulted in no improvement. She had poor understanding of instructions and commands. Her speech continued to deteriorate. She was re-evaluated at 6½ years of age due to episodes of awakening during sleep, agitated and unaware of her surroundings. She had no recall of the events in the morning. A diagnosis of night terrors was suggested. Shortly after this, she developed more obvious seizures with twitching of the left side of her face, accompanied by incontinence and post-ictal headache. An EEG at 6³/⁴ years of age revealed multifocal epileptiform discharges, with right hemispheric predominance, and was thought to be consistent with perinatal cerebral hypoxic-ischemic injury despite a normal perinatal history. Her motor skills remained normal. Next, she developed episodes of nocturnal awakening with her lower limbs being rigid, head turned to the left and clonic movements lasting for about 10 minutes, occurring three times a week. She was also reported to have had multiple other types of clinical episodes. Sodium valproate was commenced but the attacks continued. At 7 years of age, lamotrigine was added. Her understanding appeared to deteriorate further and she seemed to be disconnected from her surroundings. A pediatric neurologist diagnosed an acquired language abnormality with mixed receptive and expressive problems, with a marked receptive deficit. All investigations were normal, apart from the EEG. Clobazam was commenced and her language improved for 1 week but then deteriorated again. Steroids were given at 50 mg per day for 14 days followed by slow reduction. Within 5 days there was dramatic improvement. There were no seizures. She gained skills. Her understanding improved but she was still unable to express herself in spoken language. Two months later the seizures increased again and carbamazepine was started. When she was 7¾ years of age, vigabatrin was prescribed and this appeared to improve seizure control but the language deteriorated further. Her understanding remained very poor and she was highly dependent on others. A PET scan revealed hypometabolism involving the left parietal and temporal regions. A sodium amytal test demonstrated that the epileptiform discharges on the right side stopped with injection but not on the left. When she was evaluated at 8 years of age, she was aphasic and the overnight EEG revealed more than 85% of slow-wave sleep being replaced with spike-wave discharges consistent with electrical status epilepticus of slow-wave sleep (ESES). She had already been referred to a neurosurgeon who performed multiple subpial transections when she was 8 years and 2 months of age. She uttered the word "mummy" for the first time in several months, as she woke from the anaesthetic. Within 3 months her speech was improving and the seizures were controlled. The overnight EEG was improved. Her speech continued to improve and her entire persona changed dramatically because she was able to interact verbally with those around her, becoming more lively, vivacious, smiling, happy, and interactive.

DIAGNOSTIC APPROACH

The Landau-Kleffner syndrome (LKS), also known as acquired epileptic aphasia, is a rare syndrome and was initially described in 1957. Typical cases present between 3 and 8 years of age and are characterized by normal early development, including early normal language development, followed by a verbal agnosia, which can extend to an auditory agnosia, implying that the individual fails not only to understand speech but also fails to comprehend the significance of environmental sounds (for example, bird song). The verbal agnosia can result in an inability of the individual to understand his or her own speech, with a consequent partial or complete expressive aphasia. It is not surprising that the verbal/auditory agnosia is often accompanied by behavioral difficulties, sometimes including features of autism or attention deficit hyperactivity disorder.

LKS is one of the manifestations of the broader syndrome of status epilepticus of slow-wave sleep (ESES) or continuous spike-weight been so-wave sleep (CSWS). The International League Against Epilepsy has reclassified epilepsies of this type as epileptic encephalopathies with spike-wave activation in sleep EE-SWAS or, depending on the situation, developmental encephalopathies with spike-wave activation in sleep DEE-SWAS, although this classification has been subject to some debate. The syndromes of EE-SWAS and DEE-SWAS can present with other forms of cognitive deterioration than verbal agnosia. They are rare, perhaps 0.2% –0.5% of all child-hood epilepsies. LKS is not a homogeneous syndrome. It has been estimated that 8%–20% have mutations in the *GRIN2A* gene but that 80% or more do not have any identifiable genetic mutation. There have been various proposals for the classifica-tion of LKS, emphasizing the heterogeneity of the syndrome. For example, three subgroups have been identified:

• Rapid or fluctuating performance, usually with seizures, and recovery is usually rapid.
• Progressive aphasia or repeated episodes of aphasia after a seizure; recovery may take months or years.
• Gradual marked auditory comprehension deficit, with few or no seizures, followed by variable rates and degrees of recovery.

About 20% present with aphasia and an abnormal EEG but with no prior history of seizures. Some cases may mimic self-limited epilepsy with centrotemporal spikes (benign Rolandic epilepsy) at presentation, but the course is anything but benign with the development of ESES/EE-SWAS and aphasia.

TREATMENT STRATEGY

The treatment of this condition has been the subject of much debate over the years. A recent Cochrane review concluded that there was no evidence from trials to sup-port or refute the use of pharmacological treatment. A recent general review also concluded that there was a lack of evidence, from long-term follow-up studies, for the efficacy of surgical treatment.

These conclusions do not, however, necessarily imply that treatment in individual cases will be ineffective. It is difficult to obtain reliable data on a rare, heterogeneous syndrome that does not have a single cause, is of variable severity and has a fluctuat-ing course with a very wide range of outcomes. There have been several studies sug-gesting efficacy of many different treatments. After applying inclusion and exclusion criteria, van den Munchkin et al. analyzed 112 studies with a total of 575 patients and reported an improvement in cognition or EEG as follows: surgery ($N=62$) 90%, steroids ($N=166$) 81%, benzodiazepines ($N=171$) 68% and antiseizure medica-tions (ASMs) ($N=495$) 49%. Sanchez-Fernandez et al. collected 232 surveys from members of the American Epilepsy Society indicating that the preferred first-choice medications to decrease "sleep-potentiated epileptiform activity" were high-dose benzodiazepines (47%), valproate (26%), and corticosteroids (15%). The preferred second choice medications were valproate (26%), high-dose benzodiazepines (24%), and corticosteroids (23%). The preferred high-dose benzodiazepine was diazepam 1 mg/kg for one night, followed by 0.5 mg/kg/day and the preferred steroid was oral prednisolone 2 mg/kg/day.

Other suggested treatments have included sulthiame, ethosuximide, levetirace-tam, amantadine, and the ketogenic diet. The preferred surgical treatment is multiple subpial transections, introduced by Morrell, in which transection around the epileptic focus prevents spread of the epileptiform discharge but leaves eloquent brain tissue relatively intact. Other forms of surgery have been undertaken.

Decisions about whether to undertake surgical treatment are, perhaps, the most challenging, because of the conflicting nature of the issues involved. Knowing that some patients might not recover speech without surgical treatment might suggest that early intervention is important but by contrast, knowing that other patients will recover spontaneously, could imply that surgery might be undertaken unnecessarily.

The situation is further complicated by the lack of agreement about the efficacy of surgery. A recent review has suggested that there is no significant additional benefit for most children above the natural recovery that can occur over time. If there were clear biomarkers or other indicators to predict prognosis, the decision regarding whether to undertake early surgery or, indeed, whether to undertake surgery at all, might be easier.

These relatively unfavorable assessments of surgery are in sharp contrast to the published results of the original series by Morrell, indicating marked improvements in speech in most patients treated with multiple subpial transections. Subsequent studies have failed to replicate such favorable outcomes. However, there is no doubt that the patient presented in this case report improved dramatically, not only in terms of speech function but also in terms of her whole persona. Even if the ultimate cognitive outcome were the same between waiting for improvement on one hand or carrying out surgical intervention on the other hand, if such improvement were delayed in a growing and developing child, would this have had unfavorable long-term psychological sequelae?

LONG-TERM OUTCOME

With so many uncertainties about the cause(s), prognoses, and treatment(s) of this rare syndrome, how should the clinician manage cases in practice? Because the psychological and other consequences of leaving a child with aphasia for extended periods of time are likely to be unfavorable, there might be a strong argument for treating promptly.

In practice, many clinicians are likely to treat with steroids or high-dose benzodiazepines, although other ASMs have been prescribed with apparent success. Despite the difficulty in replicating the very favorable results of the original Morrell series of multiple subpial transections, this does appear to be an effective treatment in a proportion of cases that are resistant to treatment with medication.

Until more definitive data – perhaps with information on biomarkers or other determinants of prognosis – become available, it would seem reasonable to treat with the favored medications, as indicated earlier, followed by multiple subpial transections if there is an unsatisfactory response to medication.

CLINICAL PEARLS

- LKS is one of the manifestations of the broader syndrome of ESES/ CSWS now known as epileptic encephalopathy with spike-and-wave activation in sleep (EE-SWAS).
- Verbal agnosia can extend to auditory agnosia, implying that the individual fails not only to understand speech but also fails to comprehend the significance of environmental sounds (for example, bird song).
- About 20% may present with aphasia and an abnormal EEG but with no history of seizures.

SUGGESTED REFERENCES

Besag F., Gobbi G., Aldenkamp A., Caplan R., Dunn D.W., Sillanpää M. Psychiatric and Behavioural Disorders in Children with Epilepsy (ILAE Task Force Report): Behavioural and psychiatric disorders associated with epilepsy syndromes. *Epileptic Disorders* 2016;18:S37–S48.

Clark M., Holmes H., Ngoh A., Siyani V., Wilson G. Overview of Landau–Kleffner syndrome: Early treatment, tailored education and therapy improve outcome. *Paediatr Child Health* 2021;31:207–19.

Deonna T., Beaumanoir A., Gaillard F., Assal G. Acquired aphasia in childhood with seizure disorder: A heterogeneous syndrome. *Neuropadiatrie* 1977;8:263–73.

Landau W.M., Kleffner F.R. Syndrome of acquired aphasia with convulsive disorder in children. *Neurology* 1957;7:523–30.

Moresco L., Bruschettini M., Calevo M.G., Siri L. Pharmacological treatment for continuous spike-wave during slow wave sleep syndrome and Landau-Kleffner Syndrome. *Cochrane Database Syst Rev* 2020;11:CD013132.

Morrell F., Whisler W.W., Bleck T.P. Multiple subpial transection: A new approach to the surgical treatment of focal epilepsy. *J Neurosurg* 1989;70:231–9.

Sánchez Fernández I., Chapman K., Peters J.M., Klehm J., Jackson M.C., Berg A.T., Loddenkemper T. Treatment for continuous spikes and waves during sleep (CSWS): Survey on treatment choices in North America. *Epilepsia* 2014;55:1099–108.

Van Den Munckhof B., Van Dee V., Sagi L., Caraballo R.H., Veggiotti P., Liukkonen E., Loddenkemper T., Fernández I.S., Buzatu M., Bulteau C., Braun K.P.J., Jansen F.E. Treatment of electrical status epilepticus in sleep: A pooled analysis of 575 cases. *Epilepsia* 2015;56:1738–46.

38 Developmental/Epileptic Encephalopathy with Spike-and-Wave Activation in Sleep (D/EE-SWAS)

Kevin Chapman
University of Arizona College of Medicine

CONTENTS

CASE PRESENTATION

An 8-year-old male presents with a 3-year history of seizures associated with head deviation to the left and with left-sided clonic activity lasting less than 2 minutes. His initial awake EEG demonstrated frequent spikes and sharp waves arising independently from the left frontal and right central head regions. A noncontrast brain MRI was normal. The patient was started on oxcarbazepine but continued to have brief monthly seizures. During this time, family members, as well as teachers, noted worsening school performance and increasing irritability. He was switched from oxcarbazepine to valproic acid, which led to mild improvement in seizure control; however, his school performance and neurobehavioral problems persisted. A repeat EEG included a brief period of sleep associated with a significant increase in spike activity. An overnight EEG demonstrated nearly continuous high-amplitude spike–wave activity during sleep, with only occasional spikes while awake (Figure 38.1). He was diagnosed with developmental epileptic encephalopathy with spike-and-wave activation in sleep (D/EE-SWAS) and treated with high-dose oral prednisone

DOI: 10.1201/9781003296478-42

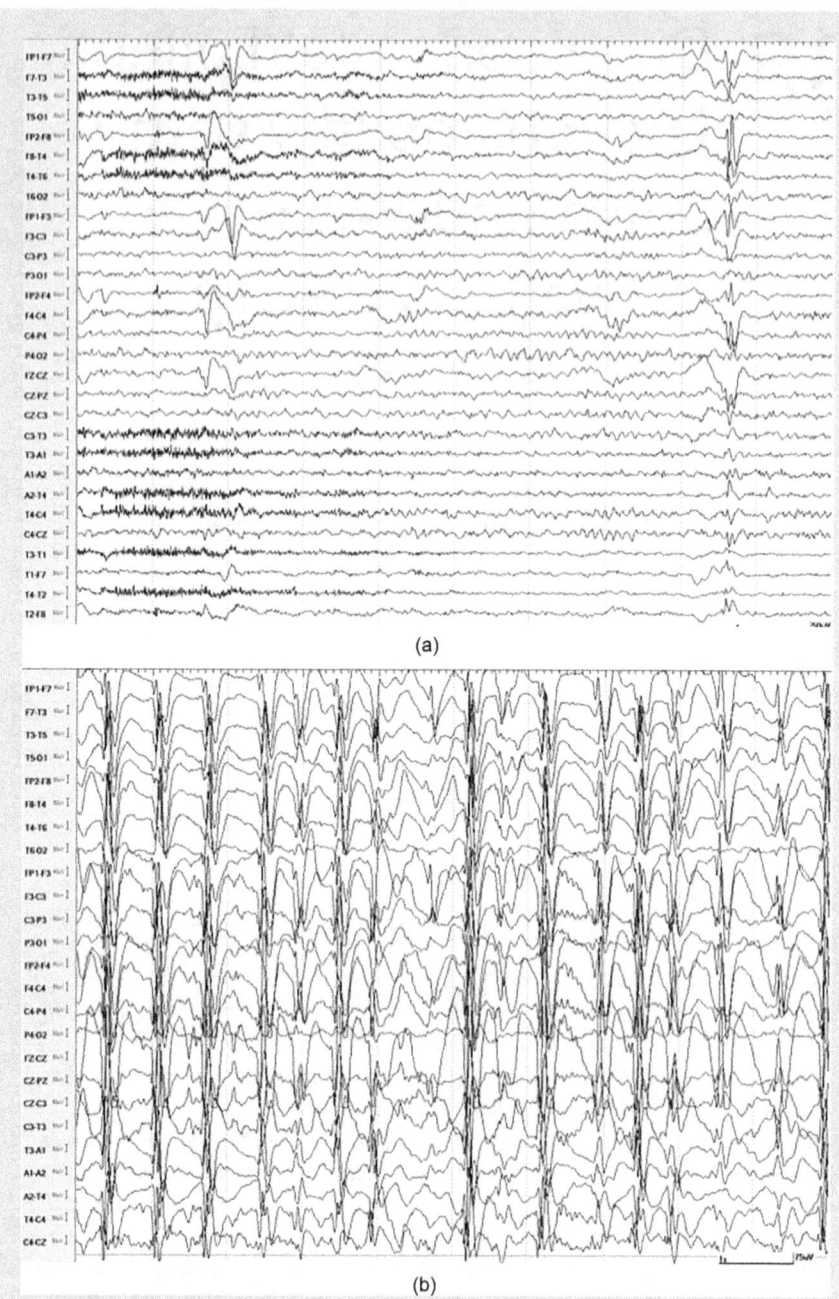

FIGURE 38.1 (a) Electroencephalogram (EEG) recorded during the awake state demonstrating a single generalized spike discharge. (b) EEG recorded during sleep demonstrating nearly continuous generalized 1.5–2 Hz spike–wave activity.

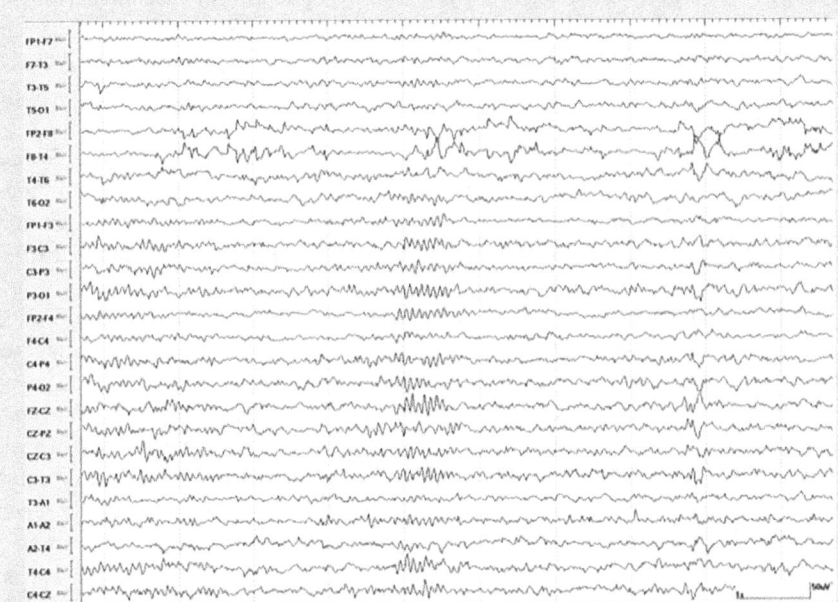

FIGURE 38.2 A repeat EEG recorded during sleep demonstrating normal sleep architecture and lack of spike–wave activity.

in addition to his valproic acid. On this regimen, his teachers and parents noted improvement, but he did not return to his previous cognitive baseline. The continuous spike–wave activity during sleep improved (Figure 38.2). A 2-deoxy-2-[18F] fluoro-D-glucose positron emission tomography (FDG-PET) scan was normal. Prednisone was tapered and discontinued on two occasions with a worsening of his school performance. Lamotrigine was substituted for valproic acid without any clinical improvement. Currently, he exhibits only rare seizures on prednisone and lamotrigine therapy with persistent mild difficulty in school.

DIFFERENTIAL DIAGNOSIS

In the differential diagnosis, two aspects of D/EE-SWAS should be considered: the typical EEG findings during sleep associated with the acute onset of cognitive and behavioral regression or stagnation. Lennox–Gastaut syndrome (LGS) may also show nearly continuous slow spike-and-wave discharges during sleep (see Chapter 35). However, the EEG of patients with LGS often have generalized paroxysmal fast activity and are often developmentally delayed from early childhood. They usually do not have an abrupt regression as seen in D/EE-SWAS. Further, LGS patients often exhibit a combination of myoclonic, tonic-clonic, atonic, and atypical absence seizures that are difficult to control, something not typically seen in D/EE-SWAS.

Another syndrome characterized by abundant epileptiform discharges during sleep is self-limited epilepsy with centrotemporal spikes (SeLECTS; aka, benign Rolandic epilepsy). Clinically, these patients may have learning disability or ADHD, but significant regression is not seen. Patients with SeLECTS may rarely transition to EE-SWAS.

Finally, a subgroup of EE-SWAS is Landau–Kleffner syndrome (LKS; see Chapter 37), which is characterized by focal, not generalized, nearly continuous sleep-activated spike–wave discharges, seen primarily in the dominant temporal lobe. Furthermore, patients with LKS have significant language regression, but sparing of other cognitive abilities.

Epilepsy syndromes that are associated with regression include the progressive myoclonus epilepsies, such as Lafora body disease or Unverricht–Lundborg disease. In these cases, the regression is often associated with worsening generalized myoclonic seizures which were not present in the representative case above. Neuronal ceroid lipofuscinoses may also present with similar symptoms, but this set of progressive myoclonus epilepsies is often associated with visual impairment. Cognitive slowing may be a side effect of antiseizure medications (ASMs), particularly when administered at high doses, irrespective of the epilepsy syndrome.

DIAGNOSTIC APPROACH

The clinical entity of D/EE-SWAS has undergone many changes in nomenclature. It was initially described by Patry et al. in 1971 as electrical *status epilepticus* of sleep (ESES) and later termed continuous spike-and-wave during sleep (CSWS). The syndrome is diagnosed based on the percentage of the sleep EEG recording containing spike–wave activity. The traditional definition requires that the spike–wave index is greater than 85% during slow-wave sleep, but lower percentages associated with regression have been reported. In addition to the EEG criteria, patients with EE-SWAS have normal development and have associated neuropsychological regression during the period of sleep-activated spiking. D/-EE-SWAS occurs in children with preexisting neurodevelopmental disorders. Some patients may only experience a developmental plateau associated with the spike-and-wave activation in sleep. However, caution should be used in ascribing a lack of expected skills in patients with preexisting conditions to frequent spiking during sleep.

The incidence of D/EE-SWAS is estimated to be less than 1% of childhood epilepsy but may be more commonly recognized given the increased use of continuous video-EEG monitoring. The initial seizure is usually nocturnal and occurs at a peak age of 4–6 years. The syndrome D/EE-SWAS demonstrates broad clinical heterogeneity, and as such, there may be a variety of seizure types encountered with this condition, including focal unaware seizures, generalized tonic-clonic, myoclonic, and absence seizures. Absence status epilepticus may occur at some point in these patients.

Spike activation during sleep is required for the diagnosis of D/EE-SWAS, but there is a lack of clear diagnostic criteria. The classic spike–wave index (SWI) of 85% is considered too restrictive when clear regression is observed. More commonly a spike–wave index of at least 50% is considered consistent with SWAS, though some studies have used lower percentages.

Different duration of sleep evaluation for SWI determination exists from 100 seconds of sleep to entire night-time recordings. Automated SWI calculation methods may allow for improved consistency and more efficient workflows in busy clinical practices. The spikes are often focal or multifocal during awake and REM sleep, with anterior foci being slightly more frequent than posterior. The spike–wave activity becomes more frequent and may generalize during non-REM sleep, particularly in the early stages of the sleep cycle. Normal sleep architecture may be absent or difficult to distinguish due to the abundant abnormal epileptiform activity. The spike–wave index may vary during the natural history of the disease and with treatment.

Neuropsychological testing may demonstrate a variable pattern of dysfunction, although most patients exhibit declines in their IQs or developmental quotients. Language regression, visuospatial disturbances, motor impairment, and memory difficulties may be seen in patients with D/EE-SWAS, and these may depend somewhat on the sites of maximal epileptiform activity. Behavioral disturbances including aggression, psychosis, anxiety, and attention deficit hyperactivity disorder may be significant, requiring further evaluation with a child psychiatrist or psychologist. Children with preexisting conditions can be particularly difficult to assess reliably depending on their level of development and parental rating scales may need to be employed for children with low levels of function.

Neuroimaging with MRI should be performed to evaluate for structural abnormalities that provide insight into an underlying etiology. Structural abnormalities may be seen in 25%–50% of patients and may include malformations of cortical development, porencephaly, and hydrocephalus. FDG-PET scanning may identify areas of hypermetabolism corresponding to regions with increased spike activity seen on EEG. Single photon emission computed tomography (SPECT) has demonstrated areas of hypoperfusion in regions with increased spike–wave activity in some patients. Some genetic etiologies, such as *GRIN2A*, have been associated with D/EE-SWAS, and evaluation with a genetic epilepsy panel is recommended for children without a clear structural abnormality.

TREATMENT STRATEGY

Patients are typically brought to medical attention due to clinical seizure activity and initially may be treated with a variety of ASMs prior to the diagnosis of D/EE-SWAS. Most studies evaluating treatment are retrospective in nature with very limited prospective randomized treatment trials. Treatments typically consist of one of the three categories: ASMs, benzodiazepines (separately), and hormones (corticosteroids and the peptide adrenocorticotropic hormone or ACTH).

A variety of ASMs have been studied including levetiracetam, valproic acid, lamotrigine, and ethosuximide without clarity about relative efficacy rates. High-dose diazepam and clobazam have been studied and found effective, though comparative effectiveness trials are lacking. Corticosteroids (including oral and intravenous formulations) and ACTH have been used effectively in patients with D/EE-SWAS. Given the varied dosing protocols and types of hormones/steroids used, it is challenging to recommend a specific medication or regimen. Relapse is common upon discontinuation. A 2015 pooled analysis of mostly retrospective treatment studies for ESES determined that corticosteroids were more effective than benzodiazepines, which were more effective than ASMs.

Epilepsy surgery was the most effective but had considerably fewer patients. In addition, epilepsy surgery appeared to be focused on seizure control and should be considered carefully in the context of D/EE-SWAS alone. Carbamazepine and oxcarbazepine should be tapered if there is a worsening of the EEG during sleep and regression in neurocognitive functioning.

In some patients, the development of broadly distributed spike–wave activity during sleep may represent secondary bilateral synchrony, suggesting that a single epileptiform focus could be the cause of D/EE-SWAS. Use of imaging modalities, such as MRI, PET, SPECT, and magnetoencephalography, may allow for more accurate localization of the ictal onset zone and evaluation of a resective surgical option. Other treatment modalities, such as ketogenic diet, vagus nerve stimulation, and intravenous gamma globulin, have been attempted with limited strong data to support their routine use.

LONG-TERM OUTCOME

The prognosis in D/EE-SWAS is guarded even though nearly all patients experience resolution or significant reduction of the EEG pattern during adolescence. Epileptic seizures remit in most patients, but nearly half continue with significant neuropsychological impairment. As is common in other epileptic encephalopathies, the duration of D/EE-SWAS, early treatment, and premorbid conditions, such as developmental delay, may impact the likelihood of clinical recovery.

PATHOPHYSIOLOGY/NEUROBIOLOGY OF DISEASE

The neuropsychological deterioration seen in D/EE-SWAS is assigned to the nearly continuous epileptiform activity during sleep. This attribution is supported by clinical improvement with the resolution of this activity through either medical treatment or the eventual maturation of the individual. However, the actual mechanisms through which this syndrome occurs are not known.

Generalized and focal spike–wave discharges may cause a transitory cognitive impairment during specialized testing, with the type of impairment dependent on the lateralization of the discharge. Memory consolidation is thought to occur during sleep and may be negatively impacted by the frequent spike–wave discharges. In addition, D/EE-SWAS occurs during a period of peak synaptogenesis, and the frequent spike–wave activity may interfere with the normal creation and pruning of synapses.

There is increasing evidence that the thalamus may play a crucial role in the generation of D/EE-SWAS. The regulation and generation of sleep by thalamocortical networks may explain the sleep activation of spikes and the presumed secondary bilateral synchrony that occurs in some patients. Neuroimaging with MRI has demonstrated thalamic injury in a significant number of individuals with D/EE-SWAS, while some PET studies have demonstrated thalamic hypometabolism.

CLINICAL PEARLS

- D/EE-SWAS should be considered in children with a neuropsychological decline associated with epilepsy.
- In addition to neuropsychological challenges, the diagnosis requires an EEG demonstrating spike-and-wave activity occupying >50% of the sleep recording. An overnight EEG may increase the sensitivity of the study.
- Treatment with ASMs often has little impact on the EEG findings in D/EE-SWAS, while treatment with steroids and high-dose benzodiazepines has been shown to be effective.
- The long-term neuropsychological prognosis for D/EE-SWAS is guarded with nearly 50% of patients experiencing continued difficulties despite resolution of the EEG pattern during adolescence.

SUGGESTED REFERENCES

Galanopoulo A.S., Bojko A., Lado F., Moshé S.L. The spectrum of neuropsychiatric abnormalities associated with electrical status epilepticus in sleep. *Brain Dev* 2000;22(5):279–95.

Guzzetta F., Battaglia D., Veredice C., Donvito V., Pane M., Lettori D., Chiricozzi F., Chieffo D., Tartaglione T., Dravet C. Early Thalamic injury associated with epilepsy and continuous spike-wave during slow sleep. *Epilepsia* 2005;46(6):889–900.

Nieuwenhuis L., Nicolai J. The pathophysiologic mechanisms of cognitive and behavioral disturbances in children with Landau-Kleffner syndrome or epilepsy with continuous spike-and-waves during slow-wave sleep. *Seizure* 2006;15(4):249–58.

Specchio N., Wirrell E.C., Scheffer I.E., Nabbout R., Riney K., Samia P., Guerreiro M., Gwer S., Zuberi S.M., Wilmshurst J.M., Yozawitz E., Pressler R., Hirsch E., Wiebe S., Cross H.J., Perucca E., Moshé S.L., Tinuper P., Auvin S. International League Against Epilepsy classification and definition of epilepsy syndromes with onset in childhood: Position paper by the ILAE Task Force on nosology and definitions. *Epilepsia* 2022;63(6):1398–442.

van den Munckhof B., van Dee V., Sagi L., Caraballo R.H., Veggiotti P., Liukkonen E., Loddenkemper T., Sánchez Fernández I., Buzatu M., Bulteau C., Braun K.P., Jansen F.E. Treatment of electrical status epilepticus in sleep: A pooled analysis of 575 cases. *Epilepsia* 2015;56:1738–46.

39 Epilepsy with Eyelid Myoclonia (Jeavons Syndrome)

Ifrah Zawar
UVA Health

Elia Pestana Knight
Cleveland Clinic

CONTENTS

CASE PRESENTATION

A 17-year-old right-handed female with a history of premature birth due to a twin pregnancy presented with seizures at age 4 years. Seizure semiology was described as a blank stare and unresponsiveness lasting 20–30 seconds occurring daily up to weekly and more commonly in the morning. Family also reported multiple episodes of eyelid myoclonia described as frequent eye-flickering movements upon awakening or when going to bed at night, especially when the lights in her room were dim. At that time, she was diagnosed with childhood absence epilepsy. Seizures have been difficult to control. Generalized tonic-clonic seizures began at the age of 15 years and have recurred at a frequency of 2–4 per year despite multiple trials of antiseizure medications. One of these seizures occurred while the patient drove under a canopy of trees. At times, the eyelid myoclonia clusters would last from 15 minutes to 1 hour during which time she would become confused and clumsy. Her development was described as borderline normal, but just a little late compared to her twin sister. She had an Individualized Educational Plan since first grade and now is completing high school. She has also been diagnosed with attention deficit hyperactivity disorder (ADHD) and depression. A recent EEG showed a photoparoxysmal response and frequent episodes of eyelid myoclonia and eye closure sensitivity. There were frequent generalized 3–4 Hz spike-and-wave complexes often mixed with polyspike discharges. During sleep, there were abundant generalized polyspikes and independent spikes were seen in the right and left occipital and temporal head regions. Thus, the diagnosis was revised to epilepsy with eyelid myoclonias (Jeavons syndrome). Initial treatment with levetiracetam had dramatically reduced seizure frequency but she only had intermittent periods of seizure freedom. Further, in the ensuing years, she failed to respond to valproate, clonazepam, perampanel, and topiramate. Seizures were better controlled on lorazepam, zonisamide, lamotrigine, and lacosamide with only eyelid myoclonic present upon awakening.

DIFFERENTIAL DIAGNOSIS

The differential diagnosis of epilepsy with eyelid myoclonias or Jeavons syndrome (JS) includes other genetic generalized epilepsies such as Childhood Absence Epilepsy (CAE), Juvenile Absence Epilepsy (JAE), Juvenile Myoclonic Epilepsy (JME) and Generalized Tonic-Clonic Seizures Upon Awaking. Other considerations in this regard are reflex epilepsy, sunflower syndrome, idiopathic occipital lobe epilepsy, benign myoclonic epilepsy in infancy, epilepsy with myoclonic absences, Lennox–Gastaut syndrome, Dravet syndrome, and progressive myoclonic epilepsy. Some patients may even be mistaken to have nonepileptic conditions such as tic or behavior disorders.

Jeavons syndrome is an under-recognized condition that can result in diagnostic delays of several years or even a misdiagnosis. Studies have shown that anywhere from 77% to 89% of the patients may not be clinically diagnosed with JS despite meeting the clinical diagnostic criteria. JS patients may be misdiagnosed as CAE because eyelid myoclonia in JS can be difficult to distinguish from subtle eyelid fluttering which may be observed during absence seizures in CAE.

Eyelid myoclonia can also be mistaken for eye blinking seen as a part of some focal seizures or it could be thought of as a tic or behavior disorder. JS patients have an older age of onset, female predominance and more commonly have other seizure types in addition to absence seizures when compared with CAE. JS may often be confused with JME because of overlapping features. However, JS tends to have an earlier age of onset and is more likely to have absence seizures as a predominant feature of clinical presentation compared to JME which presents with generalized myoclonic seizures as the predominant seizure type.

DIAGNOSTIC APPROACH

JS is a childhood genetic generalized epilepsy (GGE) syndrome that accounts for around 2.7% of all epilepsies and 7.3%–12.9% of GGEs. Mean age of onset is around 6.5–7 years (range: 6 months to 14 years) and there is a female predominance. It is characterized by the diagnostic triad of (1) eyelid myoclonia (with or without absence seizures) which are considered the hallmark of the disease, (2) eyelid closure-induced EEG paroxysms characterized by interictal generalized epileptiform discharges or seizures, and (3) photosensitivity (Figure 39.1).

JS is thought to have a genetic etiology. Between 33% and 83% of patients may demonstrate a positive family history of epilepsy. Mode of inheritance is unclear and thought to involve complex genetic heterogeneity. Genetic mutations have been reported in *KCNB1, CHD2, NAA10, KIAA2022,* and some other genes.

In 2017, the International League against Epilepsy (ILAE) recognized JS as a separate childhood epilepsy syndrome called "Epilepsy with Eyelid Myoclonias".

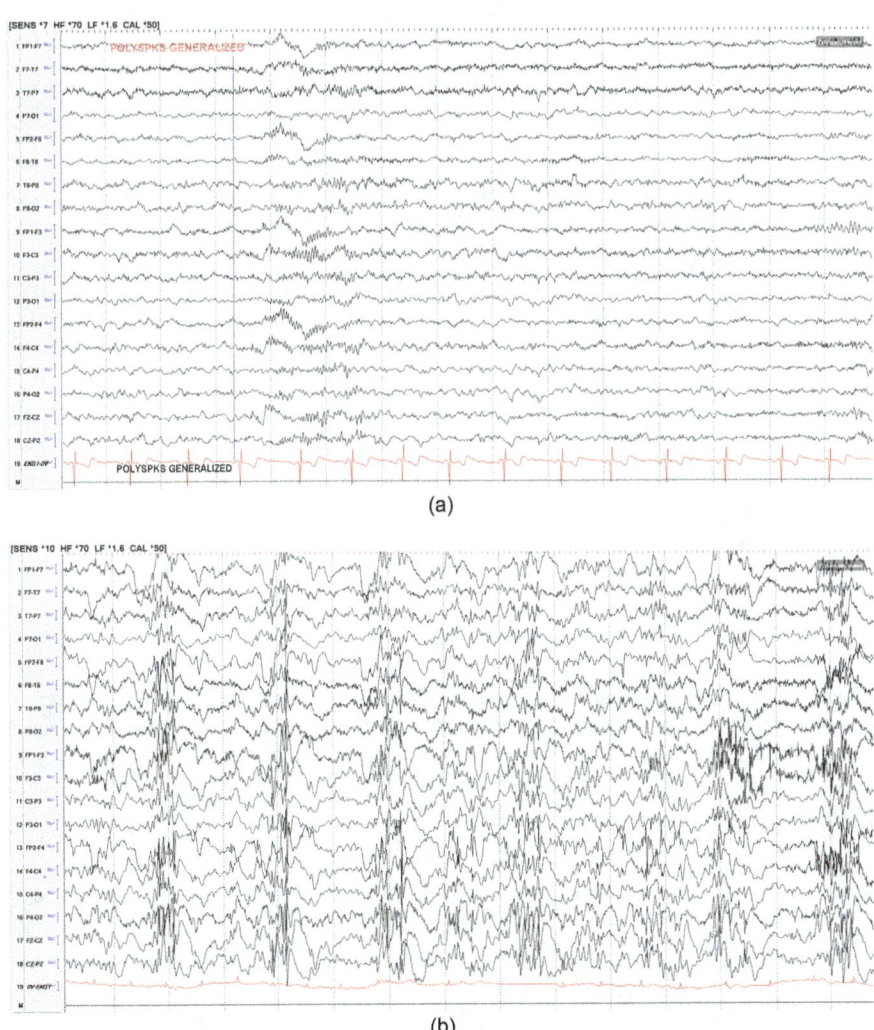

(a)

(b)

FIGURE 39.1 *Continued*

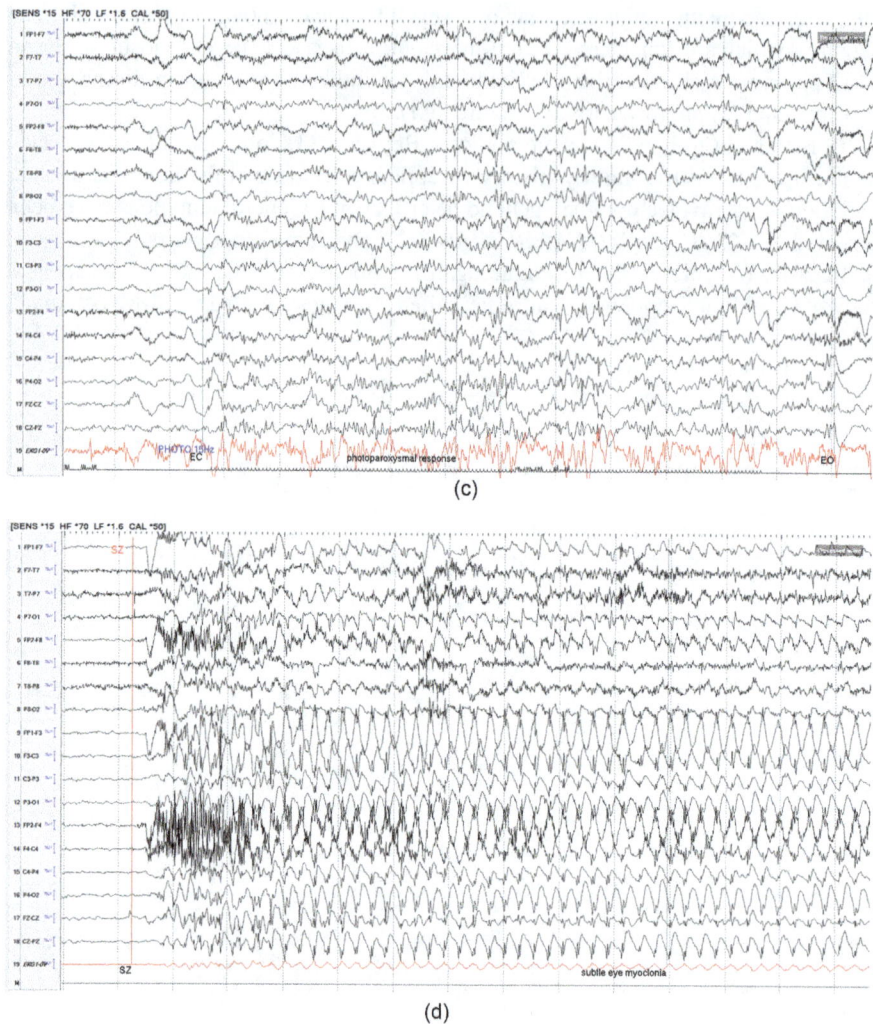

(c)

(d)

FIGURE 39.1 Electroencephalogram (EEG) findings in Epilepsy with Eyelid Myoclonias (Jeavons syndrome): (a) Generalized polyspikes; (b) Eye closure sensitivity. Note the posterior dominant polyspike activity seen with each eye blink; (c) Photoparoxysmal response. Note the generalized polyspike activity seen with 15 Hz intermittent photic stimulation; (d) Eyelid closure-induced seizure. Note the eye blink at the onset of seizure which leads to a seizure.

While eyelid myoclonias (a hallmark finding in 100% of patients) and absence seizures (up to 80%–100% of patients) are the predominant seizure types, other seizure types include GTC seizures (up to 60%–70% of patients), generalized myoclonic seizures (33%–49% of patients) and other generalized seizures like tonic and atonic seizures (3%–13% of patients). A subset of patients may also have co-existing focal epilepsy. Eyelid myoclonia *status epilepticus* has also been described especially if seizures remain untreated.

TABLE 39.1

Interictal and Ictal Findings That May Be Seen in Epilepsy with Eyelid Myoclonias

Interictal findings:

1. Generalized polyspikes or spike–wave complexes (3–6 Hz)
2. Eye closure-induced EEG paroxysms (SWC or PSP complexes 3–6 Hz)
3. Photoparoxysmal response: photic-induced EEG paroxysms
4. Hyperventilation-induced EEG paroxysms
5. Sharply contoured posterior alpha activity, which may spread to frontal regions (more common in females)
6. Focal posterior epileptiform discharges
7. Frontal predominant epileptiform activity (more common in males)
8. Sleep-related amplification of duration, frequency, and amplitude of discharges
9. Fixation-off sensitivity

Ictal findings:

1. Eyelid myoclonia (following slow eyelid closure). Three different patterns have been described in the literature.
2. In addition, absence seizures may or may not be present.
3. Brief preceding posterior dominant discharges may be seen before generalized epileptiform activity.
4. Photic stimulation-induced ictal phenomenon (eyelid myoclonia, absence seizures, and/or myoclonic jerks).
5. Hyperventilation-induced ictal phenomenon (eyelid myoclonia, absence seizures, and/or myoclonic jerks).
6. Eyelid myoclonia *status epilepticus.*

Source: Adapted from Zawar et al. (2021).
EEG, Electroencephalography; PSP, Polyspikes; SWC, Spike-and-wave complexes.

Generalized polyspikes or spike–wave complexes are the most common interictal finding. Other interictal and ictal EEG findings that may be seen in JS are detailed in Table 39.1. MRI findings are either normal or nonspecific. Most patients with JS (68%–88%) are cognitively normal. Mild intellectual disability may be present in a minority of patients.

TREATMENT STRATEGY

No randomized controlled trials have been conducted and the literature on antiseizure medication (ASM) treatment for JS is limited. Treatment decisions are based on expert opinion, case reports, and anecdotal evidence. Typically, broad-spectrum medications are tried and the mechanisms for their efficacy are unknown. ASMs that have been found to be most effective include levetiracetam, valproic acid, ethosuximide, and benzodiazepines. However, the use of valproic acid may be limited in the female population because of its teratogenic potential and other side effects. One open-label pilot study of levetiracetam in JS found an 80% responder rate with acceptable tolerability. In addition, levetiracetam has antimyoclonic properties and it has been shown to reduce the photic stimulation response on EEG, making it a suitable medication for JS patients.

Other medications found to be effective to some degree in various studies include lamotrigine, topiramate, lacosamide, and phenobarbital (especially in GTC seizures). Carbamazepine, oxcarbazepine, gabapentin, phenytoin, tiagabine, and vigabatrin are contraindicated as they may exacerbate generalized seizures. Cannabidiol has been reported to worsen eyelid myoclonias in a case series and therefore should be used with caution in this patient population. Data regarding the use of dietary therapies in JS is limited. A few studies have shown at least some response to the ketogenic diet, modified Atkins diet, and low-glycemic index treatment. Therefore, dietary interventions may be considered for patients who are pharmaco-resistant. With respect to less commonly tried therapies, Blue Lens therapy was found to be effective in 72.7% of the patients who attempted this.

Information on the use of neuromodulation is scarce but encouraging; this approach may be considered for select JS patients with debilitating and drug-resistant seizures. Vagus nerve stimulation (VNS) was found to be effective in 50%–75% of patients in two studies. One report of a JS patient treated with centromedian, ventrolateral thalamic responsive neurostimulation (RNS) demonstrated absence seizure reduction from 60 to less than 10 per day.

LONG-TERM OUTCOME

Just like juvenile myoclonic epilepsy, JS tends to be life-long and drug-resistant. Between 60% and 80% of the patients have been shown to be refractory to medical treatment. Due to its propensity for persisting throughout life and remaining medically intractable, both pediatric and adult neurologists tend to manage these patients. The presence of any seizures other than absences (notably, GTC seizures), female sex, persistence of eyelid closure sensitivity, and photosensitivity or photoparoxysmal response have been found to be predictors for drug refractoriness and seizure persistence. EEG findings of occipitally predominant generalized epileptiform discharges also may have an association with drug resistance. In contrast, a positive family history of epilepsy, male sex, and presence of frontally predominant generalized epileptiform discharges on EEG have been shown to have an association with seizure freedom.

PATHOPHYSIOLOGY/NEUROBIOLOGY OF DISEASE

Researchers have emphasized the role of the occipital lobe in JS. The visual occipital cortex is thought to play a role in seizures induced by eyelid closure and photosensitivity. "Spiky" posterior alpha activity and occipital predominant epileptiform discharges often seen in JS may be a manifestation of alpha rhythm generator malfunction in the visual cortex. Photic stimulation and eyelid closure are thought to synchronize neurons in the occipital cortex. The degree of epileptogenic occipital cortex activated, and the level of excitability may be affected by the light intensity. Eyelid myoclonia is produced when this hyperexcitability spreads to the brainstem.

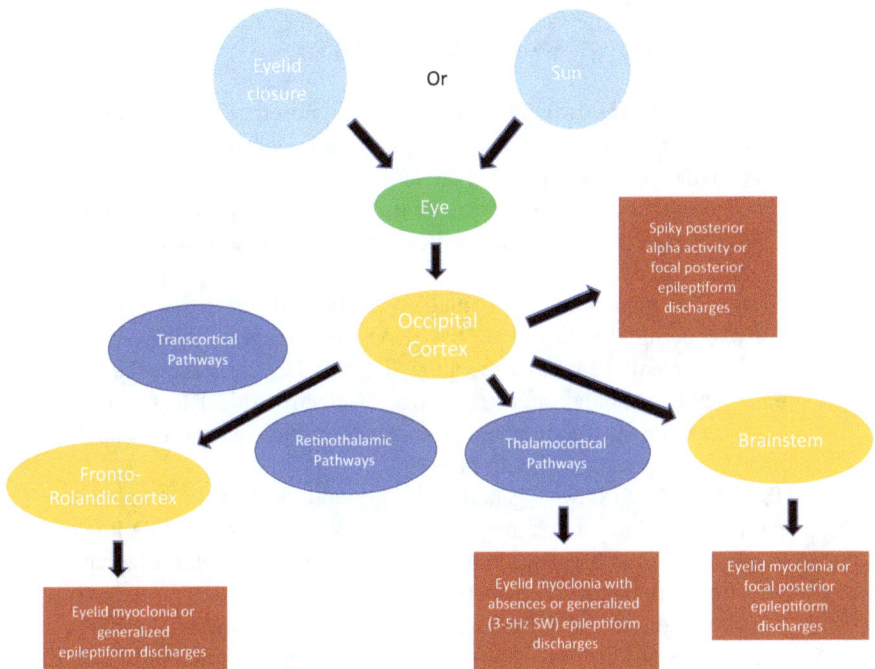

FIGURE 39.2 Neuronal Pathways involved in the pathogenesis of epilepsy with eyelid myoclonias. (Jeavons syndrome; Adapted from Zawar et al., 2020.)

Next, epileptiform discharges extend to the frontocentral cortex via either transcortical or thalamocortical pathways. This results in the generation of generalized discharges associated with JS (Figure 39.2).

Studies have reported focal occipital seizures in a subset of JS patients. Focal posterior temporal seizures have also been reported. These studies further support the role of the occipital cortex in JS and suggest that the network involved may even extend beyond the occipital lobe to involve the posterior temporal lobe. The hypothesis that the altered function of posterior quadrant plays a major role in the generation of epileptiform activity in JS is further supported by a functional MRI study. This report compared JS patients with other generalized epilepsies and healthy controls, and found greater blood oxygenation level-dependent signal with eyelid closure in the posterior thalamus and occipital cortex. Gray matter concentration at the visual cortex and thalamic pulvinar were observed to increase.

Recently, it has been postulated that the frontal lobe may have a role in the pathogenesis of JS as well. Frontally predominant generalized epileptiform discharges are often observed, and a subset of patients may even demonstrate focal frontal epileptiform activity. Moreover, as seen in frontal lobe epilepsy, tonic or clonic eye deviation and eye rolling during seizures have been frequently described in JS.

A study assessing the connectivity of neuronal electrical activity in JS patients showed reduced physiologic alpha over the occipital cortex and reduced physiologic beta over the frontal lobe during the resting state. Beta activity increased over the

CLINICAL PEARLS

- Epilepsy with eyelid Myoclonias or Jeavons syndrome (JS) is a common childhood genetic generalized epilepsy with female predominance.
- It is characterized by the triad of (1) eyelid myoclonias with or without absence seizures, (2) eye closure induced electroencephalographic (EEG) paroxysms (epileptiform discharges and/or seizures), and (3) photosensitivity.
- Neurodevelopment and neuroimaging are typically normal.
- Despite being recognized by the ILAE as a separate syndrome in 2017, JS remains an under-recognized entity. Understanding the disease pathophysiology and knowledge of electroclinical features are important for the treating neurologist and/or epileptologist for appropriate management of the disease.
- JS is thought to have a genetic etiology and about a third or more patients may have a positive family history of epilepsy. While it is a generalized epilepsy, occipital and less commonly frontal lobe have also been implicated in the pathophysiology.
- Literature on medical treatment is scarce. Broad-spectrum ASMs such as levetiracetam, valproic acid, lamotrigine, and benzodiazepines are typically used for treatment.
- However, many patients develop drug-resistant epilepsy. Therefore, randomized control trials and more effective treatments are needed to treat this difficult-to-control epilepsy.

frontal as well as parieto-occipital cortex immediately following eye closure. These findings provide additional evidence of abnormal occipital and frontal lobe activity in JS.

SUGGESTED REFERENCES

Smith K.M., Youssef P.E., Wirrell E.C., Nickels K.C., Payne E.T., Britton J.W., Shin C., Cascino G.D., Patterson M.C., Wong-Kisiel L.C. Jeavons syndrome: Clinical features and response to treatment. *Pediatr Neurol* 2018;86:46–51.

Zawar I., Knight E.P. Epilepsy with eyelid myoclonia (Jeavons Syndrome). *Pediatr Neurol* 2021;121:75–80.

Zawar I., Pestana Knight E.M. An overview of the electroencephalographic (EEG) features of epilepsy with eyelid myoclonia (Jeavons Syndrome). *Neurodiagn J* 2020;60:113–27.

Zawar I., Toribio M.G.G., Xu X., Alnakhli R.S., Benech D., Valappil A.M.N., Wyllie E., Burgess R., Kotagal P., Lachhwani D., Gupta A., Knight E.P. Epilepsy with Eyelid myoclonias – A diagnosis concealed in other genetic generalized epilepsies with photoparoxysmal response. *Epilepsy Res* 2022;181:106886.

40 Anti-NMDA Receptor Encephalitis

Jennifer Yang
UC San Diego

Jennifer Graves
Rady Children's Pediatric MS Center

CONTENTS

CASE PRESENTATION

A 15-year-old previously healthy girl presented with 2 weeks of confusion, difficulty speaking, orofacial dyskinesias, and new-onset focal seizures. An MRI of the brain was normal, and continuous video-EEG monitoring showed continuous clinical seizures with electrographic correlate consistent with epilepsia partialis continua, as well as persistent left hemispheric focal slowing. Additional hyperkinetic movements of the face and arms were not correlated with seizure activity on EEG monitoring. Her cerebrospinal (CSF) studies showed normal white blood cell count, normal total protein, and positive oligoclonal bands. She was found to have a positive anti-N-methyl-D-aspartate receptor (NMDAR) antibody titers in both the serum and CSF. She received 5 days of IV methylprednisolone 1,000 mg daily, intravenous immunoglobulins (IVIG) 2 g/kg, and two doses of rituximab 750 mg/m² spaced 2 weeks apart. Malignancy screening with pelvic ultrasound and body MRI did not reveal any concerning neoplastic processes. Her seizures were treated with levetiracetam and fosphenytoin in the hospital, and she continued maintenance levetiracetam after discharge. At her outpatient follow-up, her seizures were controlled, and her encephalopathy improved over the course of 1 month after immunotherapy. However, she required an individualized education plan for a modified academic schedule for over 6 months and continued to struggle with migraine headaches and anxiety. She had an acute worsening of her neuropsychiatric symptoms 11 months after the initial episode that improved with repeat rituximab dosing.

DIFFERENTIAL DIAGNOSIS

Anti-N-methyl-D-aspartate receptor (NMDAR) encephalitis is the most common autoimmune encephalitis. It was first described in 2007 and occurs more than four times as frequently as herpes simplex virus 1 (HSV), West Nile virus (WNV), or varicella zoster (VZV) according to data from the California Encephalitis Project.

Anti-NMDAR encephalitis typically presents in young females (children, adolescents, and young adults) due to its association with ovarian teratomas. The classic clinical presentation is a subacute onset of behavioral changes, short-term memory loss, altered mental status, psychiatric symptoms (aggression, hallucinations, delusions), seizures, movement disorder (orofacial dyskinesias, dystonia or apraxia), and insomnia or hypersomnia that may progress to catatonia, autonomic instability, and central hypoventilation. Pediatric patients – especially prepubertal patients – present with less clinically defined syndromes and may present with more nonspecific neuropsychiatric symptoms.

The differential diagnosis for anti-NMDAR encephalitis may be narrowed by the presenting clinical syndrome and initial diagnostic testing. For example, patients with predominantly neuropsychiatric symptoms often first present for psychiatric evaluations. In these patients, the initial differential may include primary psychosis, schizophrenia, or depression with psychotic features. Infectious processes, especially viral infections such as herpes simplex virus (HSV), should be evaluated at the same time as symptoms can mimic anti-NMDAR encephalitis including temporal lobe T2 hyperintensities on MRI.

It should be noted that there is a known association between anti-NMDAR encephalitis and HSV encephalitis; therefore, patients with acute worsening of neuropsychiatric symptoms or seizures weeks after HSV encephalitis should be evaluated for anti-NMDAR encephalitis. Inflammatory demyelinating disorders such as acute disseminated encephalomyelitis and antimyelin oligodendrocyte glycoprotein antibody disease may be considered depending on neuroimaging and CSF profiles.

Other inflammatory brain disorders that may mimic anti-NMDAR encephalitis include primary central nervous system (CNS) angiitis, which presents with headache, cognitive dysfunction, behavioral changes, and seizures, and Rasmussen encephalitis is a chronic inflammatory disease consisting of refractory focal seizures leading to progressive unilateral hemispheric atrophy. Rheumatological disorders such as systemic lupus erythematous and neurosarcoidosis can present with subacute onset neuropsychiatric symptoms as well as T2 changes on MRI and CSF abnormalities. In these cases, a careful review of systems can help determine whether there should be an expanded diagnostic work-up.

In the case of neurosarcoidosis, cranial nerve and spinal cord are often involved, which would be atypical for anti-NMDAR encephalitis. CNS tumors such as gliomas or lymphomas can present with new-onset seizures with temporal lobe involvement on MRI, though the neuroimaging features are different for tumors compared to autoimmune encephalitis. While contrast enhancement, diffusion restriction, and hemorrhage may be present in tumors, these features would be atypical for anti-NMDAR encephalitis.

Finally, patients with mitochondrial disease and other inborn errors of metabolism can present with new-onset seizures, confusion, and stroke-like events, especially in the setting of an acute infection. However, there is typically a history of chronic multiorgan system involvement, which is not expected in anti-NMDAR encephalitis.

DIAGNOSTIC APPROACH

Several diagnostic evaluations are routinely recommended when anti-NMDAR encephalitis is suspected. A lumbar puncture prior to neuroimaging should be performed to evaluate for cell count, total protein, and glucose as these can help differentiate autoimmune from infections and other demyelinating disorders. In anti-NMDAR encephalitis, the CSF profile can be normal, but 60%–80% of patients have a lymphocytic pleocytosis with moderately elevated white blood cell count (usually <100/μL). Glucose is typically normal, and total protein is either normal or mildly elevated. A mildly elevated IgG index or presence of CSF-specific oligoclonal bands may be seen in approximately 50%–60% of cases based on retrospective studies with pediatric data.

A comprehensive viral panel should be sent to differentiate viral encephalitis from autoimmune encephalitis including HSV, VZV, and WNV, with the caveat that anti-NMDAR encephalitis can occur secondary to HSV encephalitis. Other autoantibodies should be checked along with anti-NMDAR antibodies as there is an increasing number of newly discovered autoantibodies that present with similar symptoms. Therefore, a comprehensive autoimmune encephalopathy antibody panel should be sent from both serum and CSF. For anti-NMDAR antibodies, the sensitivity in serum is 85% and close to 100% in the CSF though some other autoantibodies have more sensitivity in the serum. The most reliable antibody detection method is the cell-based assay, which is used in most commercially available antibody panels.

A brain MRI should be obtained, though this can be normal early in the disease. Other findings include bilateral or unilateral T2 hyperintensities in medial temporal lobes or more rarely multifocal T2 hyperintensities involving gray and white matter (Figure 40.1). Neuroimaging in these cases can help narrow down the differential diagnosis.

EEG is rarely specific, although up to 85%–96% of pediatric and adult patients demonstrate some form of abnormality, either generalized or focal slowing, epileptiform discharges, or clinical/subclinical electrographic seizures. Extreme delta brushes have been reported in anti-NMDAR encephalitis cases, but the prevalence of this finding in pediatric anti-NMDAR encephalitis varies (Figure 40.1). Retrospective studies reported frequencies of extreme delta brushes as low as 6% in all patients with first-time EEG (adult and pediatric) and as high as 30% in another cohort with

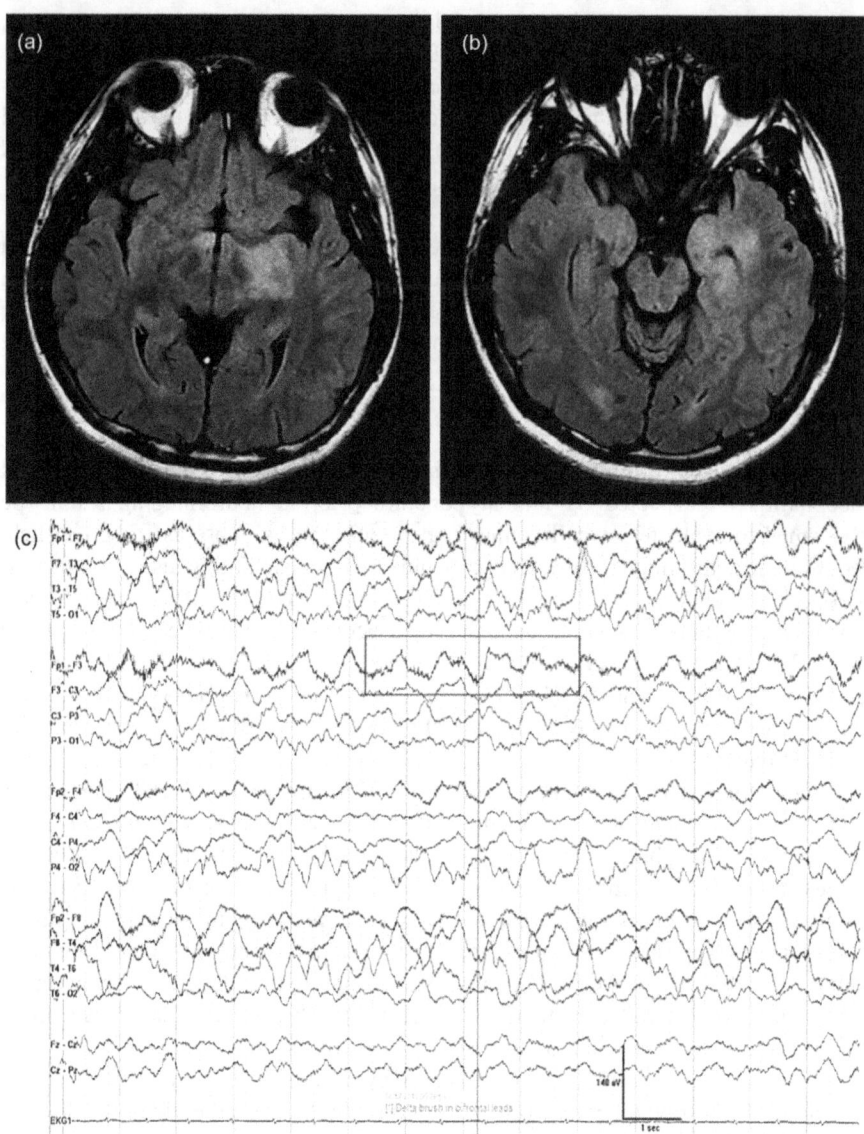

FIGURE 40.1   (a and b) MRI brain demonstrating T2 hyperintensity in the left hypothalamus and mesial temporal lobe with mild extension to the contralateral structures; C: EEG tracing showing extreme delta brush pattern. (EEG tracing courtesy of Grace Gombolay, MD. Reprinted with permission from Elsevier.)

continuous EEG monitoring. Additionally, disrupted sleep patterns may be present on prolonged video-EEG in the early stages of anti-NMDAR encephalitis, and non-REM sleep can be reduced or increased. Since approximately 90% of pediatric patients present with some form of movement disorder, which are often hyperkinetic (orofacial dyskinesias, chorea, stereotypies, myoclonus), video-EEG monitoring can help discern whether certain clinical events are epileptic or nonepileptic in nature.

Finally, screening for ovarian teratomas in female patients and testicular tumors in male patients should be obtained whenever anti-NMDAR encephalitis is suspected. A paraneoplastic association is rarer in prepubertal patients, but screening is still recommended. Screening methods include ovarian/testicular ultrasound or MRI of the abdomen and pelvis. There is no clear superiority between ultrasound and MRI for tumor screening, but the transvaginal ultrasound is more sensitive than the transabdominal ultrasound for female patients. In the case of a negative result and given association of these autoantibodies with small tumors, it may be prudent to repeat these screenings 1–2 years after onset. In severe cases or when patients fail to improve with initial treatment, further evaluation with other imaging modalities such as PET scan can be considered in collaboration with oncology and radiology.

TREATMENT STRATEGY

Currently, there is lack of Class 1 evidence for immunotherapy treatment for anti-NMDAR encephalitis. However, based on several large-scale cohort studies over the last decade, there are several consensus expert recommendations on acute treatment strategies.

If a primary tumor is identified, tumor removal should be performed as soon as it is safe for the patient to undergo surgery. Regardless of tumor presence, acute immunotherapy is recommended. First-line immunotherapy typically includes high dose IV methylprednisolone 30 mg/kg/day (max 1,000 mg) daily for 3–5 days and IVIG 2 g/kg divided over 3–5 days. For severe disease, plasmapheresis for 3–5 courses is recommended to be given before IVIG with close monitoring for autonomic instability.

If the patient does not improve after 1–2 weeks, a second-line agent should be considered. The most commonly used second-line agent is rituximab, a monoclonal antibody against CD20+ B cells. Typical dosing for rituximab is 375 mg/m^2 (max 1,000 mg) weekly for four doses or 750 mg/m^2 (max 1,000 mg) given 2 weeks apart. Another second-line agent is cyclophosphamide 500–1,000 mg/m^2 (max 1,500 mg) monthly for up to six doses. An emerging second-line therapy is tocilizumab, which is a monoclonal antibody targeting interleukin (IL)-6, which is elevated in many cases of anti-NMDAR encephalitis and has a more tolerable safety profile than cyclophosphamide.

The treatment for seizures varies among providers but typically follows standard recommendations for new-onset seizures and/or status epilepticus. While levetiracetam is a popular first-line antiseizure medication (ASM), patients should be monitored for any worsening neuropsychiatric symptoms. Other commonly used medications include carbamazepine derivatives as they may help with behavior and dyskinesias.

For symptomatic treatment of psychiatric symptoms, collaboration with a child and adolescent psychiatrist is recommended if available. Typically, long-acting benzodiazepines (lorazepam, clonazepam), alpha-adrenergic agents (clonidine), and atypical antipsychotics (quetiapine, olanzapine) are used for both neuropsychiatric symptoms and sleep. Rehabilitation after acute treatment followed by long-term physical, occupational, and speech therapies can often help improve functional recovery.

LONG-TERM OUTCOME

Compared to other subtypes of autoimmune encephalitis, patients with anti-NMDAR encephalitis overall have better long-term prognoses. Treatment outcomes from two large systematic reviews of adult and pediatric patients with anti-NMDAR encephalitis reported that 90% of patients had a "good outcome" defined by the modified Rankin scale score ≤2, which focuses on motor function recovery. However, more recent studies suggest that despite good functional outcomes, patients can have persistent cognitive and neuropsychological symptoms. A systematic literature review demonstrated that 36% of pediatric onset anti-NMDAR encephalitis had ongoing psychiatric symptoms at long-term follow-up that are associated with abnormal initial EEGs and persistent cognitive impairments.

Clinical relapses are reported in 12%–25% of cases, which may occur months to 2–3 years after the initial episode. The use of second-line immunotherapy, specifically rituximab, may reduce relapse risk, though this has not been studied prospectively. Risk factors associated with relapsing disease are still unclear, but the rate of relapse has reduced in more recent years (closer to 15%) due to the increasing use of second-line immunotherapy during the acute treatment period.

Based on several retrospective cohort studies, most anti-NMDAR encephalitis patients are able to wean off ASMs after 1–2 years unless they have a preexisting risk for epilepsy. However, any return of seizure activity should prompt reevaluation of a potential clinical relapse and need for chronic immunotherapy.

PATHOPHYSIOLOGY/NEUROBIOLOGY OF DISEASE

The generation of anti-NMDAR autoantibodies is thought to be triggered by an infection, typically viral, or a paraneoplastic phenomenon associated with an identified tumor. However, in many cases, the trigger is unknown. The proposed pathophysiology involves a peripheral activation of T helper lymphocytes and B cells that undergo differentiation and initiate autoantibody production. The antibodies then cross the blood–brain barrier to reach the central nervous system where activated B cells undergo further differentiation to create intrathecal autoantibodies along with microglial activation. The antibodies bind to the GluN1 subunit of the NMDA receptor expressed on neuronal cell surfaces leading to cross-linking and internalization of the antigen–antibody complex that alter NMDA receptor-mediated synaptic neurotransmission.

The NMDA receptor is an ionotropic glutamate receptor important for neuroplasticity, learning, behavior, and memory. Seizures associated with anti-NMDAR antibodies may be due to early excitotoxicity from antibody binding to open synaptic NMDA receptors prior to internalization of the NMDA receptor complex.

The internationalization of the receptor likely underlies the other behavioral and cognitive changes, sleep disruption, and autonomic dysfunction observed in

CLINICAL PEARLS

- Anti-NMDAR encephalitis presents with subacute onset of neuropsychiatric symptoms, new-onset seizures, encephalopathy with or without movement disorders, sleep disturbance, and dysautonomia.
- Evaluation should include CSF studies, serum and CSF autoimmune encephalopathy antibody panels, EEG, MRI, and malignancy screening.
- Early acute immunotherapy leads to improved clinical outcomes. First-line immunotherapies include IV methylprednisolone, IVIG, and plasmapheresis. Patients not responsive to first-line therapy should be treated with second-line therapy, most commonly rituximab.
- Anti-NMDAR encephalitis generally has a good prognosis compared to other subtypes of autoimmune encephalitis.
- Despite good motor outcomes, long-term symptoms are common including cognitive dysfunction, depression/anxiety, migraine headaches, and fatigue that require ongoing monitoring and support.

anti-NMDAR encephalitis, and movement disorders likely reflect the downregulation of NMDA receptors. The slow internalization of the NMDA receptor also explains why earlier treatment with immunotherapy leads to better outcomes as treatment becomes more difficult with reduced cell surface expression. Although the internalization of NMDA receptor is reversible, this process takes time, which is why clinical recovery can take several months or even years.

SUGGESTED REFERENCES

Cellucci T., Van Mater H., Graus F., Muscal E., Gallentine W., Klein-Gitelman M.S., Benseler S.M., Frankovich J., Gorman M.P., Van Haren K., Dalmau J., Dale R.C. Clinical approach to the diagnosis of autoimmune encephalitis in the pediatric patient. *Neurol Neuroimmunol Neuroinflamm* 2020;7(2):e663.

Dalmau J., Armangué T., Planagumà J., Radosevic M., Mannara F., Leypoldt F., Geis C., Lancaster E., Titulaer M.J., Rosenfeld M.R., Graus F. An update on anti-NMDA receptor encephalitis for neurologists and psychiatrists: Mechanisms and models. *Lancet Neurol* 2019;18:1045–57.

Graus F., Titulaer M.J., Balu R., Benseler S., Bien C.G., Cellucci T., Cortese I., Dale R.C., Gelfand J.M., Geschwind M., Glaser C.A., Honnorat J., Höftberger R., Iizuka T., Irani S.R., Lancaster E., Leypoldt F., Prüss H., Rae-Grant A., Reindl M., Rosenfeld M.R., Rostásy K., Saiz A., Venkatesan A., Vincent A., Wandinger K.P., Waters P., Dalmau J.A. clinical approach to diagnosis of autoimmune encephalitis. *Lancet Neurol* 2016;15:391–404.

Nguyen L., Yang J.H., Goyal S., Irani N., Graves J.S. A systematic review and quantitative synthesis of the long-term psychiatric sequelae of pediatric autoimmune encephalitis. *J Affect Disord* 2022;308:449–57.

Nosadini M., Thomas T., Eyre M., Anlar B., Armangue T., Benseler S.M., Cellucci T., Deiva K., Gallentine W., Gombolay G., Gorman M.P., Hacohen Y., Jiang Y., Lim B.C., Muscal E., Ndondo A., Neuteboom R., Rostásy K., Sakuma H., Sharma S., Tenembaum S.N.,

Van Mater H.A., Wells E., Wickstrom R., Yeshokumar A.K., Irani S.R., Dalmau J., Lim M., Dale R.C. International consensus recommendations for the treatment of pediatric NMDAR antibody encephalitis. *Neurol Neuroimmunol Neuroinflamm* 2021;8(5):e1052.

Zekeridou A., Karantoni E., Viaccoz A., Ducray F., Gitiaux C., Villega F., Deiva K., Rogemond V., Mathias E., Picard G., Tardieu M., Antoine J.C., Delattre J.Y., Honnorat J. Treatment and outcome of children and adolescents with N-methyl-D-aspartate receptor encephalitis. *J Neurol* 2015;262:1859–66.

41 Nonconvulsive *Status Epilepticus*

Sonali Sen and James J. Riviello, Jr.
Baylor College of Medicine

CONTENTS

CASE PRESENTATION

A 6-year-old girl was admitted for evaluation of increasing seizure activity, consisting of generalized tonic-clonic seizures and staring spells. The seizure onset had been approximately 1 year previously. Her first EEG showed generalized spike-and-wave activity, and brain MRI was normal. She was subsequently treated with phenobarbital, valproic acid, topiramate, and lamotrigine, and despite this, her seizures continued and were actually increasing in frequency. On the day of hospital admission, she was noted to have frequent staring spells and myoclonic movements in addition to frequent generalized tonic-clonic seizures with persistent altered awareness in the post-ictal state. The initial EEG is shown in Figure 41.1.

DOI: 10.1201/9781003296478-45

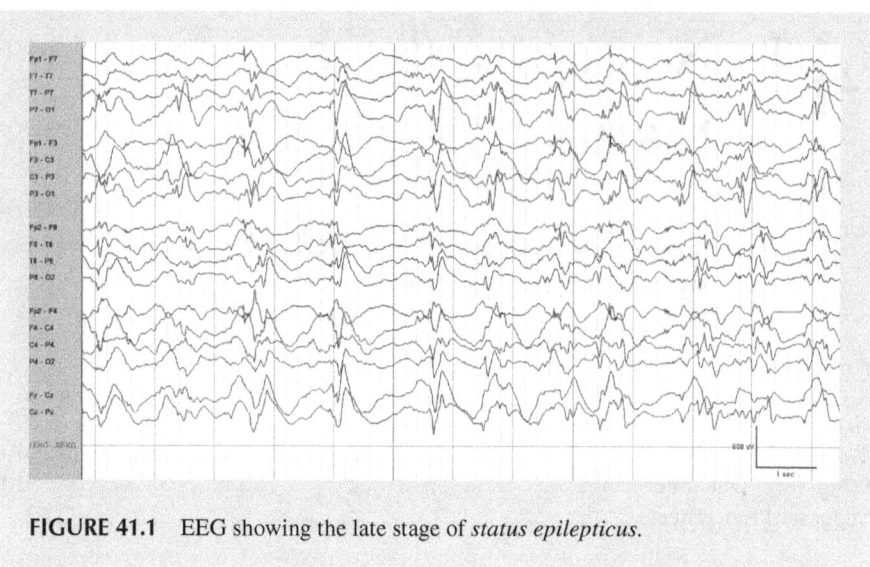

FIGURE 41.1　EEG showing the late stage of *status epilepticus*.

DIFFERENTIAL DIAGNOSIS AND DIAGNOSTIC APPROACH

This case involves a child with a history of staring spells and myoclonus, generalized tonic-clonic seizures, and persistent altered awareness after control of the convulsive movements. Could this represent a case of ongoing *status epilepticus* (SE)? Using a semiological classification system, SE is divided into convulsive SE (CSE) versus nonconvulsive SE (NCSE). NCSE is defined as altered awareness associated with electrographic seizure activity and may occur in either a generalized or focal epilepsy. While clear tonic or clonic activity is not seen, there may be subtle movements associated with the electrographic seizure. The EEG confirms NCSE in this case.

In children, there are several types of NCSE: NCSE after CSE, with generalized epilepsies (absence SE), with focal epilepsies (focal SE), and with the entity referred to as autonomic epilepsy. CSE itself is easily recognized and typically does not require EEG confirmation for diagnosis. However, in patients with CSE in whom the convulsive movements are successfully treated with benzodiazepines, the persistence of altered awareness raises the question of NCSE. This occurs infrequently after the treatment of SE and requires EEG confirmation. Electrographic seizures occur in 10%–40% of critically ill children. A retrospective multicenter cohort study including 550 children in the pediatric intensive care unit (PICU) who underwent continuous EEG monitoring found that 30% of patients were found to have nonconvulsive seizures (NCS) and 11% had NCSE.

In this case without overt CSE, but with frequent seizures without a return to baseline mental status, NCSE must be considered. This may initially present with intermittent nonconvulsive seizures, which may then evolve along a continuum from isolated NCS with increased duration and increasing frequency, ultimately merging as continuous NCSE. With NCSE, the continuous electrographic seizures are thought to be the cause of the altered awareness. However, with NCS, it is unclear if the NCS are the cause of the altered awareness, result from the underlying cause of epilepsy, or both.

If either NCSE is seen after the treatment of CSE, NCSE occurs in the presence of an acute encephalopathy, or if NCS are possibly responsible for persistent altered awareness, then additional antiseizure therapy is needed. If the electrographic SE or NCS resolve and mental status improves, then the epileptiform activity was likely causative of the altered awareness. Unfortunately, we may not be able to predict this in advance.

An EEG is necessary for the identification of NCSE or NCS. Indications for emergency EEG have been proposed and include:

- Unexplained altered awareness (with or without motor activity).
- No return to baseline mental status within 30 minutes after control of CSE.
- The use of neuromuscular paralysis in an acute encephalopathy or patient with a seizure disorder.
- Refractory SE that requires pentobarbital, or other high-dose, suppressive medications.

However, it is relatively uncommon for there to be a full return to baseline mental status after the control of CSE. We usually use clinical assessment, such as an improvement in mental status, with some responsiveness, or at least a response to noxious stimuli as indicators excluding NCSE, which may also have some accompanying subtle motor movements.

In persistent altered awareness without preceding CSE, absence, focal, or autonomic SE must be considered. In children, absence SE almost exclusively occurs in a child with known absence epilepsy, and therefore, would typically have a history of increasing absence seizures with ongoing altered awareness. Absence SE has been referred to as spike-wave stupor. Although EEG is needed to absolutely confirm absence SE, presumptive treatment could be administered in a child with known absence epilepsy and altered awareness.

The entity of autonomic epilepsy has recently been delineated. The majority of childhood cases occur with the Panayiotoupolos syndrome although autonomic symptoms may occur in other childhood and adult epilepsy syndromes. SE is estimated to occur in over 40% of these children. This is a subtype of focal SE. The typical case develops out of sleep, feeling sick, followed by retching and vomiting, and frequently accompanied by pallor, tachycardia, bradycardia, and mydriasis. This is then followed by fluctuating altered awareness and may progress to overt convulsive activity.

Nonconvulsive focal SE occurs when there is altered awareness associated with focal electrographic seizure activity on EEG. The clinical manifestations include altered awareness, staring, eye deviation, automatisms, crying, lip smacking, amaurosis, and decreased visual tracking and recognition. This may be more likely to occur in the critically ill child with acute symptomatic etiology. Risk factors for electrographic seizures include younger age, prior history of epilepsy, initial presentation with clinical seizures, and acute brain injury. This suggests that NCSE and NCS should be strongly considered in patients with unexplained altered awareness, particularly in the presence of acute intracranial pathology or previous seizures.

TREATMENT STRATEGY

Is the treatment of CSE different from NCSE? The treatment of NCSE is similar to CSE. Benzodiazepines remain the first-line therapy as previously discussed in Chapter 8. Fosphenytoin, valproic acid (VPA), levetiracetam (LEV), and phenobarbital are second-line options. IV VPA has especially been used for absence SE.

Recommended dosing for IV VPA is 40 mg/kg (maximum 3,000 mg) and LEV 60 mg/kg (maximum 4,500 mg). The TRENdS study demonstrated noninferiority of IV lacosamide (400 mg) to IV fosphenytoin (20 mg/kg; maximum 1,500 mg) in the treatment of NCS, with a similar adverse effect profile. A single-center prospective observational study of 131 children with NCS demonstrated resolution in 38% after one antiseizure medication (ASM) and 73% after two ASMs. Anesthetics should be considered if NCSE persists.

LONG-TERM OUTCOME

As in CSE, the outcome of NCSE is related to the underlying etiology. This is especially so with acute encephalopathies associated with NCSE or NCS. Although not as severe as in CSE, cerebral hemodynamic alterations also occur in NCSE. In critically ill children, increased NCS burden is independently associated with neurological decline. One recent study demonstrated a maximum seizure burden of 20% per hour, above which the probability of neurological decline rose sharply.

Another prospective observational study collected long-term follow-up data on 60 previously developmentally normal children who had NCSE in the setting of an acute

---

CLINICAL PEARLS

- NCSE may develop after the control of the convulsive movements in CSE.
- In patients with unexplained alteration of awareness, especially in the PICU or emergency department, NCSE should be considered, and an EEG performed. A preexisting history of epilepsy as well as acute brain injury increases the likelihood of NCSE or NCS.
- Treatment for NCSE typically begins with a benzodiazepine.
- The outcome of absence SE or autonomic SE is generally favorable while the outcome of NCSE is related to the underlying cause.
- Increased NCS burden is independently associated with neurological decline.
- Autonomic SE is likely a focal disorder and ictal EEG may have rhythmic delta or theta activity with admixed spikes, rather than overt spike and wave or focal spike discharges.
- We recommend that the child with epilepsy carry some sort of identification so that if altered awareness occurs without an available historian, the medical providers are aware of this possibility.

neurologic disorder. NCSE but not isolated NCS was associated with unfavorable long-term global outcomes, lower health-related quality of life, and increased risk of subsequent development of epilepsy.

SUGGESTED REFERENCES

Abend N.S., Arndt D.H., Carpenter J.L., Chapman K.E., Cornett K.M., Gallentine W.B., Giza C.C., Goldstein J.L., Hahn C.D., Lerner J.T., Loddenkemper T., Matsumoto J.H., McBain K., Nash K.B., Payne E., Sánchez S.M., Fernández I.S., Shults J., Williams K., Yang A., Dlugos D.J. Electrographic seizures in pediatric ICU patients: Cohort study of risk factors and mortality. *Neurology* 2013;81:383–91.

Beniczky S., Hirsch L.J., Kaplan P.W., Pressler R., Bauer G., Aurlien H., Brøgger J.C., Trinka E. Unifies EEG terminology and criteria for nonconvulsive *status epilepticus*. *Epilepsia* 2013;54(Suppl 6):S28–9.

DeLorenzo R.J., Waterhouse E.J., Towne A.R., Boggs J.G., Ko D., DeLorenzo G.A., Brown A., Garnett L. Persistent nonconvulsive *status epilepticus* after the control of generalized convulsive status epilepticus. *Epilepsia* 1998;39:833–40.

Fung F.W., Jacobwitz M., Vala L., Parikh D., Donnelly M., Xiao R., Topjian A.A., Abend N.S. Electroencephalographic seizures in critically ill children: Management and adverse events. *Epilepsia* 2019;60:2095–104.

Husain A.M., Lee J.W., Kolls B.J., Hirsch L.J., Halford J.J., Gupta P.K., Minazad Y., Jones J.M., LaRoche S.M., Herman S.T., Swisher C.B., Sinha S.R., Palade A., Dombrowski K.E., Gallentine W.B., Hahn C.D., Gerard E.E., Bhapkar M., Lokhnygina Y., Westover M.B.; Critical Care EEG Monitoring Research Consortium. Randomized trial of lacosamide versus fosphenytoin for nonconvulsive seizures. *Ann Neurol* 2018;83:1174–85.

Panayiotopoulos C.P. Autonomic seizures and autonomic *status epilepticus* peculiar to childhood: Diagnosis and management. *Epilepsy Behav* 2004;5:286–95.

Payne E.T., Zhao X.Y., Frndova H., McBain K., Sharma R., Hutchison J.S., Hahn C.D. Seizure burden is independently associated with short term outcome in critically ill children. *Brain* 2014;137:1429–38.

Privitera M.D., Strawsburg R.H. Electroencephalographic monitoring in the emergency department. *Emerg Med Clin North Am* 1994;12:1089–100.

Tay S.K.H., Hirsch L.J., Leary L., Jette N., Wittman J., Akman C.I. Nonconvulsive *status epilepticus* in children: Clinical and EEG characteristics. *Epilepsia* 2006;47:1504–9.

Wagenman K.L., Blake T.P., Sanchez S.M., Schultheis M.T., Radcliffe J., Berg R.A., Dlugos D.J., Topjian A.A., Abend N.S. Electrographic *status epilepticus* and long-term outcome in critically ill children. *Neurology* 2014;82:396–404.

42 Febrile Infection-Related Epilepsy Syndrome (FIRES)

Rima Nabbout
University of Paris cite

Sara Matricardi
Children's Hospital "G. Salesi"

CONTENTS

CASE PRESENTATION

A previously healthy 8-year-old boy presented to the emergency room because of recent onset of two focal motor seizures each lasting less than 2 minutes. He presented 1 week before fever with an upper respiratory tract infection and associated fatigue. He was admitted for work-up and developed increasing frequency of focal seizures that rapidly progressed to status epilepticus (SE) characterized by left or right focal motor and focal to bilateral seizures. SE was refractory to levetiracetam, phenytoin, and high doses of midazolam. The patient was treated after SE lasting over 24 hours (refractory SE) with propofol in addition to ASM. He received empiric treatment with acyclovir and ceftriaxone.

In the first 48 hours, he underwent blood and serum testing, including electrolytes, complete blood count, C-reactive protein, viral and bacterial serology and cultures, and toxicology screening that were all unrevealing. The cerebrospinal fluid (CSF) analysis showed mild pleocytosis (10 cells/μL) and a slightly increased protein level. PCR for common viral and bacterial causes in CSF and serum were negative. Inborn errors of metabolism, including mitochondrial disorders were ruled out within the first few days, and serum and CSF autoimmune antibody panels returned negative after 10 days. A next-generation sequencing panel for genetic epilepsies was performed within 2 weeks and did not subsequently reveal any pathogenic variants in the assessed genes. He underwent continuous EEG monitoring which showed a

DOI: 10.1201/9781003296478-46

background characterized by monomorphic diffuse delta activity with spikes-and-wave discharges over the frontotemporal head regions. Ictal discharges of focal fast rhythmic activity were recorded in both temporal regions in an alternate fashion. Two days after SE onset, the first brain magnetic resonance imaging (MRI) with gadolinium contrast study was normal. On day 10 after SE onset, a second brain MRI showed mild T2/FLAIR hyperintensities in the mesial temporal regions. Subsequent trials with antiseizure medications (ASMs), including valproate, lacosamide, cannabidiol, and ketamine were unsuccessful during the first 72 hours. Ketogenic diet was started through a nasogastric tube within 48 hours of the SE onset. At 72 hours of onset, first-line immunotherapy was initiated, including intravenous steroids for 2 days associated with intravenous immunoglobulins (IVIg) 2 g/kg for 3 days without efficacy. At 10 days, Anakinra was introduced in addition to KD and ASMs. At 2 weeks, refractory status epilepticus (RSE) resolved. Seizures were persistent but occurred with a decreased frequency. Sedation was decreased without recurrence of the SE. At 3 weeks, the patient was completely weaned from sedation and mechanical ventilation. At 2 months, he had sporadic seizures on KD, anakinra, cannabidiol, and lacosamide. At 4 months, he had normal tone and was able to say some words, but his communication was mostly non-verbal. He was autonomous in some daily life activities at the rehabilitation center but often needed adult help or supervision. He was left with a major cognitive impairment affecting executive function and short-term memory. Brain MRI showed bilateral hippocampal atrophy with slight cortical atrophy which was prominent in temporal and frontal lobes. Positron emission tomography scan revealed a large area of hypometabolism across bilateral orbitofrontal and temporoparietal regions.

DIFFERENTIAL DIAGNOSIS AND DIAGNOSTIC APPROACH

Febrile infection-related epilepsy syndrome (FIRES) is an epilepsy syndrome characterized by new onset of refractory *status epilepticus* (RSE) without a clear acute or active structural, toxic, or metabolic cause. According to the consensus definition, FIRES is considered a subcategory of new-onset refractory *status epilepticus* (NORSE), and the diagnosis requires prior febrile infection starting between 2 weeks and 24 hours before the onset of RSE (with or without fever at the onset of SE). Both sexes are affected. The FIRES definition applies to all age groups, even though the prevalent ages at FIRES presentation are during childhood and early adulthood. FIRES has no identified etiology but growing evidence suggests a major role of non-antibody-mediated neuroinflammation in its pathophysiology.

At onset, focal seizures increase in frequency and the patient enters super refractory status epilepticus often within 2 weeks of onset. The duration of the status may be highly variable, lasting from few days to several months. Seizures are multifocal and can evolve to bilateral tonic-clonic seizures. EEG during the acute phase shows a slow background with highly frequent multifocal seizures. After this acute phase, the patient enters, without a seizure-free period, a chronic phase characterized by drug-resistant focal epilepsy with a variable degree of intellectual disability or cognitive impairment. Imaging excludes structural etiologies and shows edema of both hippocampal and temporal regions that can evolve to atrophy in the chronic phase in almost half of the patients.

The diagnostic work-up must rule out bacterial and viral encephalitis, toxic etiologies, autoimmune encephalitis, and metabolic diseases including mitochondrial diseases. No genetic etiology was identified but genetic testing in addition to CSF and DNA collection should be performed for research purposes whenever possible.

TREATMENT STRATEGY

FIRES is a life-threatening epilepsy syndrome with a challenging management during the acute and chronic phases. Diagnosis should be recognized early after ruling out possible identifiable causes amenable to specific treatments.

The acute phase of FIRES management is life-threatening and highly challenging, and should be carried out by neurointensivists with the epileptologist and a multidisciplinary team. Once infectious, metabolic, toxic, and structural etiologies are excluded within the first 48–72 hours, the diagnosis should be raised, and immunomodulatory therapies should be initiated. The ketogenic diet, in addition to ASMs, has reported efficacy in the acute phase in some series. Partial efficacy of cannabidiol was reported in a few cases. Anakinra and tocilizumab are the two immunomodulatory molecules reported with efficacy although there are yet no controlled studies. Neuropsychological assessment and intensive programs for cognitive and motor rehabilitation are pivotal during the chronic phase.

Future research should address early diagnosis, better insight into the pathogenesis, and the development of more tailored therapies. Multicenter international efforts, including clinical registry and biobank, as well as clinical interventional trials, should be promoted.

CLINICAL PEARLS

- FIRES is an epilepsy syndrome characterized by new onset of RSE without a clear acute or active structural, toxic, or metabolic cause.
- FIRES is considered a subcategory of new-onset refractory *status epilepticus* (NORSE).
- FIRES has no identified etiology but growing evidence suggests a major role of non-antibody-mediated neuroinflammation in its pathophysiology.
- Immunomodulation and ketogenic diet should be considered early and are recommended to be continued in the postacute phase if effective.

SUGGESTED REFERENCES

Gaspard N., Hirsch L.J., Sculier C., Loddenkemper T., van Baalen A., Lancrenon J., Emmery M., Specchio N., Farias-Moeller R., Wong N., Nabbout R. New-onset refractory *status epilepticus* (NORSE) and febrile infection-related epilepsy syndrome (FIRES): State of the art and perspectives. *Epilepsia* 2018;59:745–52.

Hirsch L.J., Gaspard N., van Baalen A., Nabbout R., Demeret S., Loddenkemper T., Navarro V., Specchio N., Lagae L., Rossetti A.O., Hocker S., Gofton T.E., Abend N.S., Gilmore E.J., Hahn C., Khosravani H., Rosenow F., Trinka E. Proposed consensus definitions for new-onset refractory *status epilepticus* (NORSE), febrile infection-related epilepsy syndrome (FIRES), and related conditions. *Epilepsia* 2018;59:739–44.

Koh S., Wirrell E., Vezzani A., Nabbout R., Muscal E., Kaliakatsos M., Wickström R., Riviello J.J., Brunklaus A., Payne E., Valentin A., Wells E., Carpenter J.L., Lee K., Lai Y.C., Eschbach K., Press C.A., Gorman M., Stredny C.M., Roche W., Mangum T. Proposal to optimize evaluation and treatment of febrile infection-related epilepsy syndrome (FIRES): A report from FIRES workshop. *Epilepsia Open* 2021;6:62–72.

Nabbout R. FIRES and IHHE: Delineation of the syndromes. *Epilepsia* 2013;54(Suppl 6):S54–6.

Nabbout R., Vezzani A., Dulac O., Chiron C. Acute encephalopathy with inflammation-mediated *status epilepticus*. *Lancet Neurol* 2011;10:99–108.

van Baalen A., Vezzani A., Häusler M., Kluger G. Febrile infection-related epilepsy syndrome: Clinical review and hypotheses of epileptogenesis. *Neuropediatrics* 2017;48:5–18.

43 New-Onset Refractory *Status Epilepticus* (NORSE)

Steven Yang and Jerry Shih
UC San Diego School of Medicine

CONTENTS

CASE PRESENTATION

A 17-year-old girl with no past medical history presented with several weeks of behavioral changes, lethargy, and worsening headaches. Over several days, she became restless and anxious with new hallucinations. She then developed generalized tonic-clonic seizures and was started on levetiracetam. The seizures increased in frequency and progressed to convulsive status epilepticus (SE) requiring escalation of antiseizure medications (ASMs), sedation, and ventilation in the intensive care unit. Complete blood count, comprehensive metabolic panel, thyroid panel, rheumatologic panel, toxicology screen, and blood and urine cultures did not reveal clinically significant abnormalities. Chest, abdominal, pelvis, and brain imaging on presentation were normal. Cerebrospinal fluid (CSF) was not consistent with infection. Autoimmune antibody panel from CSF and serum did not identify a causative antibody or pathogen. Continuous EEG showed generalized periodic epileptic discharges at 1–2 Hz that frequently developed into generalized seizures. Her seizures were very difficult to control requiring multiple ASMs and anesthetics. Given a presumed autoimmune etiology, she was treated with immunotherapy including corticosteroids, intravenous immunoglobulin (IVIG), plasma exchange and subsequently anakinra, rituximab, and tocilizumab. Because she continued to have daily seizures, therapy with bilateral deep brain stimulation to anterior thalami was implemented. Over the subsequent 2 months, her seizure frequency decreased and she was able to be weaned off sedatives. She eventually was able to be discharged to the rehabilitation service.

DOI: 10.1201/9781003296478-47

317

DIFFERENTIAL DIAGNOSIS

When either clinical or electrographic seizures continue after initial treatment with first and second-line ASMs, the episode is often termed refractory *status epilepticus*. A new-onset seizure progressing to *status epilepticus* in an adolescent without a history of epilepsy should always raise concern for a provoked seizure.

Careful history taking, neurologic examination, and basic laboratory tests and neuroimaging might identify the most common etiologies of seizures, such as intoxication, central nervous system (CNS) infections, acute metabolic disturbances, alcohol withdrawal, or structural brain injury. Up to 20% of patients with refractory *status epilepticus* have a negative initial workup. Such cases have been referred as new-onset refractory status epilepticus (NORSE), which describes a clinical presentation, not a specific diagnosis, in a patient without active epilepsy or other pre-existing relevant neurological disorders. Patients do not have an identifiable acute or active structural, toxic, or metabolic cause. This includes patients with viral or autoimmune causes.

A subset of NORSE termed febrile infection-related epilepsy syndrome (FIRES) requires a prior febrile infection, with fever starting between 2 weeks and 24 hours prior to onset of refractory *status epilepticus*, with or without fever at onset of *status epilepticus*. Previous studies found that an etiology could ultimately be identified in 48% of cases, the most common being autoimmune encephalitis (37%) and viral infections (8%). More than half of the cases remained cryptogenic despite extensive, although variable work-ups.

DIAGNOSTIC APPROACH

The diagnosis and treatment of NORSE/FIRES are typically delayed until after an extensive search for underlying causes. However, initial investigation (blood tests, brain imaging, CSF analysis, and EEG), within 24–48 hours of onset, can easily exclude treatable and reversible structural, rheumatologic, infectious, metabolic, or toxic causes of refractory *status epilepticus*.

CSF analysis typically shows nonspecific mild pleocytosis (<10 cells/μL) and slightly elevated protein. Subsequent investigations may identify rare causes. After initial evaluation, we recommend evaluating serum and CSF for paraneoplastic and autoimmune epilepsy or encephalopathy antibodies. The brain MRI scan may show nonspecific abnormalities, most commonly hyperintensities in medial temporal lobes and limbic areas, but is often normal. Later, the MRI may show hippocampal and cortical atrophy. EEG is essential to monitor seizure activity and guide treatment.

There is currently no specific EEG marker for NORSE. Most studies reported periodic discharges and multiple seizure patterns (generalized, focal, and multifocal). Brain biopsy is rarely reported unless there is suspicion of other neuroinflammatory processes, with little evidence to support its routine use in the evaluation of NORSE.

Additional investigations may be pursued for inborn errors of metabolism and genetic testing for genes such as *SCN1A*, *SCN2A*, *SCN10A*, *KCNT1*, *CACNA1*, and

IlIRN. Malignancy screening should be considered in patients with cryptogenic NORSE or positive autoantibodies, and should include chest, abdomen, and pelvic CT, testicular/ovarian ultrasound, and whole-body positron emission tomography (PET)-CT if initial screening is negative.

TREATMENT STRATEGY

In the acute management of refractory status epilepticus, we prioritize the control of seizures over the diagnosis and treatment of the underlying etiology. Patients with NORSE are best managed in a neurologic intensive care unit with access to advanced diagnostic tools such as continuous EEG monitoring. Management by staff with epilepsy and neuroimmunology expertise is ideal. As detailed elsewhere in this volume, we recommend following treatment protocols for refractory *status epilepticus* with ASMs (e.g., levetiracetam, phenytoin, valproate, lacosamide, phenobarbital), anesthetics agents (e.g., midazolam, propofol, ketamine), and if needed, barbiturates to control seizures in acute setting. Some studies suggest that sodium channel blockers can be more effective than other ASMs.

Given the possible causal role of inflammation in NORSE/FIRES, immune therapies should be started within the first 72 hours of seizure onset, and if needed second-line immune therapy should be started within 7 days of seizure onset. First-line agents include corticosteroids, IVIG, and plasma exchange. Second-line immunotherapy agents include tacrolimus (interleukin-6 or IL-6 inhibitor), rituximab (antibody against CD20), cyclophosphamide, and anakinra (interleukin-1 or IL-1 receptor antagonist). To be effective, immunotherapy should be used for at least 3 months.

Current evidence does not support the use of cannabidiol or hypothermia as first-line therapy. The ketogenic diet (KD) may be beneficial in treating status epilepticus and has been used in cases of NORSE. The KD is a high-fat, low-carbohydrate diet that exerts both antiseizure activity and antiinflammatory effects. Case reports have shown improvement in seizure control once patients reach a state of ketosis. Neuromodulation through deep brain stimulation or vagus nerve stimulation is increasingly being used to treat refractory *status epilepticus* and may provide benefits in NORSE.

LONG-TERM OUTCOME

Most NORSE cases become super refractory requiring aggressive anesthetics which carry an increased risk of complications and poor outcomes. The median stay in the intensive care unit for adults is 15 days and 20–40 days for children. Mortality in children is ~12% and in adults is 16%–27%. The functional outcome is usually poor, with half to two-thirds having cognitive and functional impairment and most having refractory epilepsy. Longer duration of status epilepticus and a higher score on the Status Epilepticus Severity Scale are associated with poorer outcomes. In addition, cryptogenic NORSE is associated with higher rates of drug-resistant epilepsy and permanent cognitive impairment. As many patients are healthy prior to developing NORSE and some have good functional outcomes, aggressive treatment is justified.

The mortality rate in NORSE can be as high as 11%–30% and intellectual disability was 66%–100% of survivors in prior studies. Patients should be screened for sleep, cognitive and psychiatric disorders. Poor cognition has been shown to be associated with longer duration of anesthesia in patients with NORSE. All patients had subsequent epilepsy after discharge. Up to 15% became seizure free in long-term follow-up studies.

Malignancy screening should be repeated annually for 5 years in patients with positive autoantibodies or recurrence of symptoms. Adults with cryptogenic NORSE should also have malignancy screening repeated annually for 5 years.

Relatives of patients with NORSE face a tremendous and sudden life change as patients are typically young and previously healthy, and have now suffered a devastating neurologic illness, with an uncertain prognosis. Ongoing conversations with family about treatment plans and prognosis during the hospitalization are crucial. After the hospitalization and acute rehabilitation phase, families are faced with physical, emotional, and financial challenges in caring for a loved one who may have significant physical, cognitive, and behavioral dysfunction. A multidisciplinary outpatient team may be the best model to provide ongoing care. More information can be found at www.norseinstitute.org.

PATHOPHYSIOLOGY/NEUROBIOLOGY OF DISEASE

NORSE typically presents in healthy people with a prodrome of mild, nonspecific influenza-like illness with headache, gastrointestinal or upper respiratory symptoms. Prodromal symptoms can precede seizures by 1–14 days, sometimes with an asymptomatic interval in between. This is followed by rapidly progressive onset of seizures and encephalopathy that evolve into refractory *status epilepticus*. While no unifying mechanism has been found, there is speculation that NORSE/FIRES may be caused by an inflammatory response in the CNS. Several studies have found overproduction of intrathecal proinflammatory cytokines and chemokines in children with FIRES compared to control groups, some of which have proconvulsant activity. This accumulation of inflammatory factors could be due to activation of T cells, perivascular cells, and glia and take several days, perhaps explaining the latency between a febrile episode and the onset of *status epilepticus*. However, it is still unclear whether intrathecal inflammation is a cause or consequence of prolonged episode of refractory *status epilepticus*.

The most common cause identified in adults is autoimmune or paraneoplastic encephalitis. Antibodies against the N-methyl-D-aspartate (NMDA) receptor and the voltage-gated potassium channel complex are the most common causes of NORSE in adults. In children, there is no antibody consistently associated with NORSE/FIRES. Series testing in UK and Europe in epilepsy genes did not find any causative mutations in patients with NORSE/FIRES. Children with FIRES may have increased CSF concentrations of proinflammatory cytokines (IL-6, TNF-alpha, and chemokines). A Japanese study found mutation in IL-1 receptor antagonist gene in children with FIRES.

CLINICAL PEARLS

- NORSE is a clinical presentation, not a specific diagnosis, in a patient without active epilepsy or other preexisting relevant neurological disorder, who has new-onset refractory *status epilepticus* without a clear acute or active structural, toxic, or metabolic cause.
- FIRES is a subcategory of NORSE, applicable to all ages, that requires a prior febrile infection starting between 2 weeks and 24 hours prior to onset of refractory *status epilepticus*, with or without fever at onset of status epilepticus.
- Management of NORSE includes investigating the underlying cause, controlling *status epilepticus*, treating presumed inflammatory or immune-mediated processes.
- We recommend treating *status epilepticus* aggressively and consider immunotherapy as some cases have good outcomes despite prolonged SE for up to several months.
- More information can be found at the NORSE Institute (www.norseinstitute.org).

SUGGESTED REFERENCES

Gaspard N., Foreman B.P., Alvarez V., Kang C.C., Probasco J.C., Jongeling A.C., Meyers E., Espirnera A., Haas K.F., Schmitt S.E., Gerard E.E., Gofton T., Kaplan P.W., Lee J.W., Legros B., Szaflarski J.P., Westover B.M., LaRoche S.M., Hirsch L.J. New-onset refractory status epilepticus: Etiology, clinical features, and outcome. *Neurology* 2015;85:1604–13.

Gaspard N., Hirsch L.J., Sculier C., Loddenkemper T., van Baalen A., Lancrenon J., Emmery M., Specchio N., Farias-Moeller R., Wong N., Nabbout R. New-onset refractory status epilepticus (NORSE) and febrile infection-related epilepsy syndrome (FIRES): State of the art and perspectives. *Epilepsia* 2018;59:745–52.

Hirsch L.J., Gaspard N., van Baalen A., Nabbout R., Demeret S., Loddenkemper T., Navarro V., Specchio N., Lagae L., Rossetti A.O., Hocker S., Gofton T.E., Abend N.S., Gilmore E.J., Hahn C., Khosravani H., Rosenow F., Trinka E. Proposed consensus definitions for new-onset refractory status epilepticus (NORSE), febrile infection-related epilepsy syndrome (FIRES), and related conditions. *Epilepsia* 2018;59:739–44.

Khawaja A.M., DeWolfe J.L., Miller D.W. New-onset refractory status epilepticus (NORSE) - The potential role for immunotherapy. *Epilepsy Behav* 2015;47:17–23.

Sakuma H., Tanuma N., Kuki I., Takahashi Y., Shiomi M., Hayashi M. Intrathecal overproduction of proinflammatory cytokines and chemokines in febrile infection-related refractory status epilepticus. J *Neurol Neurosurg Psychiatry* 2015;86:820–2.

Wickstrom R., Taraschenko O., Dilena R., Payne E.T., Specchio N., Nabbout R., Koh S., Gaspard N., Hirsch L.J.; International NORSE Consensus Group. International consensus recommendations for management of New Onset Refractory Status Epilepticus (NORSE) incl. Febrile Infection-Related Epilepsy Syndrome (FIRES): Statements and supporting evidence. *Epilepsia* 2022;63:2840–64.

Wu J., Lan X., Yan L., Hu Y., Hong S., Jiang L., Chen J. A retrospective study of 92 children with new-onset refractory status epilepticus. *Epilepsy Behav* 2021;125:108413.

44 Low-Grade Developmental and Epilepsy Associated Brain Tumors

Christie Becu and Angus Wilfong
Barrow Neurological Institute at Phoenix Children's

CONTENTS

CASE PRESENTATION

A 13-year-old right-handed girl presented with chronic episodes that were thought to be panic attacks, which first occurred when she was 11 years old. She described an unusual sensation lasting about 30–60 seconds as if someone was behind her, leading to piloerection and anxiety. This was followed by eye widening, difficulty speaking, lip smacking, drooling, and both hands alternating between pronation and supination. The seizures were associated with loss of awareness and postictal confusion and aggression. Occasionally, she would strike out and hit family and friends. She would be able to talk within 1 minute but was amnestic of all events except the anxiety-provoking aura. Seizures first occurred about twice a month but eventually became daily, especially when she was sleepy. She was started on the antiseizure medication (ASM) levetiracetam but this did not control the seizures. Brain MRI showed a cystic lesion in the left superior temporal gyrus, suspicious for a dysembryoplastic neuroepithelial tumor (DNET; Figures 44.1–44.5). Due to ongoing seizures, oxcarbazepine was added as adjunctive therapy. However, the seizures remained refractory to medication.

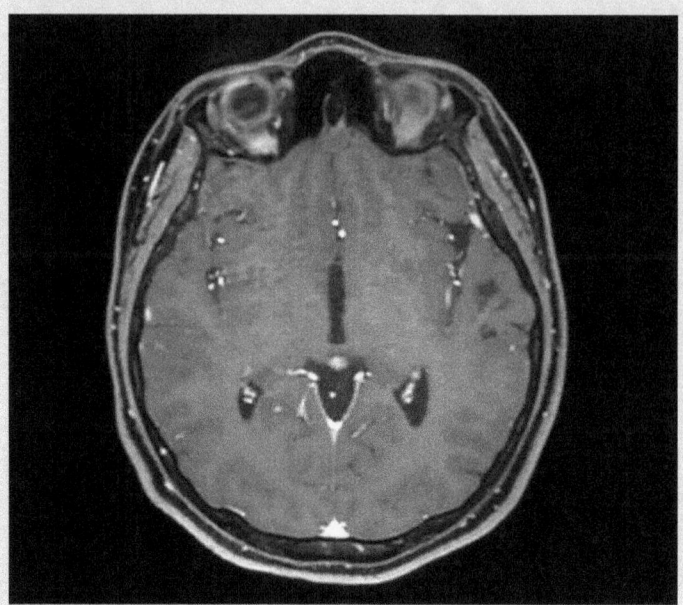

FIGURE 44.1   MRI T1 axial postcontrast image with nonenhancing lesion in the left superior temporal gyrus.

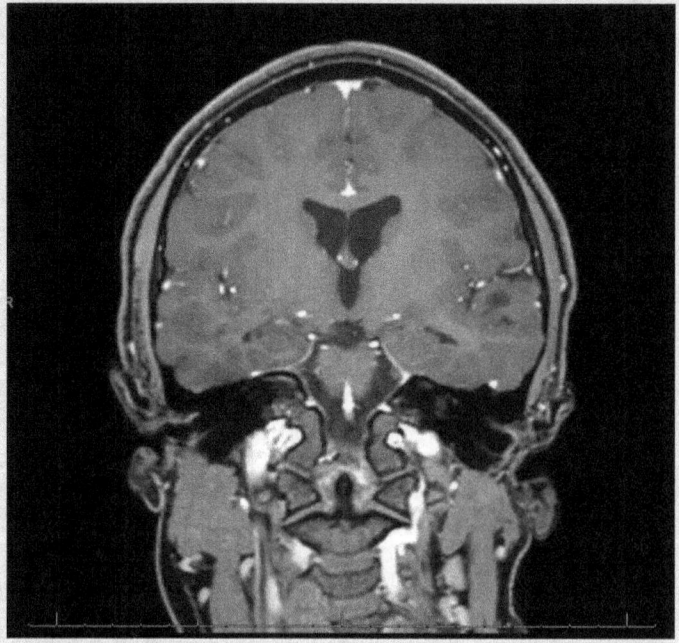

FIGURE 44.2   MRI T1 coronal postcontrast image with nonenhancing lesion in the left superior temporal gyrus.

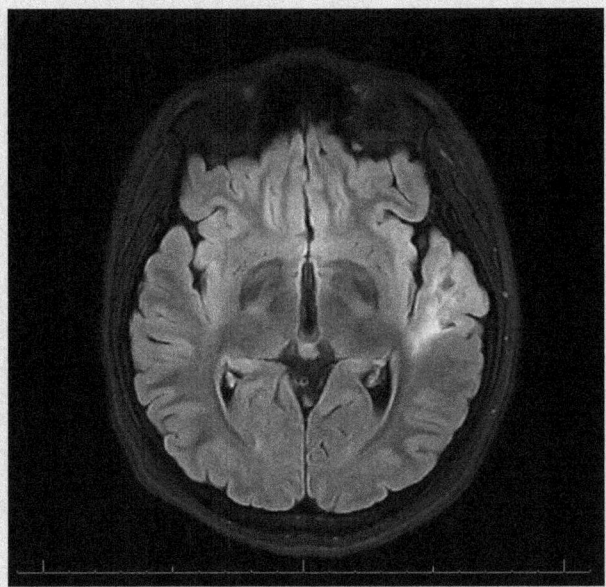

FIGURE 44.3   MRI T2 FLAIR axial image with hyperintensity in the left superior temporal gyrus.

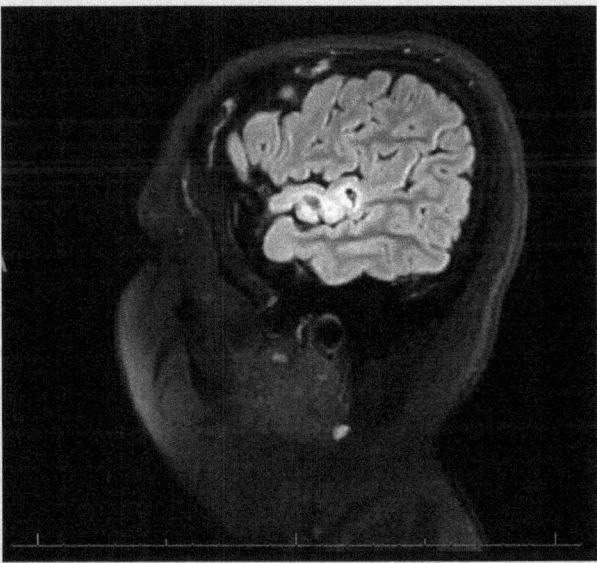

FIGURE 44.4   MRI T2 FLAIR sagittal image. There is a T2 hyperintense nonenhancing ill-defined lesion within the midportion of the left superior temporal gyrus involving both the cortex and subcortical white matter.

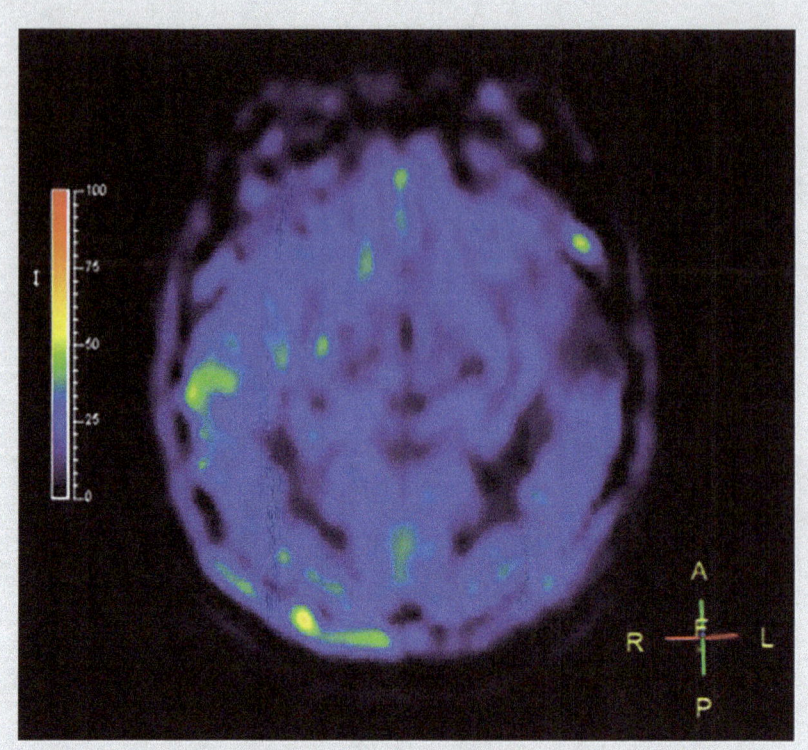

FIGURE 44.5   MR Perfusion showing hypoperfusion in the area of the tumor.

DIFFERENTIAL DIAGNOSIS

FOCAL SEIZURES

Seizures are classified into focal onset, generalized onset, and unknown onset. Seizures with focal onset may be idiopathic (genetic) or may be due to structural etiologies such as tumors, brain malformations, or gliosis (Table 44.1).

Focal seizures are further categorized as occurring with impaired awareness or without impaired awareness. Focal seizures with impaired awareness may present as staring spells, but their interruption in awareness is less complete compared to absence seizures. Patients with focal seizures with impaired unawareness may be partially responsive and may follow simple commands. The seizures are more likely to be associated with motor automatisms and are typically followed by confusion and drowsiness in the postictal state.

Most focal seizures last 1–2 minutes in duration and rarely occur more than a few times per week or month. Some children may experience an aura (focal seizure without impaired awareness) before losing awareness. The character of the aura may suggest the region of the brain where the seizure begins. Children may come to

TABLE 44.1

Etiologies of Focal Epilepsy in Children

Genetic (normal MRI, normal development, characteristic spikes on EEG)	Self-limited epilepsy with centrotemporal spikes (Benign Rolandic Epilepsy)
	Self-limited epilepsy with autonomic seizures (Panayiotopoulos Syndrome)
	Childhood Occipital Visual Epilepsy
	Photosensitive Occipital Lobe Epilepsy
Structural (abnormal MRI)	
NEURODEVELOPMENTAL	Focal cortical dysplasia
	Schizencephaly
	Periventicular nodular heterotopias
	Hemimegalencephaly
	Polymicrogyria
	Pachygyria
	Arteriovenous malformations
NEUROCUTANEOUS	Tuberous sclerosis complex
	Sturge-Weber syndrome
	Neurocutaneous melanosis sequence
NEOPLASTIC	Low-grade developmental and epilepsy associated tumors (ganglioglioma, DNET, etc.).
POSTTRAUMATIC	Focal brain injury following trauma to the brain, particularly if hemorrhagic. Also, poststroke, postmeningitic, postencephalitic, post-hypoxia-ischemia
METABOLIC DISEASES	Inborn errors of metabolism
AUTOIMMUNE	Rasmussen's disease, antiphospholipid antibody syndrome, etc.

medical attention when a focal seizure evolves into a bilateral tonic-clonic seizure, which often frightens parents or caregivers.

LOW-GRADE DEVELOPMENTAL AND EPILEPSY ASSOCIATED BRAIN TUMORS

Brain tumors are the second most frequent structural etiology in patients with focal seizures before 18 years of age, following focal cortical dysplasia. Primary central nervous system (CNS) tumors are organized according to their histopathology based on neuronal or glial morphological characteristics and architectural growth patterns, or genetically.

Low-grade developmental, epilepsy associated brain tumors (LEATs) are a group of morphologically and genetically heterogenous, low-grade, and slowly growing tumors comprised of neuronal and glial cells with pediatric onset and are a common cause of epilepsy in children (Table 44.2).

LEATs are thought to be more epileptogenic than other primary or metastatic tumors of the CNS due to their slow growth and low-grade nature, leading to longer survival as well as their strong association with focal cortical dysplasia. Most patients with a LEAT experience a seizure prior to tumor treatment with a minority first experiencing a seizure within 2 weeks after surgery or later.

TABLE 44.2

Low-Grade Developmental and Epilepsy Associated Brain Tumor Types

Ganglioglioma

Dysembryoplastic neuroepithelial tumor (DNET)

Pilocytic astrocytoma

Isomorphic diffuse glioma

Angiocentric glioma

Multinodular and vacuolated neuronal tumor

Papillary glioneuronal tumor

Polymorphous low-grade neuroepithelial tumor of the young

Low-grade neuroepithelial tumors (not otherwise specified)

Seizures typically occur by 13 years of age and are more likely to occur if tumors are located supratentorially, involve the gray matter, and have certain histological patterns such as DNET and ganglioglioma. Temporal lobe tumors comprise 77% of LEATs and they can be associated with focal cortical dysplasia. Patients may present with a seizure semiology that does not reflect the location of the brain tumor due to secondary generalization of seizure activity.

DIAGNOSTIC APPROACH

After clinical presentation of seizures, a routine EEG is obtained to help identify seizure type as well as localization of seizure onset. However, some children with epilepsy do not have any spikes on a routine EEG and not all children with spikes on their EEG will experience seizures or develop epilepsy. If the nature of the spells remains unclear after a thorough history, physical examination, and routine EEG, then a more prolonged EEG/video monitoring study may be indicated. This allows the clinical events to be recorded and time-synchronized EEG to be reviewed.

Most children with focal seizures and localization-related spikes on EEG require the higher spatial resolution of MRI to search for underlying structural abnormalities that may not be seen on CT. These include brain tumors, scars or gliosis from a remote injury, arteriovenous malformations, and abnormalities of cortical development such as focal cortical dysplasias.

Other techniques may be employed to identify focal brain abnormalities, such as ^{18}F-fluorodeoxyglucose positron emission tomography (FDG-PET) may demonstrate an area of hypometabolism. Single-photon emission computed tomography (SPECT) may show interictal hypoperfusion associated with the abnormality, along with increased perfusion during the seizure (ictal-SPECT). Magnetoencephalography (MEG) allows for co-localization of interictal abnormalities and brain MRI and may be useful in poorly localized scalp EEG findings.

TREATMENT APPROACH

The patient described in this case required intervention due to the intractable nature of her seizures. The seizures place her at risk for accidents and injuries, may impair cognition and academic performance, and may have major deleterious psychoemotional effects, particularly when seizures occur at school.

ASMs are used to manage seizures until definitive treatment of the tumor, or in some cases, if tumor treatment does not resolve seizures. There has been an ever-growing list of newer ASMs and nonpharmacologic therapies available to practitioners who manage childhood epilepsy. Traditionally, the medications have been separated into "older" and "newer" groups based upon their historic regulatory approval and appearance in the US marketplace.

Typically, when a medication is first approved for epilepsy, it receives an "on-label indication" for add-on (adjunctive) therapy for partial (i.e., focal)-onset seizures in adults. Then, as experience grows and other studies are done, the use of the drug may expand to other seizure types and younger age groups as deemed appropriate. As a broad generalization, most practitioners who specialize in epilepsy (epileptologists) would now prefer to initiate ASM therapy with one of the newer medications.

Research studies and clinical experience have shown that the newer ASMs are not more efficacious than the older drugs, but they do appear to be safer, better tolerated, and have fewer drug-to-drug interactions. The ASM chosen for initial therapy should be one that is highly effective for a particular seizure type or epilepsy syndrome and be safe and well tolerated. Single drug therapy (monotherapy) is the goal of epilepsy treatment as it is associated with better compliance, fewer adverse effects, less potential for teratogenicity during pregnancy, and lower cost than polytherapy. Drug interactions are also avoided, and the pharmacokinetics are simplified. Although surgery is the treatment of choice for LEATS, it is important to note that newer ASMs are preferred in the treatment of epilepsy due to brain tumors due to their limited interactions with chemotherapeutic agents.

However, as in the patient's case above, seizures tend to be drug-resistant and continue until definitive treatment of the tumor, which includes resection, chemotherapy, radiation, or laser interstitial thermal therapy (LITT). Surgeries include total and partial resections, and extent of surgical resection is determined on a case-by-case basis depending on the size and location of the tumor. During surgery, electrocorticography may be performed to monitor electrophysiologic brain activity and to minimize postsurgical deficits. LITT targets a focus of seizure onset using real-time MRI to implant a catheter and guide a laser that delivers ablative thermal energy. Ablation is a minimally invasive approach for smaller tumors.

Presurgical evaluation was initiated. The patient was admitted to the epilepsy monitoring unit and her EEG showed intermittent slowing over the left temporal region, interictal spikes from the left mid-anterior temporal field, and one seizure was recorded with left-sided onset with rapid generalization (Figures 44.6 and 44.7). A task-based functional MRI was obtained for language localization in relation to the tumor and revealed that she was predominantly left hemisphere dominant for both English and Spanish and had trace language activation demonstrated on the right. The patient underwent gross tumor resection and excision of the epileptogenic focus.

During surgery, electrocorticography initially revealed significant spiking discharges that resolved following resection of the tumor and the epileptogenic focus. Pathology confirmed an angiocentric glioma WHO grade 1 tumor with an abnormal rearrangement of the *MYB* gene. Following the resection, she no longer had any auras

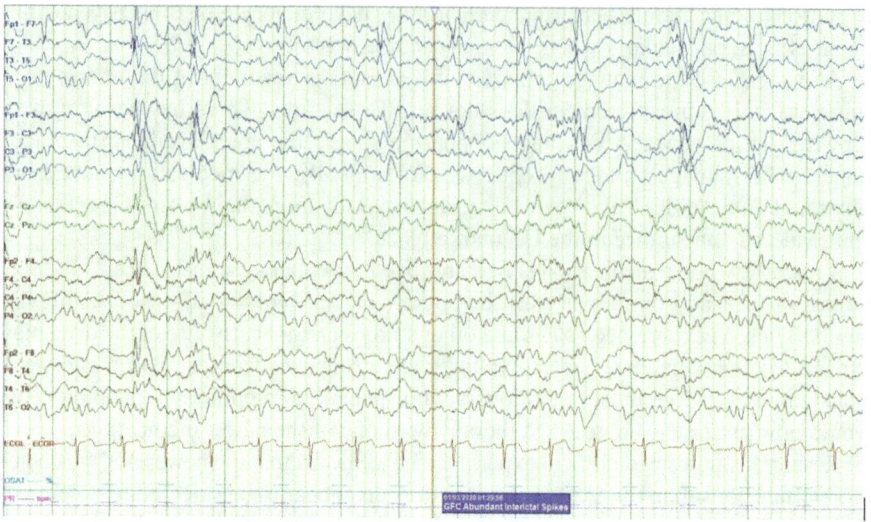

FIGURE 44.6 Electroencephalogram: abundant interictal spikes predominantly in the left anterior temporal field.

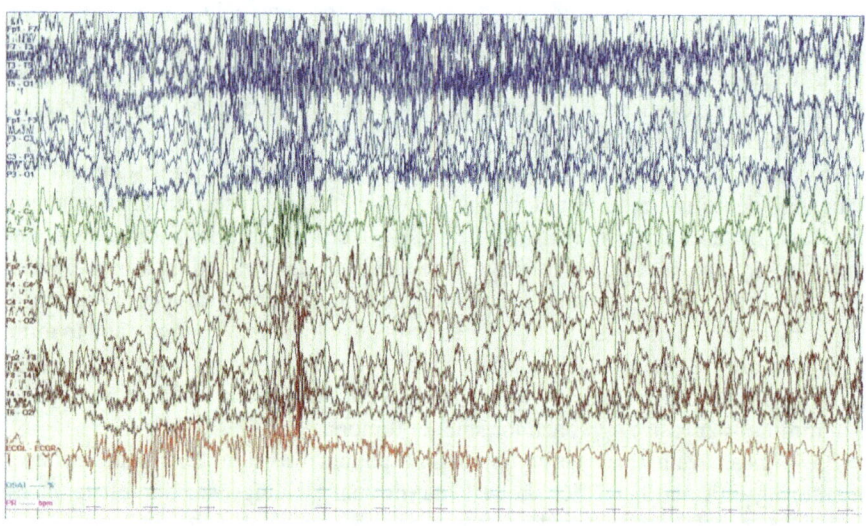

FIGURE 44.7 Electroencephalogram: electroclinical seizure with generalized electrical activity.

or seizures. She did not have any change in her speech or language function and reported no issues regarding speech fluency, word finding, or difficulty understanding what others say. Her motor functions also remained intact without any deficits.

Postoperative MRIs remained stable without tumor recurrence. Nine months following the resection, a repeat routine EEG was obtained which was completely normal with no epileptiform activity. She was weaned off oxcarbazepine, followed 1 year later by levetiracetam. Two years after surgery, she remained seizure free and off ASMs.

LONG-TERM OUTCOME

The greatest factor impacting seizure outcome after tumor treatment is the presence of seizures at presentation. Patients who have seizures prior to tumor treatment (as opposed to seizures after treatment) are more likely to continue having seizures at later follow-up. An earlier study found that total or partial resection of the tumor did not influence seizure outcome; further, tumor type or histopathology of the tumor impacted ultimate seizure prognosis. Seizure outcome is assessed using Engel classification, which was established for seizure outcome after epilepsy surgery. Engel classification can range from Class 1: free of disabling seizures to Class IV: no worthwhile improvement.

Seizure outcome following tumor resection tends to be favorable with resolution or improved control of seizures in most patients. There is not a significant difference in seizure outcome in total *versus* partial resection as long as the seizure-onset zone is resected. In patients with LEATs, resection of the tumor alone may not result in resolution of seizures if the peritumoral tissue contains an epileptogenic zone, although some argue removal of the tumor leads to normalization of the surrounding tissue. Radiotherapy and chemotherapy have also shown positive effects on decreasing seizures.

Patients who experience seizure freedom following tumor treatment may be weaned off ASMs and long-term prophylaxis may not be indicated. Most who are weaned do not have recurrent seizures apart from the setting of tumor recurrence. There are no set guidelines for when or how to wean off an ASM in the setting of tumors. Some providers tend to withdraw ASMs more quickly in patients with total resections compared to patients with partial resections.

PATHOPHYSIOLOGY/NEUROBIOLOGY OF DISEASE

Brain tumors cause seizures via tumor epileptogenicity and peritumoral epileptogenicity. Tumor epileptogenicity is due to the tumor containing an abnormal distribution of cells which may release excitatory molecules, making the tumor tissue itself epileptogenic due to imbalance of inhibitory and excitatory synaptic transmissions and cytokines.

Peritumoral epileptogenicity is due to metabolic and neurotransmitter changes in peritumoral brain, morphologic changes (including malformation and cortical dysplasia), immunologic change in the peritumoral brain, and peritumoral blood products, gliosis, and necrosis which directly irritate or alter the microenvironment.

Peritumoral astrocytosis or infiltration by glial tumor cells leads to a more alkaline environment, which in turn increases Ca^{2+} conductance through N-methyl-D-aspartate (NMDA) receptors and decreased Cl^- conductance through gamma-aminobutyric acid type A ($GABA_A$) receptors, thus enabling a more hyperexcitable state. Interictal epileptiform activity or seizures promotes abnormal neuronal networks that eventually are able to independently generate interictal epileptiform activity or seizures.

CLINICAL PEARLS

- Brain tumors are the second most frequent structural etiology in children with focal seizures.
- LEATs are more epileptogenic than other primary or metastatic tumors of the central nervous system.
- Surgery is the treatment of choice for children with drug-resistant focal epilepsy due to LEATS.

SUGGESTED REFERENCES

Giulioni M., Marucci G., Martinoni M., Marliani A.F., Toni F., Bartiromo F., Volpi L., Riguzzi P., Bisulli F., Naldi I., Michelucci R., Baruzzi A., Tinuper P., Rubboli G. Epilepsy associated tumors: Review article. *World J Clin Cases* 2014;2(11):623–41.

Kahlenberg C.A., Fadul C.E., Roberts D.W., Thadani V.M., Buajrski K.A., Scott R.C., Jobst B.C. Seizure prognosis of patients with low-grade tumors. *Seizure* 2012;21:540–5.

Robert-Boire V., Desnous B., Lortie A., Caremant L., Ellezam B., Weil A.G., Perreault S. Seizures in pediatric patients with primary brain tumors. *Pediatr Neurol* 2019;97:50–5.

Sánchez Fernández I., Loddenkemper T. Seizures caused by brain tumors in children. *Seizure* 2017;44:98–107.

Slegers R.J., Blumcke I. Low-grade developmental and epilepsy associated brain tumors: a critical update 2020. *Acta Neuropathol Commun* 2020;8:27.

45 Rasmussen's Encephalitis

Maria Augusta Montenegro
UC San Diego School of Medicine

CONTENTS

CASE PRESENTATION

A 6-year-old boy was seen in the epilepsy clinic at our University Hospital after having experienced focal seizures characterized by clonic movements of the left arm and face for two months. His primary care physician had suggested the diagnosis of self-limited epilepsy with centrotemporal spikes (Rolandic epilepsy) and put him on oxcarbazepine; however, he continued to have several seizures per week and was referred to the epilepsy clinic. He was the product of an uneventful pregnancy and delivery. Developmental milestones were normal and past medical history was unremarkable. Neurological examination was normal except for a mild left arm pronator drift. He had a normal brain MRI and EEG showed only intermittent right temporal lobe slowing. Further trials of antiseizure medications (ASMs) were implemented, and a repeat brain MRI was scheduled. Over the subsequent few months, seizures remained drug-resistant, and epilepsia partialis continua emerged, affecting his left lower face. Another EEG showed continuous theta/delta waves over the right hemisphere and very frequent sharp waves in the right frontotemporal head regions. The new brain MRI showed right ventricular enlargement and T2/FLAIR cortical hyperintensity in the right perisylvian region. The diagnosis of Rasmussen's encephalitis was made, and despite multiple ASM regimens, he still had daily focal seizures and epilepsia partialis continua. Neurological examination showed progressive left hemiparesis, and 9 months after his first seizure, a hemispherotomy was performed. There was no further recurrence of seizures after surgery.

DOI: 10.1201/9781003296478-49

DIFFERENTIAL DIAGNOSIS

The differential diagnosis of Rasmussen's encephalitis includes conditions that present with drug-resistant focal epilepsy associated with unilateral hemispheric atrophy. However, during the early stage of the disease, brain MRI is normal and there is no hemiparesis or cognitive impairment. It is not uncommon that the diagnosis of self-limited epilepsy with centrotemporal spikes is considered as a possible diagnosis for some patients.

Hemiconvulsion–hemiplegia–epilepsy syndrome has its onset during early childhood and is characterized by prolonged focal *status epilepticus* associated with a febrile illness. Brain MRI shows acute unilateral hemispheric swelling that progresses to atrophy. Although the child will have hemiparesis, unilateral hemispheric atrophy, and drug-resistant focal epilepsy, the progression is faster than the one seen in Rasmussen's encephalitis.

Sturge–Weber syndrome can also present hemispheric atrophy, hemiparesis, and drug-resistant epilepsy. However, most patients have a distinct facial port wine stain, which helps in the differential diagnosis. Neuroimaging findings also show cortical calcification with a "tram track" appearance and the postcontrast sequences indicating the presence of a leptomeningeal angioma.

Perinatal stroke (ischemic or hemorrhagic) is a common cause of hemiplegic cerebral palsy. The diagnosis is easily established in the first months of life due to congenital hemiparesis. Seizures are not a mandatory diagnostic requirement. Neuroimaging usually reveals destructive vascular lesions that can be easily differentiated from the progressive hemispheric atrophy seen in Rasmussen's encephalitis. Table 45.1 lists the most common features of the conditions that should be considered in the differential diagnosis of Rasmussen's encephalitis.

DIAGNOSTIC APPROACH

The diagnosis of Rasmussen's encephalitis is based on clinical and pathological findings. Clinically, it is characterized by drug-resistant focal epilepsy with childhood

TABLE 45.1
Differential Diagnosis of Rasmussen's Encephalitis

Hemiconvulsion–Hemiplegia–Epilepsy	Sturge–Weber Syndrome	Perinatal Stroke
Onset early childhood	Congenital disease	Perinatal onset (often prenatal)
Prior normal brain MRI	Neuroimaging shows unilateral hemisphere atrophy, calcification, and leptomeningeal angioma	Hemiparesis since birth
Prior normal neurological examination		Brain MRI shows hemispheric lesion since newborn period
Status epilepticus during febrile illness		Seizures often present, but not mandatory
Acute onset, very fast progression to hemiparesis	Hemiparesis can be absent or progress slowly	
	Seizures are not always drug-resistant	

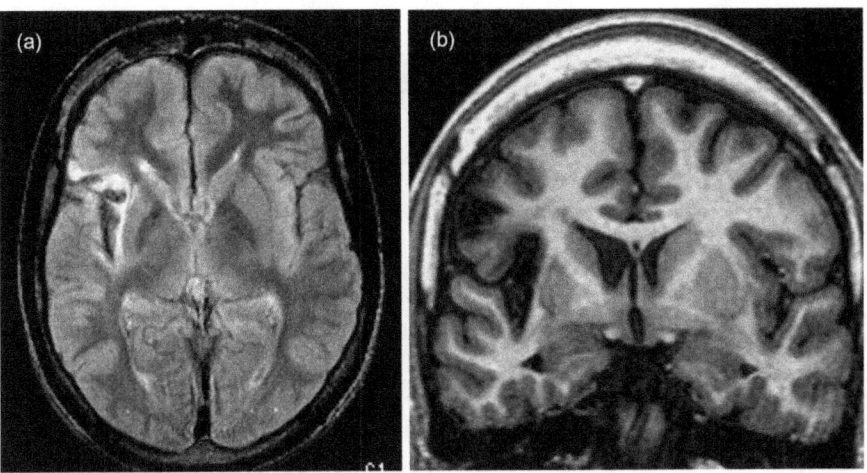

FIGURE 45.1 (a) Axial fluid-attenuated inversion recovery (FLAIR) MRI sequence showing cortical perisylvian hyperintensity. (b) Coronal T1 MRI sequence showing right lateral ventricle enlargement, right corticosubcortical perisylvian atrophy, and right caudate nucleus atrophy. Reproduced from Montenegro & Baccin, Neuropediatria Ilustrada, Revinter 2012.

onset (only 10% of the patients will present late adolescence or adult-onset). Seizure semiology is variable but suggests unilateral brain involvement, and 50% of the patients will have *epilepsia partialis continua*. It is a progressive disorder that will lead to hemiparesis, cognitive decline, and unilateral hemispheric atrophy.

EEG shows nonspecific findings, characterized by unilateral slowing and epileptiform discharges. CSF can be normal or exhibit a mildly elevated cell count (mostly lymphocytes) and protein content. Neuroimaging shows progressive cortical/subcortical hyperintensity on T2/FLAIR sequences, unilateral ventricular enlargement, and unilateral hemispheric atrophy (Figure 45.1). Although there is growing evidence that the inflammation associated with Rasmussen's encephalitis can be due to immunopathological mechanisms, there are no specific antibodies associated with the disease.

The classic neuropathologic findings after brain biopsy are confirmatory, but it should be considered only in patients that do not meet sufficient clinical criteria for the diagnosis. Neuropathology shows unilateral, multifocal inflammation mediated by T cells with activated microglial cells (typically, but not necessarily forming nodules) and reactive astrogliosis. The diagnostic criteria according to the European consensus is detailed in Table 45.2.

TREATMENT STRATEGY

ASMs are not effective in most patients, especially for *epilepsia partialis continua*. However, they can help to decrease seizure frequency and bilateral tonic-clonic seizures. Very high doses and combination therapy with multiple drugs should be avoided because these approaches will not be effective and will cause severe side effects.

TABLE 45.2

Diagnostic Criteria: All Three Criteria from Part A or Two from Part B (Bien et al., 2005)

	Part A
Clinical	Focal seizures (with or without *epilepsia partialis continua*) and unilateral cortical deficit(s)
EEG	Unihemispheric slowing with or without epileptiform activity, unilateral seizure onset
MRI	Focal cortical atrophy and at least one of the following: • Gray or white matter T2/FLAIR hyperintense signal • Hyperintense signal or atrophy of the ipsilateral caudate head

	Part B
Clinical	*Epilepsia partialis continua* or progressive cortical deficit(s)
EEG	Progressive unihemispheric focal cortical atrophy
Histopathology	T cell encephalitis with activated microglial cells (typically, but not necessarily forming nodules) and reactive astrogliosis. Exclusion criteria: numerous parenchymal macrophages, B cells or plasma cells, or viral inclusion bodies

Immunomodulatory therapy (intravenous immunoglobulin, corticosteroids, monoclonal antibodies, immunosuppressive drugs, and plasmapheresis) can temporarily improve symptoms and slow the disease progression. However, there is no evidence that any of these treatments can change the long-term prognosis. In addition, postponing surgery can lead to a worse post-surgical clinical outcome (due to limited brain plasticity in older brains), especially if the dominant hemisphere is affected. Hemispherotomy is the treatment of choice, but its timing should be carefully tailored according to the severity of epilepsy, degree of hemiparesis, and hemispheric dominance.

LONG-TERM OUTCOME

Although the timing of disease progression can vary, the clinical course of Rasmussen's encephalitis is predictable in most patients. Despite the use of ASMs and immunomodulatory therapy, the affected child will develop progressive hemiparesis, cognitive impairment, and drug-resistant focal epilepsy. Hemispherotomy is the treatment of choice with a very high rate of complete seizure control; however, its timing is controversial (especially when the left hemisphere is affected).

PATHOPHYSIOLOGY/NEUROBIOLOGY OF DISEASE

There is an increasing body of evidence that Rasmussen's encephalitis has an immunopathological basis (T cell toxicity, microglial activation, and antibody-mediated degeneration). However, the exact pathophysiology has not yet been elucidated.

CLINICAL PEARLS

- The diagnosis of Rasmussen's encephalitis should be considered in children and adolescents with progressive unilateral hemispheric atrophy, focal seizures, and hemiparesis.
- ASMs have limited efficacy in seizure control, and most patients have drug-resistant epilepsy.
- Immunomodulatory therapy can be offered as a treatment option, but this does not change the long-term outcome.
- Hemispherotomy is the surgical treatment of choice, but its timing remains controversial.

SUGGESTED REFERENCES

Bien C.G., Granata T., Antozzi C., Cross J.H., Dulac O., Kurthen M., Lassmann H., Mantegazza R., Villemure J.-G., Spreafico R., Elger C.E. Pathogenesis, diagnosis and treatment of Rasmussen encephalitis: A European consensus statement. *Brain* 2005;128:454–71.

Oguni H., Andermann F., Rasmussen T.B. The syndrome of chronic encephalitis and epilepsy. A study based on the MNI series of 48 cases. *Adv Neurol* 1992;57:419–33.

Varadkar S., Bien C.G., Kruse C.A., Jensen F.E., Bauer J., Pardo C.A., Vincent A., Mathern G.W., Cross J.H. Rasmussen's encephalitis: Clinical features, pathobiology, and treatment advances. *Lancet Neurol* 2014;13:195–205.

Section V

The Adolescent

46 Juvenile Myoclonic Epilepsy

Cornelia Drees
Mayo Clinic Arizona

CONTENTS

CASE PRESENTATION

The patient is a 14-year-old boy with normal development and no past medical history who was seen at an emergency department in the early morning hours after he was witnessed to have a seizure at a party. He was at summer camp and had stayed up longer – and slept less – than usual for most of the preceding days. His friends recalled that he yelled, stiffened, and then jerked with his whole body for about 1 minute. He had bloody frothing at the mouth and lost bladder control. Afterward, the staff at the camp was unable to arouse him for another 15 minutes and he later woke up slightly disoriented, complaining of sore muscles "all over". The patient remembered involuntary twitching of his arms, on the right more than the left, before he lost consciousness, but was amnestic to the remainder of the event. This was the first event of this kind and he and his parents denied any prior history of seizures or staring spells during infancy and childhood. However, when asked specifically, he admitted to noticing muscle twitches in his shoulders and arms for the past 6 months. They typically occurred in the morning, after getting up, and have interfered with his daily routine before leaving for school. He recalls once involuntarily throwing a toothbrush across the bathroom, and another time when a jerk made him drop his cereal bowl on the floor. His examination was completely normal.

DOI: 10.1201/9781003296478-51

DIFFERENTIAL DIAGNOSIS

A seizure in an adolescent should always raise concern for a provoked seizure, i.e., elicited by a trigger such as sleep deprivation, alcohol withdrawal after alcohol excess, and withdrawal from benzodiazepines or use of illicit drugs such as amphetamines or cocaine. Genetic generalized epilepsies (GGEs) that first manifest with seizures during the teenage years should also be considered, such as juvenile myoclonic epilepsy (JME) or juvenile absence epilepsy. Childhood absence epilepsy may present with a generalized seizure, but the age of onset is earlier in childhood, and it is unusual for associated staring spells to go undetected by parents and teachers for years, and typically seizures remit during puberty. Obviously, a seizure could have occurred due to an underlying structural lesion, such as a cortical dysplasia, a vascular malformation, or a tumor, something to always remember even when acute provocation seems most likely (e.g., from sleep deprivation or intoxication), particularly when focal features are reported, such as head turn or asymmetric stiffening or jerking of extremities.

DIAGNOSTIC APPROACH

As always, the key to the diagnosis lies in the history! This otherwise normal young man experienced vigorous myoclonic jerks while completely awake, predominantly in the morning. Myoclonic seizures have a propensity to occur in the morning. In combination with a generalized tonic-clonic seizure, the most likely diagnosis is JME – a condition with onset usually between ages 10 and 24 years. Occasionally, patients have clinical features which may suggest a focal-onset seizure, such as a warning (prodrome or "aura" seen in 24%–70%), a head turn (version) or asymmetric clonic or tonic movements during convulsions (in 35%–46%), or asymmetric myoclonic seizures (in 14%–61%).

Typical EEG findings confirm this suspicion, i.e., generalized 3–5.5 Hz spike-wave and polyspike-wave complexes, occurring spontaneously out of an otherwise normal EEG background (Figure 46.1). In about 30% of patients, these discharges are triggered by photic stimulation, in 33% they are triggered by hyperventilation, and in some, they might only appear after provocation with sleep deprivation or drinking caffeinated beverages. During a myoclonic seizure, the myoclonic jerk corresponds to a generalized polyspike-wave discharge. In contrast, other myoclonic jerks, e.g., when an individual is drifting off to sleep (also called a hypnic jerk, hypnagogic myoclonic jerk, or sleep myoclonus) or when someone is startled, are not accompanied by epileptiform activity.

It should be noted that the EEG of JME patients may exhibit focal features or focal appearing fragments in 16%–37% of cases, thus suggesting a structural abnormality or lesion in the brain. Though, neuroimaging in a typical case is not required since the brain is structurally normal in these patients. Many physicians may still obtain an MRI of the brain to rule out other reasons for seizures that may mimic the presentation of JME. A toxicology/alcohol screen should be done if there is a suspicion that drugs might be involved.

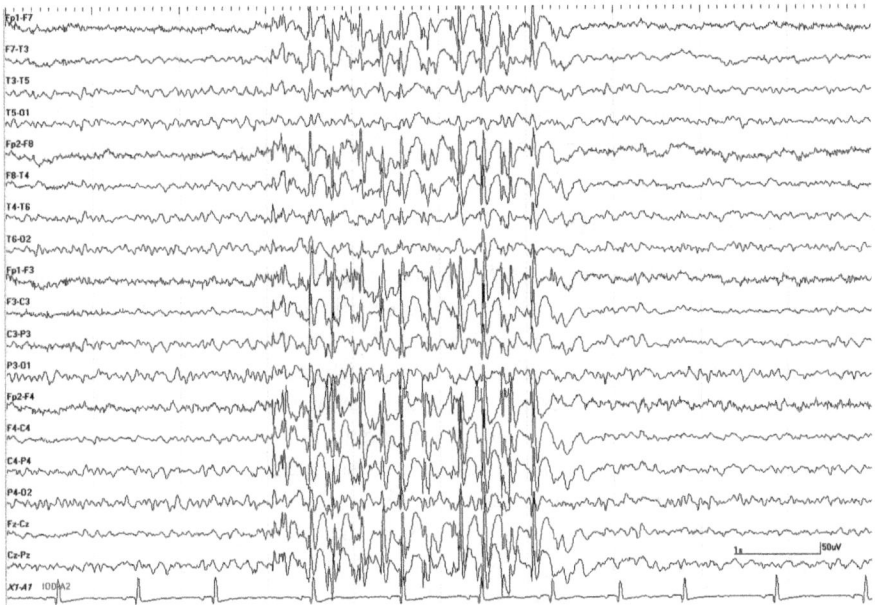

FIGURE 46.1 Burst of generalized 4–6 Hz spike-wave and polyspike-wave discharges. These are often without any clinical correlation but can be associated with clinical symptoms and signs such as jerks, staring, or behavioral arrest (especially if the bursts last for longer than 5 seconds).

TREATMENT STRATEGY

Patients with JME have a greater than 90% chance of experiencing recurrent seizures. Therefore, after diagnosis, life-long treatment with antiseizure medications (ASMs) and avoidance of possible provoking factors (e.g., alcohol, illicit drugs, sleep deprivation, and flickering lights) are recommended. About 80% of patients will have recurrent seizures when stopping ASM use. The frequency of myoclonic seizures and tonic-clonic convulsions may decline later in life (beyond age 40) and a minority of patients may no longer need treatment.

Therapeutic agents effective against seizures in GGE should be used and are usually very successful in controlling seizures. Currently, lamotrigine, levetiracetam, topiramate, zonisamide, and valproic acid (in males), are considered first-line treatment, and lacosamide and perampanel have also received regulatory approval as adjunctive therapy in GGE. Valproic acid has been shown to be the most effective drug, but it is typically avoided in young women because of teratogenicity and an increased likelihood of cognitive problems in children who were exposed to it *in utero*. In addition, valproic acid has hormonal and cosmetic adverse effects. Long-acting benzodiazepines, such as clonazepam or clobazam are also effective, but there is the potential for tolerance and addiction.

Most patients (80%–90%) are controlled with a single agent (i.e., monotherapy), but some require combination therapy. Several drugs prescribed for focal-onset seizures can exacerbate seizures, and even cause status epilepticus, in patients with JME (e.g., sodium channel blockers such as phenytoin, carbamazepine, oxcarbazepine, and gabapentin, tiagabine, and vigabatrin) and should not be used.

LONG-TERM OUTCOME

Studies on the natural history of JME indicate that about 80% of patients will have recurrent seizures after ASM treatment is discontinued. Unfortunately, this mandates that most JME patients be treated for life. Over the course of the condition, though, myoclonic seizures and convulsions diminish in frequency and about 30% of patients have no further seizures or only mild myoclonic seizures.

Patients have otherwise normal intelligence and life expectancy, although JME can have a negative psychosocial impact as it is associated with higher-than-average rates of unemployment and social isolation. With respect to inheritance, it is estimated that a mother with GGE has about a 10% risk of having a first-degree relative (child, parent, or sibling) with GGE, and about 21% of relatives are asymptomatic but will have EEG changes consistent with JME.

PATHOPHYSIOLOGY/NEUROBIOLOGY OF DISEASE

Juvenile myoclonic epilepsy has a strong genetic basis, and several genes have been implicated as causing the condition, although many people with JME do not have a positive family history or a detectable gene mutation. The family history is positive in 10%–50% of patients, but the inheritance patterns are often not clear-cut and suggest a process influenced by multiple genes and possibly other factors. The net result of one or multiple gene defects and/or a combination of factors is increased neuronal excitability, especially a tendency for thalamocortical networks to produce spike-wave and polyspike-wave-complexes seen on EEG.

Gene mutations on several chromosomes are associated with JME, and in the future, the list will continue to grow. However, the family with a monogenic form of JME is a rarity. Identified pedigrees have been studied extensively and are those that tell us something about the connection between specific gene defects and the electroclinical manifestation of epilepsy. Examples are gene defects causing "channelopathies" – conditions known to alter normal ion channel function and yield an episodic clinical phenotype such as epilepsy. For JME, mutations in genes encoding the potassium, calcium, and chloride ion channels have been identified. Another mechanism leading to hyperexcitability are mutations of the $GABA_A$ receptor which reduce GABA-induced hyperpolarizing chloride currents. For example, an autosomal dominant mutation of a gene on chromosome 5q (i.e., *GABRA1*) interferes with the production of an important $GABA_A$ receptor subunit which in turn alters the effectiveness of the inhibitory transmitter GABA on post-synaptic neurons.

An altogether different mechanism is suspected in cases with defects in a gene called *EFHC1* which changes the function of certain voltage-dependent calcium channels normally involved in neuronal apoptosis during early brain development.

CLINICAL PEARLS

- JME constitutes about 10% of all epilepsies and patients present with the following seizure types, in isolation or in combination: (1) myoclonic seizures (principal and obligate seizure type); (2) generalized tonic-clonic seizures, (3) myoclonic-tonic-clonic seizures, and – least common – (4) absence seizures. All seizure types are associated with generalized 3–5.5 Hz spike-wave and polyspike-wave discharges on EEG.
- Myoclonic seizures are an expected and early manifestation of the condition and typically occur in the morning. This feature is often overlooked until the patient has a generalized tonic-clonic seizure, and it is frequently not reported unless the patient is prompted.
- A positive family history is not uncommon and is found in 10%–50% of patients, and 21% of asymptomatic family members can have characteristic EEG findings.
- JME patients should be advised that they will most likely be on life-long treatment with one or more ASMs, though myoclonic seizures and tonic-clonic convulsions tend to decline past the fourth decade. All first-line ASMs are expected to offer seizure control and seizure freedom (in 80%–90% of patients) and thus, many patients can live a normal, independent life.
- Several narrow spectrum ASMs, including sodium channel blockers, can worsen JME and hence should be avoided.

It is thought that by *not* eliminating some cells, a hyperexcitable circuit is fostered. Furthermore, this gene participates in providing proper scaffolding for radial migration of neuronal cells during development. Disturbances can cause cortical microdysgenesis and thereby contribute to hyperexcitable networks.

SUGGESTED REFERENCES

Baykan B., Martínez-Juárez I.E., Altindag E.A., Camfield C.S., Camfield P.R. Lifetime prognosis of juvenile myoclonic epilepsy. *Epilepsy Behav* 2013;28(Suppl 1):S18–24.

Camfield C.S., Striano P., Camfield P.R. Epidemiology of juvenile myoclonic epilepsy. *Epilepsy Behav* 2013;28(Suppl 1):S15–7.

Hirsch E., French J., Scheffer I.E., Bogacz A., Alsaadi T., Sperling M.R., Abdulla F., Zuberi S.M., Trinka E., Specchio N., Somerville E., Samia P., Riney K., Nabbout R., Jain S., Wilmshurst J.M., Auvin S., Wiebe S., Perucca E., Moshé S.L., Tinuper P., Wirrell E.C. ILAE definition of the idiopathic generalized epilepsy syndromes: Position statement by the ILAE Task Force on Nosology and Definitions. *Epilepsia* 2022;63:1475–99.

Marson A.G., Al-Kharusi A.M., Alwaidh M., Appleton R., Baker G.A., Chadwick D.W., Cramp C., Cockerell O.C., Cooper P.N., Doughty J., Eaton B., Gamble C., Goulding P.J., Howell S.J., Hughes A., Jackson M., Jacoby A., Kellett M., Lawson G.R., Leach J.P., Nicolaides P., Roberts R., Shackley P., Shen J., Smith D.F., Smith P.E., Smith C.T.,

Vanoli A., Williamson P.R.; The SANAD study of effectiveness of valproate, lamotrigine, or topiramate for generalised and unclassifiable epilepsy: An unblinded randomised controlled trial. SANAD study group. *Lancet* 2007;369:1016–26.

Martínez-Juárez I.E., Alonso M.E., Medina M.T., Durón R.M., Bailey J.N., López-Ruiz M., Ramos-Ramírez R., León L., Pineda G., Castroviejo I.P, Silva R., Mija L., Perez-Gosiengfiao K., Machado-Salas J., Delgado-Escueta A.V. Juvenile myoclonic epilepsy subsyndromes: Family studies and long-term follow-up. *Brain* 2006;129:1269–80.

Santos B.P.D., Marinho C.R.M., Marques T., Angelo L.K.G., Malta M., Duzzioni M., de Castro O.W., Leite J.P., Barbosa F.T., Gitaí D.L.G. Genetic susceptibility in juvenile myoclonic epilepsy: Systematic review of genetic association studies. *PLoS One* 2017;12:e0179629.

Schneider-von Podewils F., Gasse C., Geithner J., Wang Z.I., Bombach P., Berneiser J., Herzer R., Kessler C., Runge U. Clinical predictors of the long-term social outcome and quality of life in juvenile myoclonic epilepsy: 20–65 years of follow-up. *Epilepsia* 2014;55:322–30.

Seneviratne U., Cook M., D'Souza W. Focal abnormalities in idiopathic generalized epilepsy: A critical review of the literature. *Epilepsia* 2014;55:1157–69.

Tashkandi M., Baarma D., Tricco A.C., Boelman C., Alkhater R., Minassian B.A. EEG of asymptomatic first-degree relatives of patients with juvenile myoclonic, childhood absence and rolandic epilepsy: A systematic review and meta-analysis. *Epileptic Disord* 2019;21:30–41.

Thakran S., Guin D., Singh P., Singh P., Kukal S., Rawat C., Yadav S., Kushwaha S.S., Srivastava A.K., Hasija Y., Saso L., Ramachandran S., Kukreti R. Genetic landscape of common epilepsies: Advancing towards precision in treatment. *Int J Mol Sci* 2020;21:7784.

47 Epilepsy with Generalized Tonic-Clonic Seizures Alone

Kaitlin C. James
Monroe Carell Jr Children's Hospital at Vanderbilt

Jesus Eric Pina-Garza
Centennial Children's Hospital

CONTENTS

CASE PRESENTATION

A 14-year-old female presented to the emergency room hours after experiencing an abnormal episode shortly after awakening from sleep. Parents heard a vocalization and found her next to her bed with jerking of all extremities, upward eye deviation, and urinary incontinence. The movements subsided less than 2 minutes after the initial vocalization; breathing immediately after the event was sonorous, deep, and slow. She had some bleeding in her mouth with soreness on both sides of her tongue. Parents noted that she had gone to bed late the night before and was more fatigued than usual. Retrospectively, she had a similar tongue injury noticed upon awakening 6 months earlier. Her past medical history was unremarkable. She was the product of an uneventful pregnancy and delivery without any history of brain insults (trauma or infection). The emergency department provided a rescue medication to be used as needed and she was evaluated in the neurology clinic the next day, at which point she was fully recovered with a normal exam other than healing lacerations on each side of her tongue.

DOI: 10.1201/9781003296478-52

DIFFERENTIAL DIAGNOSIS

The first step when evaluating a suspected convulsion is to determine if the event is epileptic or nonepileptic. Potential etiologies of unresponsiveness with shaking or stiffening include seizure (whether provoked or unprovoked), convulsive syncope, and psychogenic spells. Epileptic seizures tend to be highly stereotyped and sporadic, unpredictable, and brief, with the majority lasting less than 1–2 minutes. Postictal breathing after seizures is slow and labored. Urinary incontinence is much more common in epileptic seizures, and lateral tongue biting is almost pathognomonic for generalized tonic or tonic-clonic seizures.

Convulsive syncope has a classic prodrome of lightheadedness, nausea, clamminess, and darkening of vision. Syncope almost never occurs out of sleep in the absence of heart disease; patients nearly always report a positional component. Psychogenic spells vary significantly and often present as multiple distinct episodes with acute onset and drastic worsening over a few days with spells occurring multiple times per day and lasting for minutes to hours. Postictal breathing is fast in psychogenic episodes due to the physical exertion of the spell. Urinary incontinence is uncommon and tongue biting, if present, tends to be on the tip of the tongue rather than the sides.

The labored and slow postictal breathing and the location of this patient's tongue injury are consistent with a generalized tonic or tonic-clonic seizure; however, the history is not sufficient to differentiate a primary *versus* secondary generalized tonic-clonic seizure. The differential diagnosis in this patient therefore includes focal seizures that evolve to bilateral tonic-clonic seizure such as autosomal dominant nocturnal frontal lobe epilepsy *versus* a genetic generalized epilepsy (GGE) such as juvenile absence epilepsy, juvenile myoclonic epilepsy, or epilepsy with generalized tonic-clonic seizures alone (GTCA).

DIAGNOSTIC APPROACH

In this case, the patient history supports a diagnosis of generalized tonic-clonic seizure. Further history taking determined that she had never experienced any other seizure type; specifically, there was no history of myoclonic or absence seizures. Her one definite seizure was provoked by sleep deprivation and occurred shortly after awakening in the morning. Retrospectively, she noted that she was sleep deprived during one other episode when she awoke with unexplained tongue lacerations. Her younger brother had a history of febrile seizures in infancy. A maternal aunt has unspecified convulsions treated with levetiracetam. The history of isolated generalized tonic-clonic seizure shortly after awakening is highly suggestive of GTCA.

The patient's neurologist obtained an EEG which showed fragments of generalized, 4.5–5 Hz polyspike and spike-wave discharges with a normal background (Figures 47.1 and 47.2). Although the patient had a history of mild specific learning disability in reading, her overall neurological exam was normal, and brain imaging was not required.

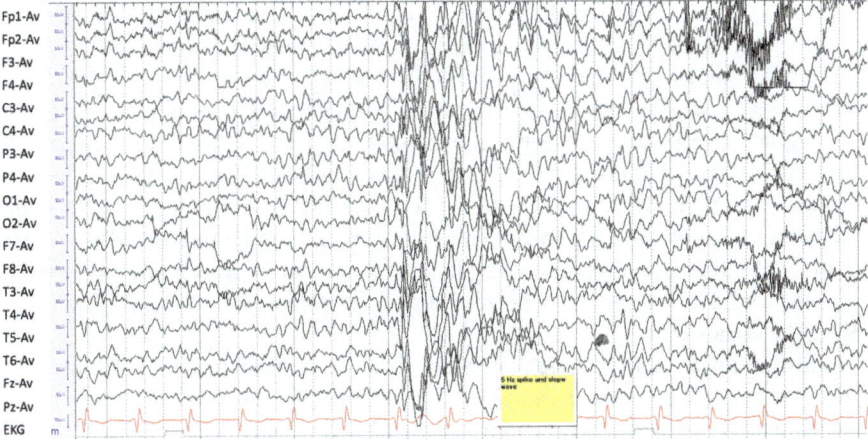

FIGURE 47.1 EEG showing fragments of generalized, 4.5–5 Hz polyspike and spike-wave discharges with a normal background.

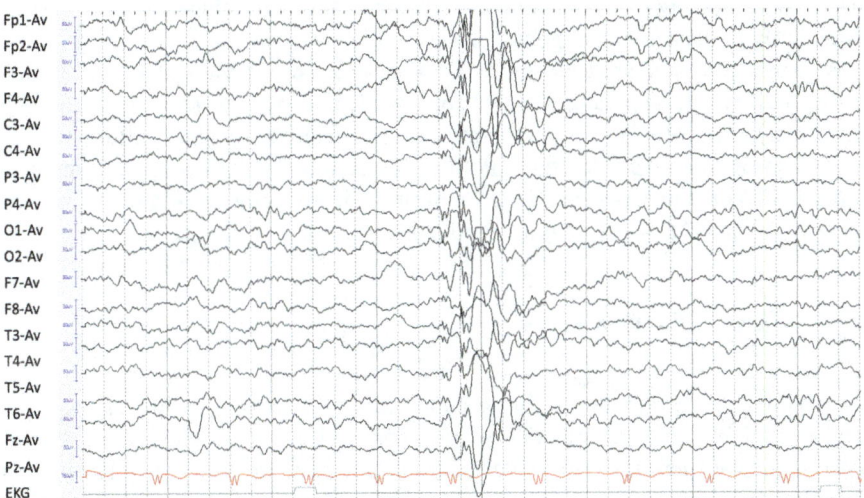

FIGURE 47.2 EEG also showing fragments of generalized, 4.5–5 Hz polyspike and spike-wave discharges with a normal background.

TREATMENT STRATEGY

Our patient has a presumed diagnosis of GTCA, an etiology that overlaps significantly with other GGE syndromes such as childhood absence, juvenile absence, and juvenile myoclonic epilepsies. Epidemiological data are limited by difficulties with terminology and diagnosis, but it is thought that GTCA accounts for up to 30% of the adolescent-onset GGEs. The differentiating characteristic is that in GTCA there are no seizure types present other than generalized tonic-clonic seizures.

There are many antiseizure medications (ASMs) that we can select based on current evidence, standard of care, and FDA indications, including lacosamide, lamotrigine, levetiracetam, perampanel, topiramate, zonisamide, and valproate. These ASMs have roughly equal efficacy at treating the GGEs; therefore, selection should be based on safety and tolerability. For our patient, we prefer levetiracetam or lamotrigine as she is a young woman approaching reproductive age. Both ASMs are thought to be safe in pregnancy, but as lamotrigine requires a prolonged titration time and can interact with hormonal contraceptives, we give a slight preference to levetiracetam.

Zonisamide, lacosamide, and perampanel are not contraindicated, but it must be stressed that their potential teratogenicity is still unclear and therefore adolescent females should be counseled regarding risks and encouraged to consider birth control options prior to initiation. The worst choices would be valproic acid and topiramate as they are known to be teratogenic; valproic acid can also cause hair loss, weight gain, and polycystic ovary syndrome, and topiramate has well-described cognitive side effects that are undesirable in a young student. Adherence to treatment is vital to successful seizure control and once-daily medications are always a better choice, particularly in the adolescent population.

All but lacosamide are available as extended-release formulations for once-daily dosing. In this regard, perampanel and zonisamide may be superior due to their long half-lives, which allow levels to remain near therapeutic for 24 hours after a missed dose. A good cognitive side-effect profile is attractive when selecting the drug, and it should be noted that lacosamide, levetiracetam, lamotrigine, zonisamide, and perampanel all have favorable cognitive profiles.

LONG-TERM OUTCOME

GTCA is not typically associated with developmental delays, regression, or encephalopathy. Several studies have indicated that individuals with GTCA experience a higher incidence of anxiety, depression, and dysfunction in specific cognitive domains such as attention or decision-making. Seizures are typically rare, but resolution of epilepsy is uncommon, and patients often require life-long treatment with ASMs.

PATHOPHYSIOLOGY/NEUROBIOLOGY OF DISEASE

Epilepsy with generalized tonic-clonic seizures alone, like other GGEs, is a complex polygenic disease with a potential environmental component. Specific causative genes have not yet been identified. A family history is suggestive, but many patients have no family history with their epilepsy presumably due to *de novo* or recessive/polygenic mutations.

CLINICAL PEARLS

- Epilepsy with generalized tonic-clonic seizures alone (GTCA) is one of the GGEs, comprising up to 30% of adolescent-onset GGEs.
- The characteristic feature is the presence of solely generalized tonic-clonic seizures.
- Seizures most often occur within 2 hours of awakening but can occur at other times.
- Patients typically respond well to ASMs that carry an indication for generalized tonic-clonic seizures, so side-effect profiles and tolerability should largely determine drug choice.

SUGGESTED REFERENCES

Berkovic S.F., Knowlton R.C., Leroy R.F., Schiemann J., Falter U.; Levetiracetam N01057 Study Group. Placebo-controlled study of levetiracetam in idiopathic generalized epilepsy. *Neurology* 2007;69:1751–60.

Biton V., Montouris G.D., Ritter F., Riviello J.J., Reife R., Lim P., Pledger G. A randomized, placebo-controlled study of topiramate in primary generalized tonic-clonic seizures. Topiramate YTC Study Group. *Neurology* 1999;52(7):1330–7.

Biton V., Di Memmo J., Shukla R., Lee Y.Y., Poverennova I., Demchenko V., Saiers J., Adams B., Hammer A., Vuong A., Messenheimer J. Adjunctive lamotrigine XR for primary generalized tonic-clonic seizures in a randomized, placebo-controlled study. *Epilepsy Behav* 2010;19:352–8.

Camfield P., Camfield C. Idiopathic generalized epilepsy with generalized tonic-clonic seizures (IGE-GTC): A population-based cohort with N20 year follow up for medical and social outcome. *Epilepsy Behav* 2010;18:61–3.

French J.A., Krauss G.L., Wechsler R.T., Wang X.F., DiVentura B., Brandt C., Trinka E., O'Brien T.J., Laurenza A., Patten A., Bibbiani F. Perampanel for tonic-clonic seizures in idiopathic generalized epilepsy A randomized trial. *Neurology* 2015;85:950–7.

Vossler D.G., Knake S., O'Brien T.J., Watanabe M., Brock M., Steiniger-Brach B., Williams P., Roebling R.; SP0982 co-investigators. Efficacy and safety of adjunctive lacosamide in the treatment of primary generalised tonic-clonic seizures: A double-blind, randomised, placebo-controlled trial. *J Neurol Neurosurg Psychiatry* 2020;91:1067–75.

48 Juvenile Absence Epilepsy

Maria Augusta Montenegro
UC San Diego School of Medicine

CONTENTS

CASE PRESENTATION

A 15-year-old girl was seen at the emergency department after presenting with a generalized tonic-clonic seizure (GTCS). The family reported that it was the first seizure that she had ever had, and that it lasted less than 1 minute. However, after careful history taking, the family and patient reported that she had presented brief episodes of staring spells lasting a few seconds over the prior few weeks. There was no history of myoclonic seizures. Neurological examination and brain MRI were normal. An EEG was ordered, and it showed generalized 3.5 Hz spike-and-wave complexes, each lasting a few seconds in length (Figure 48.1). There was no description of impaired awareness during these discharges. Hyperventilation and intermittent photic stimulation did not trigger additional epileptic discharges or seizures. Lamotrigine was started and after reaching the target dose she became seizure-free.

DOI: 10.1201/9781003296478-53

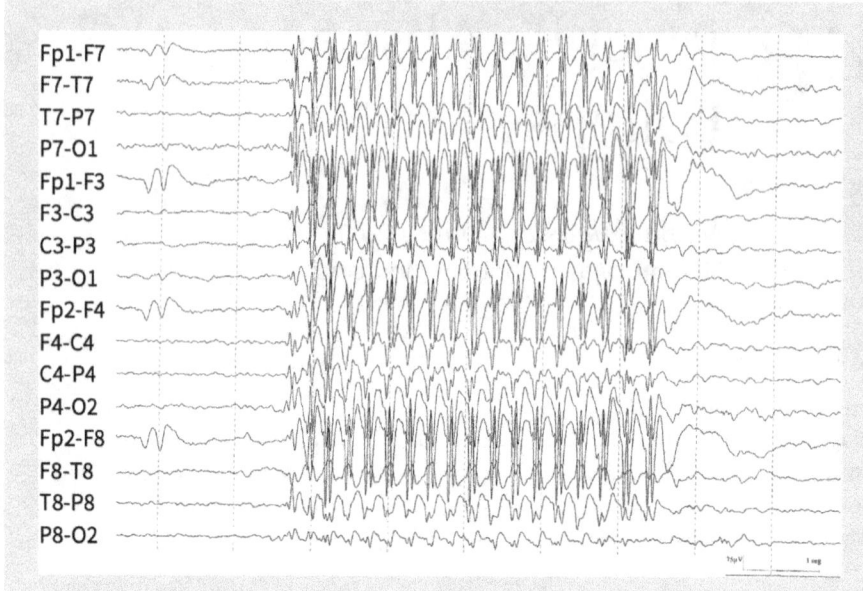

FIGURE 48.1   EEG showing generalized regular 3.5 Hz spike-and-wave complexes in a patient with juvenile absence epilepsy.

DIFFERENTIAL DIAGNOSIS

Childhood absence epilepsy (CAE), juvenile absence epilepsy (JAE), juvenile myoclonic epilepsy (JME), and epilepsy with generalized tonic-clonic seizures alone (GTCA) are classified as genetic generalized epilepsies (GGEs). As opposed to CAE where girls are more frequently affected, boys and girls are equally affected in JAE. Also, absence seizures in patients with JAE tend to be longer, less frequent, and are not as easily triggered by hyperventilation as those seen in children with CAE. The symptoms of various GGEs overlap, and Table 48.1 summarizes the main differences between each type.

DIAGNOSTIC APPROACH

The diagnosis is based on clinical and electroencephalographic (EEG) characteristics. Most patients will seek medical help only after the first GTCS, and they may not recognize and report the occurrence of absence or myoclonic seizures unless carefully interviewed during history taking. The interictal EEG shows a normal background with paroxysms of generalized regular spike-and-wave complexes at a frequency of 3–4 Hz (range of 3–5.5 Hz). It might be fragmented during drowsiness or sleep. Irregular polyspike-and-waves may also occur. As with most GGEs, intermittent photic stimulation can trigger generalized polyspike-and-wave discharges but this phenomenon is rare in JAE. During an absence seizure, the ictal EEG shows

TABLE 48.1

Characteristics of the Different Types of Idiopathic Generalized Epilepsies

Type of Epilepsy	Childhood Absence Epilepsy (CAE)	Juvenile Absence Epilepsy (JAE)	Juvenile Myoclonic Epilepsy (JME)	Epilepsy with Generalized Tonic-Clonic Seizures Alone (GTCA)
Most Common Age of Onset	4–10 years	9–15 years	10–20 years	10–20 years
Type of Seizures	Absence	Absence (longer and less frequent than in CAE) GTC	Absence GTC Myoclonic	GTC
Interictal EEG	3 Hz (2.5–4 Hz) regular SW complexes, OIRDA	3 Hz (up to 5.5 Hz) regular SW complexes (PSW complexes may occur)	3–5.5 Hz spike and irregular PSW complexes	3–5.5 Hz PSW wave complexes

GTC, generalized tonic-clonic; OIRDA, occipital intermittent rhythmic delta activity; SW, spike-and-wave; PSW, polyspike and wave.

generalized regular 3–4 Hz spike-and-wave complexes. The morphology of the discharges is identical to the ones seen in CAE; however, it can be faster (up to 5.5 Hz) in patients with JAE.

Patients with JAE often have a positive family history of epilepsy, but the type of GGE may not be concordant within the same family, with different individuals having different types of epilepsy (CAE, JAE, JME, and GTCA). GGEs are genetically linked and several genes have already been described; however, there is no genetic test available for the diagnosis of these epilepsies. That is mostly because variable expressivity (same mutation producing different phenotypes) and locus heterogeneity (same disease caused by mutations in different genes) are frequently seen in genetic epilepsies.

TREATMENT STRATEGY

Valproate, ethosuximide, and lamotrigine are the most common antiseizure medications (ASMs) used in the treatment of absence seizures. Although valproate is highly effective in the treatment of absence seizures, it should not be considered as first-line therapy in women of child-bearing age due to its association with polycystic ovary syndrome, reproductive, endocrine, menstrual disorders, and potential teratogenic effects.

Ethosuximide is effective only in the treatment of absence seizures, and it is more frequently used in the treatment of CAE. Patients with JAE often have generalized tonic-clonic seizures; therefore, ethosuximide should not be considered as the

CLINICAL PEARLS

- Seizure frequency in patients with JAE is much lower than with CAE. Later age of onset, less frequent absence seizures, and the presence of generalized tonic-clonic seizures are more in keeping with JAE.
- Myoclonic seizures in a patient with absence and generalized tonic-clonic seizures suggest the diagnosis of JME, not JAE.
- Patients with GGEs may not recognize and report the occurrence of absence or myoclonic seizures unless carefully interviewed during history taking.
- Because JAE might be a life-long condition, the choice of ASM in women of child-bearing age should be individually tailored, and with consideration of possible contraception needs or a future pregnancy.

first-line option in the treatment of patients with JAE. However, ethosuximide can be used as add-on therapy if absence seizures are not controlled.

Although lamotrigine is not as effective as ethosuximide and valproate in the treatment of absence seizures, it is not a hepatic enzyme inducer (therefore, it does not interact with other medications such as hormonal contraceptives), and it has a relatively safe teratogenic profile. Therefore, it should be considered as an option in the treatment of JAE in women of child-bearing age.

Levetiracetam, topiramate, phenobarbital, clobazam, clonazepam, zonisamide, perampanel, and brivaracetam are effective in the treatment of generalized seizures in patients with GGEs. However, these medications are usually used in patients with JAE only if first-line ASMs are ineffective.

LONG-TERM OUTCOME

Most patients with JAE will become seizure-free after introduction of an ASM, but the relapse rate can be much higher than CAE after drug discontinuation. For some patients, JAE is a life-long condition, and ASM therapies should be carefully tailored to prevent long-term adverse effects, and folic acid should be supplemented in women of child-bearing age. ASM serum levels should be closely followed during pregnancy, especially if the patient is on lamotrigine.

SUGGESTED REFERENCES

Glauser T.A., Cnaan A., Shinnar S., Hirtz D.G., Dlugos D., Masur D., Clark P.O., Capparelli E.V., Adamson P.C.; Childhood Absence Epilepsy Study Group. Ethosuximide, valproic acid, and lamotrigine in childhood absence epilepsy. *N Engl J Med* 2010;362:790–9.

Hirsch E., French J., Scheffer I.E., Bogacz A., Alsaadi T., Sperling M.R., Abdulla F., Zuberi S.M., Trinka E., Specchio N., Somerville E., Samia P., Riney K., Nabbout R., Jain S., Wilmshurst J.M., Auvin S., Wiebe S., Perucca E., Moshé S.L., Tinuper P., Wirrell

E.C. ILAE definition of the idiopathic generalized epilepsy syndromes: Position statement by the ILAE Task Force on Nosology and Definitions. *Epilepsia* 2022;63: 1475–99.

Scheffer I.E., Berkovic S., Capovilla G., Connolly M.B., French J., Guilhoto L., Hirsch E., Jain S., Mathern G.W., Moshé S.L., Nordli D.R., Perucca E., Tomson T., Wiebe S., Zhang Y.H., Zuberi S.M. ILAE classification of the epilepsies: Position paper of the ILAE commission for classification and terminology. *Epilepsia* 2017;58:512–21.

Specchio N., Wirrell E.C., Scheffer I.E., Nabbout R., Riney K., Samia P., Guerreiro M., Gwer S., Zuberi S.M., Wilmshurst J.M., Yozawitz E., Pressler R., Hirsch E., Wiebe S., Cross H.J., Perucca E., Moshé S.L., Tinuper P., Auvin S. International League Against Epilepsy classification and definition of epilepsy syndromes with onset in childhood: Position paper by the ILAE Task Force on nosology and definitions. *Epilepsia* 2022;63:1398–442.

Stephen L.J., Brodie M.J. Pharmacological management of the genetic generalized epilepsies in adolescents and adults. *CNS Drugs* 2020;34:147–61.

Trinka E., Baumgartner S., Unterberger I., Unterrainer J., Luef G., Haberlandt E., Bauer G. Long-term prognosis for childhood and juvenile absence epilepsy. *J Neurol* 2004; 251:1235–41.

Verroti A., D'Egidio C., Mohn A., Coppola G., Parisi P., Chiarelli F. Antiepileptic drugs, sex hormones and PCOS. *Epilepsia* 2011;52:199–211.

49 New-Onset Seizure in an Adolescent Female

Mary L. Zupanc
University of California-Irvine

CONTENTS

CASE PRESENTATION

A previously healthy 14-year-old adolescent girl presents with a new-onset generalized tonic-clonic seizure. She describes sitting at her computer in the early evening hours after having been to a slumber party with her friends the night before. Suddenly, she felt somewhat "dizzy" and confused. This was followed quickly by a generalized tonic-clonic seizure without focal features. The seizure lasted approximately 5 minutes and was followed by a 20-minute period of post-ictal lethargy and confusion. A witness called 911 and she was taken by ambulance to the local emergency room. Her physical examination was normal. Routine blood chemistries were performed, along with a toxicology screen. A head CT scan was also performed. All studies were normal. She was advised to be seen in follow-up by a neurologist.

DIFFERENTIAL DIAGNOSIS

This patient had a single unprovoked generalized tonic-clonic seizure while sitting in front of a computer, in the context of sleep deprivation, with possible drowsiness. The computer raises the possibility of photosensitivity, which can be seen with generalized epilepsy syndromes. However, the patient complained of dizziness prior to the onset of her generalized tonic-clonic seizure. This could represent a focal seizure with impaired awareness, followed by motor symptoms that appeared to be generalized tonic-clonic in nature. Alternatively, this could imply that the patient had a brief train of generalized or focal polyspike/spike-and-slow wave discharges, which may clinically present with dizziness and confusion. It is not surprising that she was drowsy when she had her seizure. Drowsiness and sleep deprivation are often strong precipitating factors for individuals with a predisposition for epilepsy.

Although it is most likely that the patient had her first unprovoked, epileptic seizure, one must also exclude the possibility of a cardiac dysrhythmia or vasovagal syncope as the etiology for this patient's paroxysmal event. It would be unusual for vasovagal syncope to occur when a patient is seated comfortably without a change from sitting to standing. In addition, without a prior history of heart disease or chest palpitations, it would also be unlikely that this patient had a cardiac arrhythmia. Nonetheless, prolonged QT syndrome can be insidious and should probably be excluded in this case.

To arrive at a specific diagnosis for this patient, additional diagnostic tests were ordered, including (1) EKG with rhythm strip, which was normal; (2) MRI scan of the brain (3-Tesla) with special coronal cuts through the temporal lobe, which was normal; and (3) awake and sleep EEG, which demonstrated intermittent generalized bursts of high amplitude, polyspike, spike-and-slow wave discharges at 3–6 Hz. She also had generalized discharges with photic stimulation. When the patient was seen by the pediatric neurologist, it was discovered that she had had intermittent jitteriness in the morning, which the patient and parents had attributed to clumsiness upon awakening and sleepiness.

What is this patient's diagnosis? Based on the testing and clinical history, the most likely diagnosis is juvenile myoclonic epilepsy (JME). JME is a genetic generalized epilepsy (GGE) syndrome and presents during adolescence. This patient's jitteriness in the morning was most likely myoclonic jerks associated with generalized polyspike, spike-and-slow wave discharges. Therefore, our patient has confirmed epilepsy. She has not only had a single unprovoked generalized tonic-clonic seizure but has also had daily myoclonic seizures.

JME is inherited through complex, poorly defined, genetic mechanisms. It is characterized by generalized tonic-clonic seizures, myoclonic seizures, and absence seizures. It is typically a lifelong epilepsy syndrome, although it becomes milder in the third and fourth decades. JME requires long-term treatment with antiseizure medications (ASMs). Even if a patient with JME has been seizure-free for many years, discontinuation of ASMs usually results in seizure recurrence.

When the diagnosis of epilepsy is made in an adolescent woman, there are many unique considerations, especially since she will require ASM treatment throughout her reproductive years. What advice can we give to healthcare providers who take care of adolescent women with epilepsy? Talking to the adolescent honestly and with compassion will go a long way. In addition, the adolescent needs time to discuss personal issues without a parent present. It may be the only time that a healthcare provider will learn the adolescent's most pressing concerns, which could include social/peer relationships, contraception, concerns about ASM effects on cognitive or athletic performance, driving, and other issues.

The diagnosis of epilepsy is managed best in a clinic designed for an adolescent. The checklist of topics should include (1) the need for ASM; (2) the importance of seizure control; (3) medication side effects, with emphasis on attention and concentration and cognitive processing difficulties; (4) nutrition; (5) school performance and attendance as well as participation in sports; (6) signs of depression; (7) sleep deprivation; (8) contraception; (9) use of recreational drugs and alcohol; and (10) driving a motorized vehicle (Table 49.1).

TREATMENT STRATEGIES

Medication choice should be tailored to the epilepsy syndrome. In our patient, after a careful diagnostic evaluation, she was found to have one of the most common generalized epilepsy syndromes: JME. The ASMs for use in JME syndrome include valproate, lamotrigine, and levetiracetam. Other ASMs have sometimes been used, including topiramate, zonisamide, and clobazam, but they are not as well studied.

Valproate is relatively contraindicated in women with epilepsy during their reproductive years, given the increased risk of anovulatory cycles, menstrual irregularities, polycystic ovaries, and polycystic ovarian syndrome, as well as its teratogenic effects, including neurocognitive effects on the fetus. Lamotrigine and levetiracetam are being increasingly used by pediatric neurologists as alternative choices in the treatment of JME. They appear to have a more favorable side-effect profile. However, lamotrigine does carry the risk of hypersensitivity (for a child, 0.8%; for an adult, 0.3%), but the risk of a serious allergic rash is minimized if a slow titration schedule is used. It does not affect the appetite. There is no known effect on cognitive abilities. Levetiracetam is also a reasonable choice as an ASM, as it has no known drug interactions and is renally excreted. Furthermore, there are no reported cognitive effects, and it rarely causes an allergic rash. Despite this favorable profile, levetiracetam can induce behavioral disinhibition, agitation, aggression, and depression.

In utero ASM exposure can result in teratogenic effects in the fetus. There are multiple, prospective, observational pregnancy registries that have been ongoing for several years and have provided us with good information. Neural tube defects, as

---

TABLE 49.1

Checklist for Adolescent Epilepsy Visit

- Seizure control and the need for antiseizure medication(s)
- Medication side effects: emphasis on attention and concentration, as well as cognitive processing
- Nutrition-balanced diet, folate supplementation, calcium, and vitamin D
- School performance and attendance
- Sports participation
- Signs of depression
- Sleep deprivation
- Contraception
- Recreational drugs and alcohol
- Motor vehicle driving and driver's license

well as cardiac, urogenital, and craniofacial congenital malformations, have been observed with ASMs during pregnancy, with the highest risk consistently associated with valproate, at 10.3%. Lamotrigine and levetiracetam are the ASMs with the lowest risk of fetal malformations: 2.9% and 2.8%, respectively. The risk of teratogenicity also appears to be dose-related. The lower the dosage of ASM, the lower the risk of fetal malformation. In the pregnancy registries, a valproate dose of less than 650 mg daily has been associated with a significant decrease in the risk of fetal malformations. With the most recently approved ASMs, the teratogenic risks are not fully known. We must wait for further information to be collected through the pregnancy registries. Certainly, these considerations should be fully disclosed to adolescents and their parents when discussing ASM choices.

In summary, due to complex interactions between ASMs and hormonal regulation, young adolescent women with epilepsy are at risk for reproductive and endocrine disturbances, including polycystic ovarian syndrome, anovulatory cycles, menstrual irregularities, reduced fertility, sexual dysfunction, and premature menopause. If they are taking valproate, the risks of these disturbances are higher than with other ASMs.

CONTRACEPTION

All adolescents should be presumed to be sexually active. Oral contraceptives (OCPs) are an excellent option, provided that the adolescent can be responsible and fully compliant. However, if the adolescent is started on an OCP, there is the possibility of seizure exacerbation, due to induction of the enzymes that metabolize her ASMs, such as lamotrigine. Furthermore, ASMs can have an impact on OCPs, with induction of OCP metabolism, especially by ASMs that induce the cytochrome P450 enzyme system. This can result in contraceptive failure.

For optimal contraception, OB-GYN subspecialists recommend either depot medroxyprogesterone acetate injections (Depo-Provera™) or the copper T intrauterine device that has been approved for nulliparous women. The depot medroxyprogesterone acetate injection is an excellent short-term solution, but it does carry an increased risk of osteoporosis if used chronically. In addition, just as with oral contraception, women with epilepsy who are taking CYP450 enzyme-inducing ASMs need to receive their injections more frequently than every 3 months, due to the induction of the sex steroid metabolism.

CATAMENIAL SEIZURES/EPILEPSY

Catamenial seizures can be an issue for adolescent women with epilepsy. Catamenial epilepsy is defined as at least the doubling of seizures or seizures occurring almost exclusively during specific times during the menstrual cycle. Its incidence is estimated at 33%. However, menstrual seizure exacerbations, although not meeting the criteria for catamenial epilepsy, have been reported to be as high as 70% of all women with epilepsy, including young adolescent women. During menstruation and ovulation, the estrogen-to-progesterone ratio is at its highest, favoring a proconvulsant state. Women who experience anovulatory cycles may also have menstrual-related seizures. These may be more difficult to recognize, as the seizures occur throughout the ovulatory, luteal, and menstrual phases.

There is no specific treatment for catamenial seizures that is approved by the US Food and Drug Administration (FDA). However, the Progesterone Treatment Trial ($n = 294$) was a randomized, double-blind placebo-controlled trial of natural progesterone supplements for catamenial epilepsy. This study indicated that progesterone lozenges or suppositories may be helpful in the prevention of catamenial seizures, especially in the subgroup analysis in women ($n = 63$) who had at least a tripling of their seizure perimenstrually (i.e., C1 pattern). There was a statistically significant reduction in seizures in this group, but not in the other subgroups. Synthetic progestins such as depot medroxyprogesterone acetate injections (Depo-Provera™), may significantly reduce seizures through a complete suppression of the menstrual cycle.

There are a few other small preliminary studies looking at clobazam and acetazolamide. One study ($n = 18$) investigated clobazam, with a double-blind crossover study using doses of 20 mg/day to 30 mg/day compared with placebo for a period of 10 days during peak seizure-risk time. Seventy-eight percent of these women (14/18) found the clobazam superior to placebo in improving seizure control, with minimal side effects. Another recommended treatment for catamenial seizures has been acetazolamide (Diamox™). In one small, retrospective, self-reporting study ($n = 20$), women with catamenial epilepsy, 40% of women reported a decrease in seizure frequency with doses ranging from 125 mg daily to 750 mg daily. The authors recommended a starting total daily dose of 4 mg/kg/day, maximum 1 g/day. Other proposed treatments have included the use of low-dose estrogen oral contraceptives to minimize the estrogen: progesterone ratio, or, alternatively, simply increasing the patient's primary ASM, if tolerated, to avoid catamenial seizures.

NUTRITION AND BONE HEALTH

Adolescents should be reminded of the importance of good nutrition, particularly during these growth years, with rapid bone mineralization. Daily vitamin supplementation with at least 0.4 mg of folate, maximum 5 mg, is strongly recommended. ASMs may decrease bone mineralization and predispose to osteoporosis. Therefore, calcium and vitamin D supplementation should also be discussed and encouraged.

OTHER ISSUES

Sports play an important role in many adolescents' lives. Fortunately, except for swimming restrictions, epilepsy need not alter a healthy, active lifestyle. In fact, there is no evidence that athletic competition increases the risk for breakthrough seizures. Some studies suggest regular exercise may reduce stress levels and decrease the risk of seizures. It is appropriate, however, to discourage baths and encourage showers, due to an increased risk of drowning in a bathtub.

Driving is permitted in all states after a variable period of complete seizure freedom. Typically, the waiting period is 6 months to 1 year, seizure-free on ASMs. There are a few states, such as California, which require the treating physician to file a mandatory report.

Compliance with ASM is a challenge in all patients with epilepsy, but more so during adolescence. Studies suggest that the biggest risk factor for noncompliance is the age of adolescence. While parents typically administer medication to younger children, as a child grows older, this process undergoes a transition, and the responsibility of compliance begins to shift to the adolescent.

In studies of adolescents with chronic disorders, compliance is reported to be incomplete in 50% of patients. The longer the duration of illness, less vigorous exercise, smoking and alcohol use, and more frequent seizures have been associated with poorer compliance. Strategies to improve compliance include recognizing and exploring the problem with the patient, suggesting ASDs with twice daily or once daily dosing, as well as helping the adolescent set up a routine (bedtime, mealtimes, etc.) for taking the medication. Use of wristwatch alarm reminders can also be helpful.

Lack of adequate sleep is a growing problem among American adolescents, as teens juggle rigorous academic demands, busy social lives, part-time jobs, and late nights at the computer or on their phones. Nowhere is this more relevant than for the adolescent with epilepsy, for whom sleep deprivation may provoke a seizure, as with our patient. The association between sleep deprivation and epilepsy is well documented, particularly in the setting of the genetic generalized epilepsies.

If the adolescent patient is kept as the focus of consultation rather than the parents, the patient is more likely to reveal and discuss concerns. While a specialized adolescent epilepsy clinic may not be feasible for many centers, the strategies employed are applicable to any clinical setting. The practitioner is advised to consider a comprehensive checklist for a visit involving an adolescent with epilepsy (Table 49.1).

LONG-TERM OUTCOME

Any patient who has the onset of epilepsy during adolescence should be counseled that the epilepsy is probably a chronic condition, one that is unlikely to go into remission. For our patient, JME is known as a lifelong condition. This is often very difficult for adolescents to comprehend and accept. The goal is to assist the adolescent and her family in understanding the diagnosis, focusing on the positive aspects of good seizure control, the chance of having a normal life, yet being aware of the risks of comorbid problems such as anxiety and depression. Proactive counseling can go a long way in helping the adolescent achieve an excellent quality of life.

PATHOPHYSIOLOGY/NEUROBIOLOGY OF DISEASE

JME and other epilepsy syndromes present at the onset of adolescence, during menarche and the other changes associated with puberty. Hormonal changes during the menstrual cycle can exert a significant effect on seizure activity, regardless of the seizure type or epilepsy syndrome. In addition, seizures and ASMs can have an impact on hormones, including hormonal dysregulation, altered metabolism of these hormones, and an effect on luteinizing hormone pulsativity.

In animal studies, estrogen is a proconvulsant, facilitating kindling, as well as decreasing the seizure threshold by augmenting excitatory glutamate receptor numbers and activity. Progesterone has anticonvulsant effects through allosteric modulation of the gamma-aminobutyric acid, type A (GABA$_A$) receptor conductance. The effects of estrogen and progesterone are complex and affect the brain in many ways; however, simply put, the ratio of these two hormones influences the tendency for breakthrough seizures.

With some adolescent women, the highest risk for breakthrough seizures is either at the time of ovulation or right before menses, when the estrogen:progesterone ratio is at its peak. For other adolescent women, in particular, those with anovulatory cycles, the risk for breakthrough seizures may persist throughout the cycle, because of the unopposed action of estrogen. In addition, enzyme-inducing ASMs can decrease sex steroid hormones by inducing hepatic metabolism. Valproate, an enzyme inhibitor, is associated with polycystic ovarian syndrome, probably due to multiple mechanisms, including valproate-induced weight gain, inhibition of testosterone breakdown, and possible blockade of progesterone receptors.

CLINICAL PEARLS

- Adolescent women can present with epilepsy at the onset of puberty. One of the most common epilepsy syndromes is juvenile myoclonic epilepsy.
- Adolescence is a time of great change, both physically and emotionally. If an adolescent develops epilepsy, the challenges are considerable, and there are higher risks for comorbid anxiety, depression, and suicide.
- Adolescent women with epilepsy are at risk for reproductive dysfunction, including anovulatory cycles, menstrual irregularities, polycystic ovarian syndrome, and sexual dysfunction. ASMs can increase these risks, particularly the use of valproate. As such, valproate is relatively contraindicated in women with epilepsy during the reproductive age.
- ASMs have teratogenic risks. These risks should be fully disclosed to any adolescent woman and her family during the discussion about ASM choices. Also, there is the additional risk of breakthrough seizures during pregnancy.
- ASMs have hormonal interactions. Therefore, the choice of contraceptive must be tailored for each patient. For example, the ASMs which induce the CYP450 enzyme system produce a more rapid metabolism of sex steroid hormones. Therefore, if an OCP is used in combination with these ASMs, the dose of estrogen in the OCP should be higher, i.e., at least 50 µg. If depot medroxyprogesterone acetate injections (Depo-Provera™) are used, the injections should be given more frequently. Valproate inhibits the CYP450 enzyme system and therefore, does not alter OCP metabolism. Lamotrigine blood levels may decrease when combined with OCPs.

- Catamenial seizures can occur in adolescents. There are several options for treatment, not yet FDA-approved, including optimization of the current ASM, progesterone lozenges, clobazam, and acetazolamide.
- Nutrition is generally less than optimal in adolescents, so it is vital to emphasize the importance of adequate calcium and vitamin D intake, folate supplementation, and overall good nutritional habits. Adolescent women with epilepsy may be at greater risk for osteoporosis than their peers, through a variety of mechanisms, e.g., ASMs, poor intake of calcium, and low vitamin D levels.
- Sports are not contraindicated in individuals with epilepsy.
- An adolescent clinic for patients with epilepsy is the best way to address many of the issues described above.

SUGGESTED REFERENCES

Baykan B., Wolf P. Juvenile myoclonic epilepsy as a spectrum disorder: A focused review. *Seizure* 2017;49:36–41.

Bui E. Women's issues in epilepsy. *Continuum (Minneap Minn)* 2022;28:399–427.

Carlson C., Anderson C.T. Special issues in epilepsy: The elderly, the immunocompromised, and bone health. *Continuum (Minneap Minn)* 2016;22:246–61.

Christian C.A., Reddy D.S., Maguire J., Forcelli P.A. Sex differences in the epilepsies and associated comorbidities: Implications for use and development of pharmacotherapies. *Pharmacol Rev* 2020;72:767–800.

Cohen M.J., Meador K.J., May R. Fetal antiepileptic drug exposure and learning and memory functioning at 6 years of age: The NEAD prospective observational study. *Epilepsy Behav* 2019;92:154–64.

Espinera A.R., Gavvala J., Bellinski I. Counseling by epileptologists affects contraceptive choices of women with epilepsy. *Epilepsy Behav* 2016;65:1–6.

Feely M., Calvert T., Gibson J. Clobazam in catamenial epilepsy. A model for evaluating anticonvulsants. *Lancet* 1982;2:71–3.

Forceuspst B.D., Grossman D. Folic acid supplementation for the prevention of neural tube defects: US preventive services task force recommendation statement. *JAMA* 2017;317:183–9.

Harden C.L., Hopp J., Ting T.Y. Practice parameter update: Management issues for women with epilepsy-focus on pregnancy (an evidence-based review): Obstetrical complications and change in seizure frequency report: Report of the Quality Standards Subcommittee and Therapeutics and Technology Assessment Subcommittee of the American Academy of Neurology and American Epilepsy Society. *Neurology* 2009;73:126–32.

Herzog A.G., Fowler K.M., Smithson S.D., Kalayjian L.A., Heck C.N., Sperling M.R., Liporace J.D., Harden C.L., Dworetzky B.A., Pennell P.B., Massaro J.M.; Progesterone Trial Study Group. Progesterone vs. placebo therapy for women with epilepsy: a randomized clinic trial. *Neurology* 2012;78:1959–66.

Herzog A.G., Klein P., Ransil B.J. Three patterns of catamenial epilepsy. *Epilepsia* 1997;38:1082–8.

Lim L.L., Foldvary N., Mascha E., Lee J. Acetazolamide in women with catamenial epilepsy. *Epilepsia* 2001;42:746–9.

Meador K.J., Baker G.A., Browning N. Cognitive function at 3 years of age after fetal exposure to antiepileptic drugs. *N Engl J Med* 2009;360:1597–605.

Meador K.J., Baker G.A., Browning N. Fetal antiepileptic drug exposure and cognitive outcomes at age 6 years (NEAD study): A prospective observational study. *Lancet Neurol* 2013;12:244–52.

Morrell M.J. Reproductive and metabolic disorders in women with epilepsy. *Epilepsia* 2003;44(Suppl 4):S11–20.

Morrell M.J., Flynn K.L., Seale C.G., Done S., Paulson A.J., Flaster E.R., Ferin M. Reproductive dysfunction in women with epilepsy: Antiepileptic drug effects on sex-steroid hormones. *CNS Spectrums* 2001;6:771–86.

Navis A., Harden C.A. treatment approach to catamenial epilepsy. *Curr Treat Options Neurol* 2016;18:30.

Pack A.M., Morrell M.J. Treatment of women with epilepsy. *Semin Neurol* 2002;22:289–97.

Pack A.M., Morrell M.J., Marcus R., Holloway L., Flaster E., Doñe S., Randall A., Seale C., Shane E. Bone mass and turnover in women with epilepsy on antiepileptic drug monotherapy. *Ann Neurol* 2005;57:252–7.

Pack A.M., Morrell M.J., Randall A., McMahon D.J., Shane E. Bone health in young women with epilepsy after one year of antiepileptic drug monotherapy. *Neurology* 2008;70:1586–93.

Tomson T., Battino D., Perucca E. Teratogenicity of antiepileptic drugs. *Curr Opin Neurol* 2019;32:246–52.

Woodhams E.F., Gilliam M. Contraception. *Ann Intern Med* 2019;170:ITC18–32.

Zupanc M.L. Antiepileptic drugs and hormonal contraceptives in adolescent women with epilepsy. *Neurology* 2006;66(Suppl 3):S37–45.

50 Temporal Lobe Epilepsy

June Yoshii-Contreras
UC San Diego School of Medicine

CONTENTS

CASE PRESENTATION

A 17-year-old right-handed male with a family history epilepsy (maternal uncle with seizure onset in his 20s) was referred for evaluation of seizures. The patient's seizures began at age 16 and were triggered by stress or dehydration. The stereotypic episode began with an indescribable negative feeling, déjà vu, and nausea, followed by loss of awareness, staring off, head deviation to the left, and whole-body stiffening, all lasting less than 3 minutes in duration. These have occurred at a frequency of once every 2–3 months. His neurological exam is unremarkable. Previous evaluation includes a 24-hour electroencephalogram (EEG) and a 1.5T brain magnetic resonance imaging (MRI) scan; both were interpreted as normal. Routine blood work is all within normal limits. He was placed on levetiracetam but developed irritability and depression. Mother was advised to have him follow up with a neurologist.

DIFFERENTIAL DIAGNOSIS

Temporal lobe epilepsy (TLE) is one of the most common types of focal epilepsy. According to the 2022 International League Against Epilepsy (ILAE) classification and definition of epilepsy syndromes, epilepsies are now based on the age of presentation and syndrome type, with temporal lobe epilepsies classified as epilepsy syndrome with onset at variable age. Most clinicians would differentiate mesial TLE, where the

DOI: 10.1201/9781003296478-55

onset is from the hippocampus, amygdala, and other medial structures, from lateral neocortical TLE, where the onset originates from the temporal neocortex. In this chapter, we will be discussing the most common temporal epilepsies in adolescence, including mesial temporal lobe epilepsy with hippocampal sclerosis (MTLE-HS), familial mesial temporal lobe epilepsy (FMTLE), and epilepsy with auditory features (EAF).

For completeness, it is worth mentioning that other pathologies in the temporal regions can cause temporal lobe epilepsy. These include glioneuronal tumors (such as ganglioglioma and dysembryoplastic neuroepithelial tumors), cavernous angiomas, arterial-venous formation, and malformations of cortical developmental such as focal cortical dysplasia and cerebral infections. However, the incidence of these can occur throughout a lifetime, and thus they are outside of the scope of this chapter.

According to the ILAE, mesial temporal lobe epilepsy with hippocampal sclerosis (MTLE-HS) is identified as an etiology-specific epileptic syndrome and has predominantly an acquired etiology; therefore, genetic studies are often not indicated. MTLE-HS is the most common drug-resistant focal seizure disorder with the best outcome following surgery.

DIAGNOSTIC APPROACH

The age of onset is usually in adolescence or early adulthood. Patients have normal intellectual development and neurological examination, although reduced facial movements may be noted on the contralateral side. Cognitive changes are recognized with verbal memory deficits with dominant MTLE-HS and visual memory deficits with nondominant MTLE-HS. Over 50% of patients may have a past medical history of early childhood febrile seizures or status epilepticus.

Seizures are often associated with an aura. The aura can be cognitive (*déjà vu*), emotional (fear), autonomic (tachycardia, flushing), abdominal epigastric rising, or other special sensory (olfactory or gustatory). Focal seizures with impaired awareness are commonly seen with behavioral arrest, oral automatisms, like chewing or lip-smacking, or hand automatisms. Aphasia is frequently observed when seizures arise from the dominant hemisphere. Alternatively, speech may be preserved when seizures originate from the nondominant hemisphere. The most common semiological signs with lateralizing value are dystonic posturing of the hand (contralateral to the ictal activity) and postictal nose wiping (ipsilateral to the ictal activity.) MTLE-HS seizures may progress with inappropriate amnestic behaviors (like undressing and wandering) or evolve to bilateral tonic-clonic seizure activity.

Electrographically, focal slowing over the temporal lobes may be noted during sleep or hyperventilation. Sometimes the slowing can be seen rhythmically forming a well-recognized pattern called temporal intermittent rhythmic delta (TIRDA). Interictally, the most common finding is unilateral anterior temporal lobe discharges during sleep. Bilateral independent discharges have been reported as frequently as 20%–50%. An ictal pattern of sharply contoured rhythmic theta or alpha activity (>5 Hz) over the temporal region when seen at onset (or within 30 seconds) is found to correlate with lateralization of the seizure onset to the lobe.

The most common pathology is hippocampal sclerosis, which reflects abnormal histopathological and functional changes in the hippocampus. Although sometimes used interchangeably, mesial temporal sclerosis (MTS) is defined as pathology in the hippocampus and changes in the amygdala and entorhinal cortex, occasionally extending to the parahippocampal region. Using structural MRI, hippocampal sclerosis can be detected unilateral or bilaterally by visualization of the following features:

- Hippocampal atrophy.
- Loss of definition of the internal structures of the hippocampus.
- Increased hippocampal T2-weighted signal intensity.
- Decreased T1-weighted intensity as well.

Of note, bilateral hippocampal sclerosis is common. One explanation for the bilateral disease is that pathology affects both temporal lobes, such as febrile seizures, status epilepticus, or encephalitis early in life.

PROGNOSIS AND TREATMENT STRATEGY

The first-line therapy is the initiation of an appropriately chosen antiseizure medication (ASM). The most effective ASMs are those used to treat focal-onset epilepsies. The list includes oxcarbazepine, levetiracetam, lamotrigine, topiramate, carbamazepine, perampanel, lacosamide, etc. These ASMs can be administered as monotherapy or in combination.

When choosing an ASM, it is important to consider age, history of mental illness, family planning (future pregnancies), and the side-effect profile of each medication. For patients with intractable or pharmaco-resistant MTLE-HS, presurgical evaluation is warranted. When clinical history, EEG, MRI, and neuropsychological data are all concordant, lateralizing the epileptogenic focus on the same size, one can expect a favorable outcome with epilepsy surgery. Anterior temporal lobectomy is the gold standard for the treatment of pharmaco-resistant MTLE, offering postoperative seizure freedom in 70%–80% of cases. Newer therapies have emerged with almost similar results. These are discussed in other chapters. For patients whom epilepsy surgery fails, an extratemporal seizure onset zone mimicking temporal lobe seizures can be suspected.

FAMILIAL MESIAL TEMPORAL LOBE EPILEPSY (FMTLE)

FMTLE was first identified in a community-based study involving twins. It is a genetic syndrome with a complex mode of inheritance, accounting for almost one-fifth of all newly diagnosed cases of nonlesional mesial TLE. Female predominance has been noted. Clinical recognition is facilitated through a good family history, often requiring direct questioning of relatives.

Diagnostic Approach

The age of onset is between 3 and 63 years of age, with symptoms usually starting in adolescence. Originally, it was described as a benign syndrome with normal intellectual development, normal neurological examination, and no history of febrile seizures. The key is a family history of focal seizures arising from the mesial temporal lobe.

Seizures are mild and subtle, often consisting predominantly of *déjà vu*, and less commonly nausea, perceptual distortions, and fear. Seizures may progress to impaired awareness, rarely to bilateral tonic-clonic activity. Electrographically, approximately 60% show either normal background or temporal slowing. The remaining 40% have unilateral focal epileptiform discharges. Typically, brain MRI is normal. Evidence of hippocampal atrophy or sclerosis is correlated with a poor response to medical treatment.

Prognosis and Treatment Strategy

The syndrome is associated with a benign course. Most patients become seizure free with a single ASM, and polytherapy is only occasionally required. Rarely do they become pharmaco-resistant and require epilepsy surgery.

EPILEPSY WITH AUDITORY FEATURES (EAF)

EAF is characterized by seizures with auditory symptoms or aphasia, suggesting lateral temporal lobe involvement. Appreciation of the clinical features is required for a proper diagnosis and decreases the chances of misdiagnosing EAF as a psychiatric disease. Although it mainly occurs sporadically, there is a familial form called Familial Epilepsy with Auditory Features, which has autosomal dominant inheritance with incomplete penetrance. Microdeletions in *LGI1* or *RELN* account for approximately half the cases. For this syndrome, all affected individuals must have seizures compatible with EAF.

Diagnostic Approach

The age of onset is between 10 and 30 years of age. EAF is associated with normal intellectual development and a normal neurological examination. Focal aware sensory seizures with auditory symptoms and/or receptive aphasia characterize this syndrome. Auditory symptoms include humming, buzzing, ringing, or alteration in perceived volume. Complex sounds such as voices and songs have also been described. Ictal receptive aphasia is in the absence of impairment of awareness. Reflex seizures can occur after hearing a sound. Seizures may progress to impaired awareness and to bilateral tonic-clonic activity.

The interictal EEG is often unremarkable, but focal epileptiform discharges over the temporal region are occasionally noted. Ictal EEG is rarely documented. Although the brain MRI is typically normal, in rare cases a structural lesion can be seen, and epilepsy surgery could favorably impact the outcome in those selected patients.

Prognosis and Treatment Strategy

EAF has a good response to ASMs for focal epilepsy. Outcomes can range from mild seizures with spontaneous remission to highly pharmaco-resistant seizures. Three key factors have negative effects on remission, causing poor long-term outcomes. These are:

- Early age of onset (<10 years).
- Complex auditory hallucinations.
- Focal EEG epileptiform activity.

As mentioned above, epilepsy surgery can be considered in cases of pharmaco-resistant epilepsy, with a good outcome for those with structural lesions. When considering ASM withdrawal, it is essential to counsel patients and their families that medication withdrawal often leads to clinical relapses that do not always respond to reinitiation of the treatment.

CLINICAL PEARLS

- Temporal lobe epilepsy is one of the most common causes of focal epilepsy
- Most clinicians would differentiate mesial TLE, where the onset is from the hippocampus, amygdala, and other medial structures, from lateral neocortical TLE
- The most common types of temporal lobe epilepsy are: mesial temporal lobe epilepsy with hippocampal sclerosis, familial mesia temporal lobe epilepsy, and epilepsy with auditory features.

SUGGESTED REFERENCES

Furia A., Licchetta L., Muccioli L., Ferri L., Mostacci B., Mazzoni S., Menghi V., Minardi R., Tinuper P., Bisulli F. Epilepsy with auditory features: From etiology to treatment. *Front Neurol* 2022;12:807939.

Gambardella A., Labate A., Giallonardo A., Aguglia U. Familial mesial temporal lobe epilepsies: Clinical and genetic features. *Epilepsia* 2009;50(Suppl 5):S55–57.

Kuzniecky R.I., Jackson G.D. *Magnetic Resonance in Epilepsy: Neuroimaging Techniques.* Elsevier Academic, Burlington, MA, 2nd ed., 2005, 442 p.

Riney K., Bogacz A., Somerville E., Hirsch E., Nabbout R., Scheffer I.E., Zuberi S.M., Alsaadi T., Jain S., French J., Specchio N., Trinka E., Wiebe S., Auvin S., Cabral-Lim L., Naidoo A., Perucca E., Moshé S.L., Wirrell E.C., Tinuper P. International League Against Epilepsy classification and definition of epilepsy syndromes with onset at a variable age: Position statement by the ILAE Task Force on Nosology and Definitions. *Epilepsia* 2022;63:1443–74.

51 Unverricht– Lundborg Disease

Mayank Verma and Berge A. Minassian
University of Texas Southwestern Medical Center

Danielle M. Andrade
University of Toronto

CONTENTS

CASE PRESENTATION

The patient is a 20-year-old male referred to the Epilepsy Clinic for evaluation of seizures and "gait problems". He was the product of an uneventful pregnancy and born to non-consanguineous parents from an island in the Mediterranean. Developmental milestones were attained at appropriate ages, and he had an otherwise normal development until the onset of seizures. His first generalized tonic-clonic (GTC) seizure was at the age of 11 years during a hockey game. This type of seizure recurred over the next 7 years, despite treatment with valproic acid and clonazepam, with a frequency of 2–6 per year. However, for the last 2 years, he has not had any GTC seizures. There were no clear precipitating factors, except for flashing lights. Since the onset of GTC seizures, he was also experiencing multifocal, fragmentary, stimulus-sensitive myoclonus. These were sudden, brief shock-like muscle contractions that at times generalized and interfered with activities of daily living, such as writing, swallowing, speaking, and walking. He also developed ataxia and dysarthria. These symptoms appeared insidiously and progressed slowly. His behavior also changed, and he became very introspective. Over the past few months, he exhibited occasional episodes of aggressiveness, which were never seen before and had not been reported in any of his three healthy male siblings. A clinical evaluation suggested that these episodes were nonepileptic in nature. Finally, the patient dropped out of school after doing poorly for the past two academic years. His neurological exam was significant for the presence of appendicular and truncal ataxia, dysarthria, postural and action tremor worse on the right side, and myoclonus. He required a walker given the severity of the myoclonus. He had a score of 4 on the simplified standard myoclonus rating scale (i.e., moderate-to-severe myoclonus; interference with fine movements, speech, and patient is able to stand but unable to walk without assistance). Brain magnetic resonance imaging (MRI) scan and a routine electroencephalogram (EEG) were normal. Genetic testing showed homozygous expansion of a dodecamer repeat in the promoter region of the CSTB (or EMP1) gene, thus confirming the diagnosis of Unverricht–Lundborg disease (ULD). The patient was treated with levetiracetam (which was added to valproic acid), which led to clinical improvement (score of 2 using the same myoclonus rating scale), 6 months later.

DIFFERENTIAL DIAGNOSIS

The presence of seizures, myoclonus, and progressive neurological deterioration (ataxia, dysarthria, and tremor), in addition to psychiatric symptoms (social withdrawal, depression, anxiety, aggression, and dementia), is strongly suggestive of progressive myoclonus epilepsy (PME). PME represents a group of more than 20 diseases, and although sharing common features, these diseases are distinct in terms of etiology, pathogenesis, and prognosis. The five most common and better characterized PMEs are as follows: Unverricht–Lundborg disease (ULD), Lafora disease (LD), the neuronal ceroid lipofuscinosis, sialidosis type 1, and myoclonic epilepsy with ragged red fibers (MERRF).

Onset between late childhood and late adolescence occur more commonly due to ULD or LD. Both entities are inherited in an autosomal recessive fashion. ULD and LD occur worldwide but are more prevalent in the Mediterranean region. ULD is seen with increased frequency in Finland but may be underdiagnosed in other regions. In both diseases, absence, focal impaired awareness, and focal motor seizures may occur in addition to generalized tonic-clonic and myoclonic seizures. However, in LD patients, seizures become increasingly difficult to control with antiseizure medications (ASMs). Occipital-onset seizures are suggestive of LD.

Despite progress in therapeutics, LD is universally fatal within 10–20 years after onset. In contrast, ULD patients may have a normal lifespan. Notably, in the above case, there was a paucity of seizures during the first few years after onset, and the patient was actually seizure free for the past 2 years. The relatively mild progression 9 years after clinical onset is suggestive of ULD rather than LD.

DIAGNOSTIC APPROACH

ULD usually presents between 6 and 15 years of age. It affects male and females equally. In ULD, generalized tonic-clonic seizures are the first symptom in half the cases, whereas in the other half, the presenting symptom is stimulus-sensitive myoclonus. Rare ULD patients never develop GTC seizures. Ataxia, dysarthria, and intentional tremor develop overtime. ULD patients may show a slow decline in intelligence (10 points IQ drop per decade). Their mood is labile, and depression is common.

There are no clear hallmarks of the disease via bloodwork. Biochemically, half of ULD patients present with increased urinary excretion of indicant. This is a nonspecific finding that was also reported in other disorders presenting with myoclonus and more likely due to gut dysmotility than the myoclonus. Reduction of tryptophan and 5-hydroxyindole-acetic acid (5-HIAA) was observed in the serum of ULD patients. Lastly, there is evidence of a reduction in CSF monoamines in these patients, a feature found in other myoclonus epilepsies as well. Brain MRI is usually normal or it may show nonspecific diffuse atrophy. EEGs early in the course of the disease may be within normal limits in some patients or may show abnormalities even before onset of symptoms in others. Common abnormalities include (1) slow and disorganized background activity; (2) runs of interictal epileptiform activity in the form of fast spike-and-wave or polyspike-and-wave discharges, recorded in a generalized or multifocal distribution; and (3) photoparoxysmal response (PPR), which is common and initially presents with a broad range of frequencies. The interictal epileptiform abnormalities diminish with appropriate ASM treatment. Interestingly, epileptiform abnormalities may be seen in patients who never experience clinical seizures. The stimulus-sensitive myoclonus is time locked to the cortical spikes. Cortical hyperexcitability is further demonstrated by giant somatosensory evoked potentials (SSEPs) and an enhanced long-loop (cortical) reflex.

ULD is a neurodegenerative disease without accumulation of storage material or a specific pathologic marker. Previous histopathological studies of patients who died from ULD demonstrated cerebellar granular and Purkinje cell loss, gliosis, and neuronal degeneration of the anterior, lateral, medial, and reticular nuclei of the thalamus. Such studies also reported degenerative changes in the cortex, striatum, mamillary bodies, multiple brainstem nuclei, and ventral gray matter of the spinal cord.

Prior to the discovery of the gene responsible for the great majority of ULD cases, the diagnosis was based on clinical findings, progression, and on the absence of storage material on peripheral tissue or brain biopsies. ULD is an autosomal recessive disease caused by pathogenic variants in the *EPM1* gene. This gene codes for cystatin B (CSTB). Few patients have point mutations in the coding region of the gene. The most common mutation by far is an expansion of an unstable dodecamer repeat in the promoter region of CSTB leading to a reduction in protein production. Normal alleles in this region contain two to three tandem copies of the dodecamer. ULD patients have 30–150 copies. This leads to a reduction in the CSTB protein but not a complete absence.

As a cysteine protease inhibitor, CSTB has also been implicated in the immune system as well as the bone. In a study examining the bone structure of 66 patients with ULD, several differences were noted compared to the recruited control cohort. They were found to have increased thickness of the skull bone, especially in the frontal bone (1.79 fold higher in male and 1.65 fold higher in women). In addition, osteoporotic bone structure was found on head computed tomography (CT). Additional skeletal abnormalities were found in 61% of these patients including scoliosis, large paranasal sinuses, and the presence of *os tibiale externum*. Thickening of the skull bones is a known side effect of phenytoin, but these differences were not influenced by prior phenytoin in this study. The mouse model for ULD sheds some light on the possible mechanism, which shows reduced osteoclast number and function and trabecular bone abnormalities in the *Cstb*$^{-/-}$ mouse. This was thought to be due to its effect on cathepsin K but experimental validation is pending.

TREATMENT STRATEGY

There is no specific treatment for ULD. Initially, seizures can usually be controlled with valproic acid. Clonazepam can be used as an add-on drug for both seizures and myoclonus. Zonizamide has also shown some benefits in terms of seizure control. High doses of piracetam are used to control myoclonus with moderate efficiency both in the short and long term. Levetiracetam (which is structurally related to piracetam) can also be used to control myoclonus (and possibly tonic-clonic seizures) on a long-term basis, especially in younger patients. In patients previously treated with piracetam, a switch to levetiracetam was not always possible, and a combination of piracetam and levetiracetam appeared to be the best approach. Perampanel has been shown to be effective in patients with several PMEs including ULD.

N-Acetylcysteine has been shown to improve tremor, gait, and myoclonus. The mechanism of action of N-acetylcysteine is poorly understood but is likely related to protection against oxidative stress. Interestingly, N-acetylcysteine has been shown to prevent apoptotic death of cultured neuronal cells deprived of nerve growth factors. It is tempting to speculate that N-acetylcysteine is protective against the apoptosis shown to characterize ULD neurodegeneration. Of note, phenytoin worsens the symptoms in ULD and should always be avoided. It was argued that the cerebellar neurodegeneration reported in the older literature on ULD was due to phenytoin neurotoxicity. However, animal models of ULD without phenytoin still show severe cerebellar degeneration. In one retrospective review, lamotrigine showed lack of efficacy or worsening of myoclonic jerks in five patients with ULD. Two randomized control trials for adjunctive brivaracetam showed favorable tolerability but failed to show an improvement in action myoclonus.

LONG-TERM OUTCOME

In the 1960s and early 1970s, the mean survival of ULD patients was 14 years after the onset of symptoms. At present, it is clear that clinical evolution of ULD is greatly influenced by the treatment received. In many patients, dementia can be averted, and myoclonus and seizures can be minimized. Avoidance of phenytoin is key to this goal. Phenytoin is exquisitely toxic to ULD patients and is likely a major contributor to the severity of cases described in the past. Clinical severity may vary even within families with the same genetic mutation and no genetic modifiers have yet been described.

In younger cohorts of patients, severity of functional impairment varied. Severe impairment in mobility, such as being wheelchair bound or bedridden, varied between 7% and 16% and need for help for activities of daily living varied between

30% and 38%. Seventy per cent were able to walk unassisted and 30% held a job. In all patients studied, myoclonus was mild at onset, worsened during the first 5-10 years after onset, but stabilized subsequently. Remission followed an active phase of epilepsy which occurred during the first 10 years of the disease. Serial EEGs suggested that brain activity was influenced by pharmacological treatment. Background activity tended to normalize and the photoparoxysmal response tended to abate over the years.

A recent nationwide population-based study from Finland showed severe impairment of mobility was higher in this cohort with almost 50% being wheelchair bound or bedridden and only 20% living unassisted. These patients die prematurely starting around age 40 from disease-related reasons. In a separate study, it was found that the most common cause of death for these patients was sudden unexpected death in epilepsy or SUDEP (30%), followed by complications of severe ULD (30%). There appear to be regional differences in the severity of patients with the Finnish patients being affected more severely than the Mediterranean cohort.

PATHOPHYSIOLOGY/NEUROBIOLOGY OF DISEASE

The gene responsible for ULD was identified using a positional cloning approach. The disease-causing gene, named CSTB or EPM1, is a 674 base-pair gene that contains three exons and localizes to chromosome 21q22.3. *CSTB* encodes a cysteine protease inhibitor called cystatin B (CSTB). The identification of two point mutations found in CSTB proved that this gene was responsible for ULD. To date, 17 different point mutations have been identified in EPM1. Some mutations affect conserved splice-site sequences and predict severe splicing defects. Others lead to protein truncation, and yet others affect a conserved amino acid sequence critical for cathepsins (i.e., the target proteases) binding. However, these mutations within the transcriptional unit account for less than 10% of EPM1 alleles causing ULD. More than 90% of patients have unstable expansion, described above, of a dodecamer repeat (5'CCCCGCCCCGCG-3') 175 base pairs upstream from the translation initiation codon of *CSTB*.

In contrast to some neurodegenerative disorders caused by trinucleotide repeat expansions, there is no correlation between the number of repeats and clinical severity or age of onset in ULD patients. It is suggested that once the dodecamer repeat expands beyond a critical threshold, CSTB gene expression is reduced, leading to pathological and physiological consequences. There seems to be a dosage response of CSTB deficiency as patients with lower CSTB have more severe PME and the patients lacking CSTB completely present as neonatal developmental encephalopathy.

CSTB functions as an intracellular protease inhibitor, able to inhibit cathepsins (lysosomal proteases). In humans, CSTB deficiency causes ectopic histone H3 tail cleavage in neural progenitors leading to aberrant differentiation and mitochondrial dysfunction. It has been shown that CSTB knockout mice demonstrate apoptotic cell death. These data suggest that CSTB also has a role in preventing apoptotic cell death in certain mammalian cells. The mechanisms leading to apoptosis and atrophy observed in humans and mice deficient in CSTB are poorly understood. One proposed mechanism is that cathepsins, which are inhibited by CSTB, directly activate

CLINICAL PEARLS

- ULD is the most common progressive myoclonus epilepsy.
- Seizures, ataxia, and stimulus-sensitive myoclonus are the hallmarks of this disease.
- Seizures in ULD may be easily controlled with ASMs, and some patients never develop tonic-clonic seizures.
- Phenytoin is exquisitely toxic to neurons in ULD and should be avoided.
- In ULD, there is an absence of storage material. Therefore, biopsies are negative (as opposed to the other PMEs with onset between childhood and late adolescence).
- Expansion of a dodecamer repeat in the promoter region of the *EPM1* gene is responsible for more than 90% of ULD cases.

caspases leading to the initiation of apoptosis. Another possible mechanism is that the deficiency in CSTB causes an increase in general proteolysis, thus targeting such unhealthy cells for apoptosis.

How apoptosis could lead to the clinical picture of a hyperexcitable cortex that generates seizures and myoclonus is not clear. It has been suggested that g-aminobutyric acid (GABA)ergic neurons are particularly prone to damage in *Cstb*-deficient mice. In these animals, seizure-induced cell death may be responsible for the progressive nature of the disease. It is also possible that the hyperexcitable cortex is caused by an enhancement of tryptophan metabolism in the central nervous system along the serotonin and kynurenine pathways. Neuroinflammation as a result of cell death leading to microglial activation has also been implicated.

Finally, it has been shown that in ULD patients, the thalamostriatal dopaminergic system is dysfunctional. In a small study, there was an improvement in myoclonus in patients receiving a dopamine agonist. This observation may represent a different mechanism responsible for the clinical findings. However, the exact mechanism leading to such deficiency remains to be elucidated.

SUGGESTED REFERENCES

Assenza G., Nocerino C., Tombini M., Di Gennaro G., D'Aniello A., Verrotti A., Marrelli A., Ricci L., Lanzone J., Di Lazzaro V., Bilo L., Coppola A. Perampanel improves cortical myoclonus and disability in progressive myoclonic epilepsies: A case series and a systematic review of the literature. *Front Neurol* 2021;12:1–11.

Canafoglia L., Ciano C., Panzica F., Scaioli V., Zucca C., Agazzi P., Visani E., Avanzini G., Franceschetti S. Sensorimotor cortex excitability in Unverricht-Lundborg disease and Lafora body disease. *Neurology* 2004;63:2309–15.

Kälviäinen R., Genton P., Andermann E., Andermann F., Magaudda A., Frucht S.J., Schlit A.F., Gerard D., de la Loge C., von Rosenstiel P. Brivaracetam in Unverricht-Lundborg disease (EPM1): Results from two randomized, double-blind, placebo-controlled studies. *Epilepsia* 2016;57:210–21.

Lalioti M.D., Scott H.S., Buresi C., Rossier C., Bottani A., Morris M.A., Malafosse A., Antonarakis S.E. Dodecamer repeat expansion in cystatin B gene in progressive myoclonus epilepsy. *Nature* 1997;386:847–51.

Magaudda A., Ferlazzo E., Nguyen V.H., Genton P. Unverricht-Lundborg disease, a condition with self-limited progression: Long-term follow-up of 20 patients. *Epilepsia* 2006;47:860–6.

Mancini G.M., Schot R., de Wit M.C., de Coo R.F., Oostenbrink R., Bindels-de Heus K., Berger L.P., Lequin M.H., de Vries F.A., Wilke M., van Slegtenhorst M.A. CSTB null mutation associated with microcephaly, early developmental delay, and severe dyskinesia. *Neurology* 2016;86:877–8.

Pennacchio L.A., Lehesjoki A.E., Stone N.E., Willour V.L., Virtaneva K., Miao J., D'Amato E., Ramirez L., Faham M., Koskiniemi M., Warrington J.A., Norio R., de la Chapelle A., Cox D.R., Myers R.M. Mutations in the gene encoding cystatin B in progressive myoclonus epilepsy (EPM1). *Science* 1996;271:1731–4.

Sipilä J.O.T., Hyppönen J., Kytö V, Kälviäinen R. Unverricht-Lundborg disease (EPM1) in Finland: A nationwide population-based study. *Neurology* 2020;95:e3117–23.

Suoranta S., Manninen H., Koskenkorva P., Könönen M., Laitinen R., Lehesjoki A.E., Kälviäinen R., Vanninen R. Thickened skull, scoliosis and other skeletal findings in Unverricht-Lundborg disease link cystatin B function to bone metabolism. *Bone* 2012;51:1016–24.

van Karnebeek C.D., Blydt I., Allison H., Avramovic V. Secondary biogenic amine deficiencies: Genetic etiology, therapeutic interventions, and clinical effects American College of Medical Geneticists. *Neurogenetics* 2021;22:251–62.

52 Reflex Seizures

Maria Augusta Montenegro
UC San Diego School of Medicine

CONTENTS

CASE PRESENTATION

A 12-year-old boy was followed in the pediatric epilepsy clinic for focal seizures since 9 years of age. He was the product of an uneventful pregnancy and had a history of normal developmental milestones. Trials of oxcarbazepine, valproic acid, lamotrigine, and clobazam failed to control his seizures, and he kept having weekly seizures that occurred almost exclusively during meals. Seizures were characterized by dizziness followed by impaired awareness for 1 minute, which eventually evolved into focal to bilateral tonic-clonic seizures. Neurological examination and brain MRI were normal. EEG showed independent spike-and-wave discharges over the left and right temporoparietal head regions. Hyperventilation and intermittent photic stimulation did not trigger additional epileptic discharges or seizures. He was diagnosed with eating epilepsy and despite further trials of antiseizure medications (ASMs), he did not achieve seizure freedom for any duration longer than 2 months.

DIFFERENTIAL DIAGNOSIS

The most important element in the diagnosis of reflex seizures is careful history taking. Sometimes, the patient also presents with spontaneous seizures, and the reflex component might not be appreciated or identified. Further, certain forms of reflex epilepsies (e.g., reading epilepsy) may coexist with other types of epilepsy, especially juvenile myoclonic epilepsy (JME). Since most patients can be readily diagnosed with JME, the reflex seizures might be overlooked.

In childhood, reflex seizures should be differentiated from nonepileptic events that are triggered by crying, anxiety, or movement. The most common nonepileptic events that can mimic reflex seizures are as follows:

DOI: 10.1201/9781003296478-57

- Benign myoclonus of infancy: nonepileptic jerks of the neck or upper limbs, with flexion of the head that may appear very similar to epileptic spasms. There is no loss of awareness. It may occur during meals, which might cause confusion with eating epilepsy.
- Sandifer syndrome: neck and back spasms associated with gastroesophageal reflux in infants and children. Because it frequently occurs during or after feeding, it may be diagnosed as eating epilepsy.
- Kinesigenic dyskinesias: brief episodes of dystonic posturing triggered by sudden movement. It has an autosomal dominant inheritance and has been principally linked to the *PRRT2 gene*. This is often misdiagnosed as epilepsy.
- Breath-holding spells: nonepileptic episodes triggered by crying or pain. There are two types: (1) cyanotic breath-holding spell (the child gets hypertonic with cyanosis around lips and face) and (2) pallid breath-holding spell (the child gets hypotonic and very pale, and there may be bradycardia). Because both types are triggered by pain, anger, or frustration, these can sometimes be diagnosed as reflex seizures.
- Stereotyped behaviors: repetitive movements, frequently seen in children with developmental delay or autism spectrum disorder. Sometimes, these are associated with certain activities, giving the impression that they are clinical manifestations of reflex epilepsy.

It should also be noted that some families eventually associate a specific event as a possible trigger for seizures, when in fact the association was only coincidental. It happens more frequently when the child had only a few seizures, and the family tries to find a way to explain such a traumatic event.

DIAGNOSTIC APPROACH

Reflex seizures are a group of disorders characterized by seizures consistently induced by identifiable sensory or cognitive stimuli. They can be divided according to the type of trigger:

- Simple triggers: touch, light, movement.
- Complex triggers: reading, writing, eating, doing arithmetic, listening to music, thinking about specific topics, etc.

Simple triggers usually trigger a seizure within seconds (intermittent photic stimulation), as opposed to complex triggers (eating or reading) that trigger the seizure usually after a few minutes.

A careful history can help to identify possible triggers associated with reflex seizures, and often video-EEG is needed to determine how reliably the stimulus provokes the seizure, and whether other subtle seizure types may be present. During video-EEG, the stimulus identified as the possible trigger should be applied in order to provoke a seizure.

Reflex seizures can be focal or generalized, idiopathic or symptomatic. Neuroimaging should be performed to investigate possible focal abnormalities such as focal cortical dysplasia, heterotopias, tumors, gliosis, etc. Central nervous system (CNS) structural lesions have been associated with reflex seizures, and although such events are more commonly found in the frontal or parietal lobes, other brain regions might be involved.

Photosensitivity is the most common trigger associated with reflex seizures and can be found in several types of epilepsy such as juvenile myoclonic epilepsy, photosensitive occipital lobe epilepsy, and Dravet syndrome. Some children can self-induce photosensitive seizures by actively seeking out the sun and waving their hands in front of the face to purposefully induce seizures. Table 52.1 lists the common types of reflex seizures.

TABLE 52.1
Most Common Types of Reflex Seizures

Type of Reflex Seizure/Epilepsy	Age of Onset	Trigger	EEG	Seizure Type
JME, Dravet syndrome, POLE	Childhood or adolescence	Photosensitivity, intermittent photic stimulation (including TV and video games)	Focal or generalized	Myoclonic, absence and focal seizures
CAE, JAE	Childhood or adolescence	Hyperventilation	Generalized	Absence seizures
Epilepsy with eyelid myoclonia	Childhood or adolescence	Eye closure	Generalized	Eyelid myoclonia
Reflex myoclonic epilepsy in infancy	First 2 years of life	Unexpected auditory or tactile stimuli	Generalized	Myoclonic seizures
Eating epilepsy	Adolescence or young adult	Eating	Focal	Focal seizure (staring spell, impaired awareness)
Hot water epilepsy	Adolescence or young adult	Hot bath or pouring hot water over head	Focal	Variable focal seizures, usually with sensory or autonomic symptoms
Musicogenic epilepsy	Adult	Music (specific music for each patient), even thinking or dreaming about the music	Focal	Temporal lobe seizures May be associated with hippocampal atrophy or limbic lesions
Praxis epilepsy	Childhood, adolescence or young adult	High mental activity (math, thinking, Rubik's cube, playing cards)	Focal or generalized	Myoclonic seizure, absence seizure, focal seizures May be associated with focal lesions on MRI
Reading epilepsy	Adolescence or young adult	Reading	Focal	Jaw myoclonus Focal seizures with alexia (inability to read) GTC

CAE, childhood absence epilepsy; JAE, juvenile absence epilepsy; JME, juvenile myoclonic epilepsy; POLE, photosensitive occipital lobe epilepsy.

CLINICAL PEARLS

- A careful history is one of the most important elements in diagnosing reflex seizures.
- ASM treatment should be offered for most patients.
- Avoiding the offending trigger is an important part of the treatment plan.
- Reflex seizures can be drug resistant and if a brain lesion is identified, epilepsy surgery should be considered.

TREATMENT AND LONG-TERM OUTCOME

Treatment of reflex epilepsies involves avoidance of the offending stimulus, and this strategy can be very effective for many patients. However, it may be impossible to avoid some triggers such as with eating epilepsy. Moreover, children with cognitive impairment and self-induced seizures are often noncompliant in avoiding the stimulus, possibly because the seizure is associated with a pleasurable sensation. Treatment with an ASM should be offered to most patients. The long-term outcome of reflex seizures is variable, and drug-resistant epilepsy is not uncommon. Epilepsy surgery may be considered in drug-resistant cases, especially when neuroimaging shows a focal lesion.

PATHOPHYSIOLOGY/NEUROBIOLOGY OF DISEASE

The pathophysiology of reflex seizures is poorly understood, but one possible mechanism is the activation of specialized cortical networks connected to the ictal focus by afferent stimulation. Both lesional and genetic bases for reflex seizures have been described and their pathophysiology is probably multifactorial. Several genetic causes of photosensitive reflex epilepsies have been described and include JME-related genes such as *BRD2* and *EFHC1*. However, there is not a specific mutation associated with each type of epilepsy syndrome, suggesting a complex pattern of inheritance.

SUGGESTED REFERENCES

Binnie C.D. Self-induction of seizures: The ultimate non-compliance. *Epilepsy Res Suppl* 1988;1:153–8.

Bruhn K., Kronisch S., Waltz S., Stephani U. Screen sensitivity in photosensitive children and adolescents: Patient-dependent and stimulus-dependent factors. *Epileptic Disord* 2007;9:57–64.

Radovici A., Misirliou V., Gluckman M. Epilepsie reflexe provoquée par excitations des rayons solaires. *Revue Neurologique* 1932;1:1305–8.

Verrotti A., Matricardi S., Pavone P., Marino R., Curatolo P. Reflex myoclonic epilepsy in infancy: A critical review. *Epileptic Disord* 2013;15:114–22.

53 Sleep-Related Hypermotor Epilepsy

Kevin Chapman
University of Arizona College of Medicine

CONTENTS

CASE PRESENTATION

A 10-year-old right-handed male without a significant past medical history was referred for evaluation of possible nocturnal seizures. His seizures began at 7 years of age and have occurred almost exclusively during sleep, usually within 2 hours of falling asleep. The stereotyped episodes involve rocking and bicycling motions, gagging, rolling of the eyes, and profuse sweating lasting approximately 2 minutes. These episodes have occurred on average three times per week but recently have become more frequent. He has had two similar episodes that have occurred while awake. The patient's previous evaluation included two routine sleep-deprived electroencephalograms (EEGs) and a 3T noncontrast magnetic resonance imaging (MRI) scan of the brain, all of which were interpreted as normal. Other normal laboratory tests included a complete blood count and comprehensive metabolic profile. His physical and neurologic examination is unremarkable. His family history is notable for primarily nocturnal seizures in his brother and maternal aunt that started in childhood. Ultimately, the patient was admitted for continuous video-EEG monitoring to characterize the episodes of concern. During this study, the patient had three typical clinical events identified by the family. Clinically, the patient would arouse, sit up in bed, rock, and look around the room, but did not respond. He made some occasional nonsensical vocalizations. The events lasted from 47 to 83 seconds. During the events, the EEG demonstrated a change from a normal stage II sleep recording to generalized, frontally dominant rhythmic 3 Hz high-amplitude slow activity (Figure 53.1). This activity

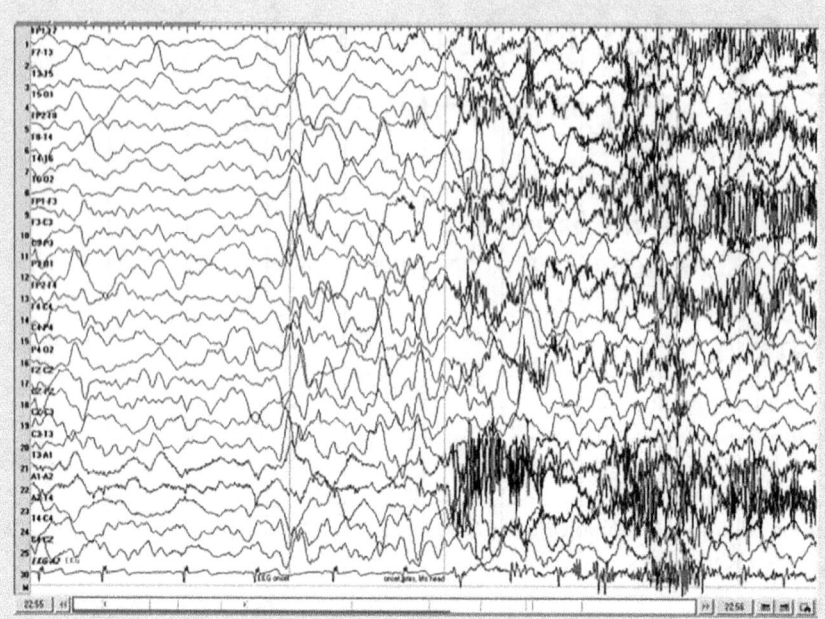

FIGURE 53.1   Electroencephalogram demonstrating rhythmic delta activity evolving over the frontal head regions.

lasted half a minute and gradually waned to a normal background rhythm without any focal slowing. Based on this video-EEG study, the diagnosis of sleep-related hypermotor epilepsy was made and the patient was started on carbamazepine. Genetic testing demonstrated a mutation in the CHRNA4 gene consistent with the diagnosis of sleep-related hypermotor epilepsy (SHE). The patient responded well to carbamazepine and would experience only rare seizures after missed doses of medication.

DIFFERENTIAL DIAGNOSIS

The unusual nocturnal behaviors seen in patients with SHE can make their diagnosis challenging. Depending on the site of origin, patients may exhibit complex automatisms, such as bicycling or rocking, vocalizations, dystonic posturing, or clonic activity, but may retain awareness. The differential diagnosis of paroxysmal nocturnal events involves distinguishing parasomnias from true epileptic seizures.

Pediatric parasomnias (e.g., night terrors, sleepwalking, and confusional arousal) occur in up to 6% of the population and may be difficult to differentiate from SHE. Night terrors (aka, *pavor nocturnus*) often occur during slow-wave sleep in the first third of the night. The patients will often make a loud cry and appear frightened. They may have thrashing movements, as if defending themselves, but these are often less stereotyped than events in SHE. During the episodes, patients are often unarousable, but may recall a frightening dream afterward. Confusional arousals often begin with simple movements or moaning that gradually progress to a more agitated and confused state that may last for 5–15 minutes. The patients are often difficult to arouse and have little recollection of the event. Sleepwalking may occur in children while asleep but is typically associated with a calm demeanor that differs from the above parasomnias or seizures. REM sleep behavior disorder may also have similar presentations but occurs later in the night and is uncommon in children. Polysomnograms demonstrate a lack of atonia during REM sleep in these patients.

Useful clues to help differentiate SHE from parasomnias include the presence of stereotyped behaviors, events occurring during periods of wakefulness, a history of clear seizures, a family history of epilepsy, later age of onset (parasomnias usually begin between 4 and 6 years of age), and multiple events per night. Seizures are less likely to occur during REM sleep and more often arise during transition from sleep to waking. The EEGs in SHE often lack clear abnormalities and may be normal despite multiple seizures per night.

DIAGNOSTIC APPROACH

Unfortunately, patients afflicted with this disorder are often misdiagnosed for many years as parasomnias, so a high index of suspicion is required to confirm SHE. SHE is a genetic focal epilepsy with a mean age of onset of around 11 years and with a slight male predominance. The medical history is often of utmost importance in proper diagnosis. The events are typically brief (<30 seconds) and may occur multiple times per night, something which is unusual for parasomnias. Secondarily generalized tonic-clonic seizures may also occur in this syndrome. SHE is transmitted in an autosomal dominant mode, with a penetrance of about 70%.

There is marked variability within affected families, with some members being more severely affected than others. Individuals appear to have normal intellect, but careful studies of neuropsychological functioning are lacking. The video-EEG in SHE can often be unrevealing and may cast doubt on the diagnosis but remains an effective tool for differentiating seizures from parasomnias.

Patients may have interictal abnormalities, seen primarily in sleep, that are frontal or bifrontal, including spikes or focal slowing. However, more than half of SHE patients do not exhibit interictal abnormalities. Typical ictal electrographic changes consist of diffuse attenuation or rhythmic slowing over the anterior regions (Figure 53.1).

Many patients may lack any clear evolving ictal changes. The seizures primarily occur out of non-REM sleep but may occur during wakefulness in about 35% of patients. About 10% of patients lack seizures during wakefulness and have normal EEGs. Polysomnographic recording may help differentiate the epileptic events from non-epileptic parasomnias, such as REM behavior disorder. Genetic testing, particularly multigene panels, can be useful in confirming the diagnosis of SHE.

TREATMENT STRATEGY

SHE often responds well to antiseizure medications (ASMs). Classically, carbamazepine has been used and appears to be particularly effective in nearly two-thirds of patients. Other ASMs, such as oxcarbazepine, phenytoin, clonazepam, valproic acid, lamotrigine, zonisamide, and acetazolamide, have been used with varying degrees of success. Interestingly, improved seizure control has been reported with tobacco use, presumably through the nicotine intake associated with smoking affecting patients with mutations in their neuronal nicotinic acetylcholine receptors. Treatment-resistant patients with mutations in *DEPDC5* may have associated focal cortical dysplasias and could be considered for epilepsy surgery.

LONG-TERM OUTCOME

While many patients respond to ASMs, one-third of patients may continue to be refractory to various medical treatments. Long-term outcome data on patients with SHE are lacking, but it has been observed that many patients experience seizures well into adulthood. Patients with *KCNT1* mutations may have a more severe disease course with associated intellectual disability.

PATHOPHYSIOLOGY/NEUROBIOLOGY OF DISEASE

SHE, originally termed autosomal dominant nocturnal frontal lobe epilepsy (ADNFLE), was the first idiopathic epilepsy syndrome linked to a specific genetic mutation – the *CHRNA4* gene. Its discovery opened the door for research into the molecular genetics of epilepsy, and further validated a class of disorders known as "ion channelopathies". SHE is most commonly due to a mutation in a gene encoding a subunit of the neuronal nicotinic acetylcholine receptor (nAChR).

Multiple mutations have been identified in three separate nAChR genes – *CHRNA4*, *CHRNB2*, and *CHRNA2*. Additional mutations in *KCNT1*, *CRH*, and *DEPDC5* have been associated with SHE, but there are limited functional data on how these mutations produce the clinical syndrome. The proposed mechanism for epilepsy associated with mutations in the nAChR gene is discussed below.

Cholinergic projections from the basal forebrain nuclei are found throughout the cortex and hippocampus and likely play a role in learning and memory. The cholinergic projections from the dorsolateral and pedunculopontine tegmentum, which are part of the reticular activating system, play an important role in the regulation of sleep and arousal through the thalamocortical system. Depolarization of these nuclei causes cortical activation and desynchronization of the EEG necessary for wakefulness. Nicotine stimulates these projections and can enhance cortical activation.

The neuronal nAChR is a pentameric ligand-gated ion channel, composed of various combinations of alpha and beta subunits, which can be opened by nicotine or acetylcholine. Permeability to various cations is dictated by the subunit combination, with the most common subtype in the mammalian brain consisting of $\alpha 4\beta 2$ subunits. nAChRs are found primarily in the presynaptic nerve terminals. Their activation leads to a brief depolarizing excitatory potential, and they can allow calcium influx leading to increased neurotransmitter release.

The pathogenic mechanisms through which mutations in nAChR subunits cause nocturnal frontal lobe seizures remain unclear. Electrophysiological studies of the specific nAChR mutations have demonstrated varying alterations of channel

---

CLINICAL PEARLS

- SHE is characterized by seizures with unusual semiology and misdiagnosis with parasomnias is common.
- Most patients respond well to carbamazepine monotherapy, but 30% may remain intractable to medical therapy.
- Video-EEG evaluations may demonstrate interictal and ictal patterns in the frontal regions, but some studies may be normal.
- Genetic testing for SHE is commercially available, but not all causative mutations have been discovered.
- The underlying pathophysiology of SHE remains unclear and continues to be an active area of research.

---

function, but increased sensitivity to acetylcholine (gain-of-function) seems common in mutations associated with SHE. This increased sensitivity may allow enhanced cortical GABAergic inhibition that may cause inhibitory hypersynchronization and seizures. It remains unclear why characteristically focal-onset (i.e., frontal lobe) seizures occur when the mutation is widely expressed throughout the brain. The important role that nAChRs play in regulating sleep may provide clues to understanding the pathophysiology of nocturnal seizures.

SUGGESTED REFERENCES

Becchetti A., Araci P., Meneghini S., Brusco S., Amadeo A. The role of nicotinic acetylcholine receptors in autosomal dominant frontal lobe epilepsy. *Front Physiol* 2015;6:1–12.

Combi R., Dalpra L., Tenchini M.L., Ferini-Strambi L. Autosomal dominant nocturnal frontal lobe epilepsy: A critical overview. *J Neurol* 2004;251:923–34.

Picard F., Makrythanasis P., Navarro V., Ishida S., de Bellescize J., Ville D., Weckhuysen S., Fosselle E., Suls A., De Jonghe P., Raina M.V., Lesca G., Depeienne C., An-Gourfinkel I., Vlaicu M., Baulac M., Mundwiller E., Couarch P., Combi R., Ferini-Strambi L., Gambardella A., Antonarakis S.E., Leguern E., Steinlein O., Baulac S. DEPDC5 mutations in families presenting as autosomal dominant nocturnal frontal lobe epilepsy. *Neurology* 2014;10:2101–6.

Provini F., Plazzi G., Tinuper P., Vandi S., Lugaresi E., Montagna P. Nocturnal frontal lobe epilepsy. A clinical and polygraphic overview of 100 consecutive cases. *Brain* 1999;122:1017–31.

Riney K., Bogacz A., Somerville E., Hirsch E., Nabbout R., Scheffer I.E., Zuberi S.M., Alsaadi T., Jain S., French J., Specchio N., Trinka E., Wiebe S., Auvin S., Cabral-Lim L., Naidoo A., Perucca E., Moshé S.L., Wirrell E.C., Tinuper P. International league against epilepsy classification and definition of epilepsy syndromes with onset at a variable age: Position statement by the ILAE Task Force on Nosology and Definitions. *Epilepsia* 2022;63:1443–74.

Scheffer I.E. Autosomal dominant nocturnal frontal lobe epilepsy. *Epilepsia* 2000;41:1059–60.

54 Psychogenic Nonepileptic Seizures

Guillermo Delgado-García and Colin B. Josephson
University of Calgary

CONTENTS

CASE PRESENTATION

A 16-year-old right-handed female was brought to the emergency department due to new-onset seizures. Her mother described three whole-body convulsions at home in the morning and one more when she was en route. Upon arrival at the hospital, the patient was back at her baseline and her vital signs were unremarkable. The patient did not recall any warning and denied any recent fever or toxin/drug/medication exposure as well as other seizure triggers. Her past history was only relevant for mild intellectual disability and long-standing, occasional self-harming behaviors. There was no family history of epilepsy or seizures. Her physical and neurological exam was unremarkable. Blood work was within normal limits including creatine kinase and serum lactate. The patient experienced another episode in the emergency department. It began with side-to-side head movements followed by arrhythmic and asynchronous jerks of all four limbs with some pelvic thrusting. Her eyes were closed, and the total duration of this episode was around 4 minutes. She had urinary incontinence but no tongue biting. The monitor showed sinus tachycardia and her peripheral oxygen saturation did not drop during the episode. Her mother witnessed this event and confirmed that it was very similar to what she saw at home. A routine electroencephalogram (EEG) was completed less than 1 hour after this episode and was reported as normal. On directed questioning, the patient stated that this year she has been struggling with bullying at school. Her mother added that for some months, she has been going through a turbulent divorce and the patient has not seen her father often.

DOI: 10.1201/9781003296478-59

After a detailed discussion, the diagnosis of probable psychogenic non-epileptic seizures (PNES) was conveyed. As her mother was not comfortable with this probable diagnosis, a short-term video-EEG was organized while in hospital, and another event was captured. The mother confirmed that was her typical semiology. The EEG was normal immediately before, during, and after this episode and, therefore, the diagnosis of PNES was documented. The patient and her mother accepted the diagnosis. Psychoeducation was started before discharge and a response plan was prepared for them. A follow-up appointment was organized, and the patient was referred to Clinical Psychology to start cognitive-behavioral therapy (CBT).

DIFFERENTIAL DIAGNOSIS

As its name implies, the main differential diagnosis for PNES is epileptic seizures. The clinical spectrum of PNES, however, is broad and this helps inform the differential diagnosis. This diversity is directly related to the different clinical phenotypes of PNES. Given that motor PNES appear to be one of the most common clinical phenotypes in pediatric patients (and a major cause of referrals), this chapter will be mainly devoted to this PNES subtype, also known as convulsive PNES.

A variety of semiological features classically described in the context of PNES have also been reported in focal epilepsies, especially in those arising from the frontal lobes, including asynchronous and thrashing movements as well as pelvic thrusting. Moreover, ictal scalp EEG can also be normal in frontal lobe seizures. Fortunately, PNES and epilepsy can be, in principle, differentiated with the aid of a few clinical clues. Frontal lobe seizures are typically (although not exclusively) nocturnal and tend to arise from sleep (especially from sleep–wake transitions), while PNES arising from EEG-confirmed sleep are exceedingly rare with only a few cases reported worldwide. In these patients, PNES occurred from stages 2 and 3 nonrapid eye movement sleep.

In addition, event duration can also be a relevant clinical discriminator in this scenario. Frontal lobe seizures are usually brief (<30 seconds) while 95% of typical epileptic seizures, especially extrafrontal, last less than 2–3 minutes, particularly those with motor manifestations. On the contrary, PNES tend to be protracted events, not uncommonly lasting 10 minutes or more. During an event, the course of PNES is more fluctuating compared to epileptic seizures and this has been termed a "stop-and-go phenomenon." Tonic posturing, especially when confirmed by a trained witness, is not expected in PNES. In contrast, forced eye closure, overt "ictal" crying/weeping, and self-protective maneuvers are positive signs pointing to PNES, especially in older adolescents and young adults. Preserved awareness (either complete or partial) during a bilateral convulsive episode as well as distractibility also suggests PNES. As a whole, the combination of different clinical findings (i.e., the overall clinical picture) suggesting PNES is more reliable than individual signs alone.

PNES should not only be considered in patients with new-onset seizures, but those with putative chronic drug-resistant epilepsies may be misdiagnosed and actually suffering from PNES (i.e., pseudo-resistance). Up to 30% of pediatric patients referred to tertiary epilepsy centers due to suspected epilepsy may not actually have this condition after a proper assessment. Event frequency might be very informative in this scenario too, as PNES tends to be markedly more explosive than epileptic seizures, and pediatric patients experiencing >190 events per month have been reported. On top of that, PNES and epilepsy are not mutually exclusive and comorbid PNES can also occur in patients with definite epilepsy. Other less frequent PNES phenotypes may have clinical presentations similar to syncope, panic attacks, some movement disorders (particularly tic disorders, choreoathetosis, and dystonias), parasomnias, or cataplexy.

DIAGNOSTIC APPROACH

PNES is not rare in clinical practice, and this is especially true for the adolescent population. For instance, a nationwide study from Denmark found an incidence rate of close to 8 cases per 100,000 person-years. Hence, PNES should always be part of the differential diagnosis when assessing an adolescent with paroxysmal events, either new-onset or long-standing. An important paradigm shift has been reframing PNES as a positive diagnosis, not simply one of exclusion, and this also applies to other functional neurological disorders.

The International League Against Epilepsy (ILAE) and International Federation of Clinical Neurophysiology strongly recommend inpatient long-term video-EEG monitoring as a means to differentiate between epileptic and nonepileptic events in patients in whom the diagnosis is not clear. The ILAE has developed a staged approach to the diagnosis of PNES. They propose four levels of diagnostic certainty based on history, witnessed events, and electrophysiological investigations (Table 54.1). While PNES are typically inducible, there is currently no consensus on the appropriateness of these techniques as a way of instigating attacks. Ideally, the neurologist is the one that should communicate this diagnosis to patients. Conveying the diagnosis is an integral part of the diagnostic and therapeutic process, and specific strategies have been proposed (e.g., Hall-Patch et al., 2010).

TREATMENT STRATEGY

The patient needs to be fully aware of this diagnosis, and prompt and structured psychoeducation should be offered as soon as the diagnosis is communicated. Patients with PNES benefit from integrated multidisciplinary management including neurologists, specialized nurses, psychiatrists, psychologists, and social workers. This management should be individualized and additionally address specific psychiatric comorbidities, which are common in pediatric patients with PNES. Ideally, patients should continue follow-up with their neurologist.

A referral to outpatient mental health services is also key in the management of these patients, as psychotherapy is a cornerstone in their treatment. In pediatric populations, there is some evidence for both top-down (e.g., CBT) and bottom-up (i.e., body-oriented) approaches, and it is currently not known if one approach is superior to the other. There is no specific pharmacological management for PNES, but these patients

TABLE 54.1

ILAE Proposed Diagnostic Levels of Certainty for PNES

Diagnostic Level	History	Witnessed Event	EEG
Possible	Consistent with PNES	By witness or self-report	Interictal routine or sleep-deprived (SD) EEG: No epileptiform activity
Probable	Consistent with PNES	By clinician in person (or on video); semiology consistent with PNES	Interictal routine or SD EEG: No epileptiform activity
Clinically established	Consistent with PNES	By clinician with experience in seizure disorders (on video or in person); semiology consistent with PNES, patient not connected to EEG	Ictal routine or ambulatory EEG during typical event: No epileptiform activity
Documented	Consistent with PNES	By clinician with experience in seizure disorders; semiology consistent with PNES, while on video-EEG	Ictal video-EEG: No epileptiform activity immediately before, during or after typical event

Source: Adapted from LaFrance et al. (2013).

may receive psychotropic medications for their psychiatric comorbidities. To avoid potential overtreatment at the emergency department, a PNES response plan should be devised together with the patient, and they should receive a written copy of it.

LONG-TERM OUTCOME

In this population, long-term longitudinal data are scarce. However, one prospective observational study recently reported that, with comprehensive and dedicated care, PNES will remit by 1 year in one-third of patients. In addition, according to the same study, close to 90% of all patients will have a notable decrease in event frequency by 1 year. Timely access to psychotherapy is crucial to ensure a good prognosis.

The importance of expeditious and comprehensive treatment should not be understated, since the adjusted hazard ratio (HR) for premature mortality compared to those without epilepsy, PNES, or conversion disorder is 5.5 (95% confidence interval [CI]: 2.8–10.8). Both natural (HR 8.1, 95% CI: 4.0–16.4) and unnatural (HR 15.3, 95% CI: 3.0–78.6) causes of death are higher than the general population, and alarmingly suicide is the leading reported cause of death (18.8%) in one nationwide population-based cohort study.

PATHOPHYSIOLOGY/NEUROBIOLOGY OF DISEASE

PNES are unconscious, unintentional, paroxysmal, and time-limited alterations in motor, sensory, autonomic, and/or cognitive function that are not caused by ictal epileptiform activity. The genesis of this condition, especially in pediatric patients,

CLINICAL PEARLS

- PNES is not rare in adolescents and should always be considered as part of the differential diagnosis.
- PNES can present with many different semiologies but is most often confused at bilateral tonic-clonic seizures, especially for the untrained witness.
- The diagnosis of PNES is based on history, witnessed events, electrophysiological investigations, and four different levels of diagnostic certainty have been described.
- PNES is a treatable condition and timely psychotherapy is key in the successful management of these patients.
- With comprehensive and dedicated care, PNES can stop or at least significantly decrease in frequency.

is better understood using a bio-psychosocial framework with multiple, closely inter-related factors.

On the one hand, PNES pathobiology and neurobiology are expanding fields, and pediatric patients with PNES exhibit a higher physiological and cortical arousal as well as a state of motor readiness to emotional signals. On the other hand, multiple psychological and social risk factors have been associated with pediatric PNES. For instance, lifetime adversities are common, with one nationwide study reporting them in over half of patients. Psychosocial stressors in pediatric patients are also typically chronic and cumulative, reinforcing the need for early and aggressive intervention.

SUGGESTED REFERENCES

Esbjörnsson J. Semiology and Classifications of Paediatric Psychogenic Nonepileptic Seizures – A Systematic Review. Degree Project in Medicine, University of Gothenburg, 2020. Available at http://hdl.handle.net/2077/66567.

Fredwall M., Terry D., Enciso L., Burch M.M., Trott K., Albert D.V.F. Outcomes of children and adolescents one year after being seen in a multidisciplinary psychogenic nonepileptic seizures clinic. *Epilepsia* 2021;62:2528–38.

Gilmour G.S., MacIsaac R., Subotic A., Wiebe S., Josephson C.B. Diagnostic accuracy of clinical signs and symptoms for psychogenic nonepileptic attacks versus epileptic seizures: A systematic review and meta-analysis. *Epilepsy Behav* 2021;121:108030.

Hall-Patch L., Brown R., House A., Howlett S., Kemp S., Lawton G., Mayor R., Smith P., Reuber M.; NEST collaborators. Acceptability and effectiveness of a strategy for the communication of the diagnosis of psychogenic nonepileptic seizures. *Epilepsia* 2010;51:70–8.

Hansen A.S., Rask C.U., Rodrigo-Domingo M., Pristed S.G., Christensen J., Nielsen R.E. Incidence rates and characteristics of pediatric onset psychogenic nonepileptic seizures. *Pediatr Res* 2020;88:796–803.

Hempel A., Doss J.L. Factors contributing to the onset of psychogenic nonepileptic seizures in children and adolescents. In: LaFrance Jr. W.C., Schachter S.C. (eds). *Gates and Rowan's Nonepileptic Seizures*, 4th ed. Cambridge: Cambridge University Press; 2018:199–206.

Higgins S., Koutroumanidis M. Psychogenic non-epileptic seizures arising almost exclusively from sleep. *Seizure* 2022;99:43–7.

LaFrance Jr. W.C., Baker G.A., Duncan R., Goldstein L.H., Reuber M. Minimum requirements for the diagnosis of psychogenic nonepileptic seizures: A staged approach: A report from the International League Against Epilepsy Nonepileptic Seizures Task Force. *Epilepsia* 2013;54:2005–18.

Velani H., Gledhill J. The effectiveness of psychological interventions for children and adolescents with non-epileptic seizures. *Seizure* 2021;93:20–31.

Zhang L., Beghi E., Tomson T., Beghi M., Erba G., Chang Z. Mortality in patients with psychogenic non-epileptic seizures a population-based cohort study. *J Neurol Neurosurg Psychiatry* 2022;93:379–85.

INDEX

For Product Safety Concerns and Information please contact our EU
representative GPSR@taylorandfrancis.com
Taylor & Francis Verlag GmbH, Kaufingerstraße 24, 80331 München, Germany

www.ingramcontent.com/pod-product-compliance
Lightning Source LLC
Chambersburg PA
CBHW060818170526
45158CB00001B/19